Diabetes and Pregnancy

Diabetes and Pregnancy

An International Approach to Diagnosis and Management

Edited by

ANNE DORNHORST

Royal Postgraduate Medical School, London, UK

DAVID R. HADDEN

Royal Victoria Hospital, Belfast, UK

John Wiley & Sons

Chichester · New York · Brisbane · Toronto · Singapore

Copyright © 1996 by John Wiley & Sons Ltd,
Baffins Lane, Chichester,
West Sussex PO19 1UD, England

National   01243 779777
International (+44) 1243 779777

Other Wiley Editorial Offices

John Wiley & Sons, Inc., 605 Third Avenue,
New York, NY 10158-0012, USA

Jacaranda Wiley Ltd, 33 Park Road, Milton,
Queensland 4064, Australia

John Wiley & Sons (Canada) Ltd, 22 Worcester Road,
Rexdale, Ontario M9W 1L1, Canada

John Wiley & Sons (Asia) Pte Ltd, 2 Clementi Loop #02-01,
Jin Xing Distripark, Singapore 0512

Library of Congress Cataloging-in-Publication Data

Diabetes and pregnancy : an international approach to diagnosis and
    management / edited by Anne Dornhorst and David R. Hadden.
        p.   cm. – (Practical diabetes series)
    Includes bibliographical references and index.
    ISBN 0 471 96204 X (hbk. : alk. paper)
    1. Diabetes in pregnancy. I. Dornhorst, Anne. II. Hadden, D. R.
III. Series: Practical diabetes (Chichester, England)
    [DNLM: 1. Pregnancy in Diabetes – diagnosis. 2. Pregnancy in
Diabetes – therapy. 3. Diabetes Mellitus – complications.   WQ 248
D53532 1996]
RG580.D5D514   1996
618.3–dc20
DNLM/DLC
for Library of Congress   96-13798
                                                                CIP

British Library Cataloguing in Publication Data

A catalogue record for this book is available from the British Library

ISBN 0-471-96204-X

Typeset in 10/11.5pt Palatino by Mackreth Media Services, Hemel Hempstead
Printed and bound in Great Britain by Biddles Ltd, Guildford
This book is printed on acid-free paper responsibly manufactured from sustainable forestation,
for which at least two trees are planted for each one used for paper production.

Contents

List of Contributors

LEONA AERTS, PhD
Department of Obstetrics and Gynaecology, Universitaire Ziekenhuizen Leuven, Herestraat 49, 3000 Leuven, Belgium

ALBERT AYNSLEY-GREEN, MA, DPhil, FRCP(Lond), FRCP(Ed)
Nuffield Professor of Child Health, Institute of Child Health, 30 Guilford Street, London WC1N 1EH, UK

JANIS BAIRD, MB ChB, MFPHM (I)
MRC Environmental Epidemiology Unit, Southampton General Hospital, Tremona Road, Southampton SO16 6YD, UK

J.S. BAJAJ, MD FRCP (Ed) FRCP (Lond) FAMS, Hon DSc (Madras), FICP, DM
All-India Institute of Medical Sciences, New Delhi 110029, India

HAYLEY J. BLANCHARD
Department of Medicine, Royal Postgraduate Medical School, Du Cane Road, London W12 0NN, UK

THOMAS A. BUCHANAN, MD
Associate Professor of Medicine, Obstetrics and Gynecology, University of Southern California School of Medicine, General Hospital, 1200 N State Street, Los Angeles, CA 90033, USA

C. ANDREW COMBS, MD, PhD
Good Samaritan Health System, 2425 Samaritan Drive, San Jose, CA 95124, USA

PETER DAMM, MD
Diabetes Centre, Department of Obstetrics and Gynaecology, Rigshospitalet, Blegdamsvej 9, DK-2100 Copenhagen, Denmark

ANNE DORNHORST, DM
Department of Medicine and Endocrinology, Royal Postgraduate Medical School, Du Cane Road, London W12 0NN, UK

ULF J. ERIKSSON,
MD, PhD,
Associate Professor, Department of Medical Cell Biology, University of Uppsala, Biomedicum, PO Box 571, 75123 Uppsala, Sweden

RICHARD G. FIRTH,
MD, FRCPI, FACP, DABIM
Consultant Physician, Mater Misericordiae Hospital, Dublin 7, Eire

JOANNA C. GIRLING,
MA, MRCP, MRCOG
Senior Registrar in Obstetrics and Gynaecology, Hammersmith Hospital, Du Cane Road, London W12 0NN, UK

DAVID R. HADDEN,
MD, FRCP
Sir George E. Clark Metabolic Unit, Royal Victoria Hospital, Grosvenor Road, Belfast BT12 6BA, UK

JANE M. HAWDON,
MA, DPhil, MRCP
Consultant Neonatologist, Neonatal Unit, University College London Hospitals, Huntley Street, London WC1E 6AU, UK

KATHLEEN HOLMANS, PhD
Department of Obstetrics and Gynaecology, Universitaire Ziekenhuizen Leuven, Herestraat 49, 3000 Leuven, Belgium

JENNIFER HUGHES,
RN
Sir George E. Clark Metabolic Unit, Royal Victoria Hospital, Grosvenor Road, Belfast BT12 6BA, UK

JOHN L. KITZMILLER,
MD
Good Samaritan Health System, 2425 Samaritan Drive, San Jose, CA 95124, USA

EVA M. KOHNER, MD
Department of Medicine, St Thomas' Hospital, Lambeth Palace Road, London SE1 7EH, UK

R. MADAN, MD, DGO,
MAMS, FAIID, FICS
Government Medical College, 78 Sector 3, Trikuta Nagar, Jammu-180-004, India

DAVID R. McCANCE,
BSc, MD, MRCP, DCH
Sir George E. Clark Metabolic Unit, Royal Victoria Hospital, Grosvenor Road, Belfast BT12 6BA, UK

ALYSON MOORE,
Senior Dietician, Royal Maternity Hospital, Grosvenor Road, Belfast BT12 6BA, UK

HEULWEN MORGAN,
FRCOG
Consultant Obstetrician and Gynaecologist, Department of Obstetrics and Gynaecology, Whittington Hospital, Highgate Hill, London N19 5NF, UK

KYPRIANOS H. NICOLAIDES, FRCOG
Professor of Fetal Medicine, Harris Birthright Research Centre for Fetal Medicine, Department of Obstetrics and Gynaecology, King's College Hospital, Denmark Hill, London SE5 8RX, UK

JEREMY J.N. OATS,
MD
The Royal Women's Hospital Melbourne, 209/300 Victoria Parade, East Melbourne, Victoria 3002, Australia

DAVID J. PETTITT, MD — *Diabetes and Arthritis Epidemiology Section, National Institute of Diabetes and Digestive and Kidney Disease, 1550 East Indian School Road, Phoenix, AZ 85014, USA*

DAVID I.W. PHILLIPS, MA, MSc, PhD, MRCP — *Clinical Scientist and Senior Lecturer in Medicine, Metabolic Programming Group, MRC Environmental Epidemiology Unit, Southampton General Hospital, Tremona Road, Southampton SO16 6YD, UK*

ROBERT PIJNENBORG, PhD — *Department of Obstetrics and Gynaecology, Universitaire Ziekenhuizen Leuven, Herestraat 49, 3000 Leuven, Belgium*

CAROLINE PIMBLETT, SRD — *Dietician, Diabetes Resource Team for Lambeth, Southwark and Lewisham, Dulwich Hospital, East Dulwich Grove, London SE22 8PT, UK*

MICHELA ROSSI, MB BS, MRCP — *Research Fellow, Department of Medicine and Endocrinology, Royal Postgraduate Medical School, Du Cane Road, London W12 0NN, UK*

DOUGLAS R. SALVESEN, MD, MRCOG — *Senior Registrar Obstetrics and Gynaecology, Queen Charlotte's and Chelsea Hospital, Goldhawk Road, London W6 0XG, UK*

JUDITH M. STEEL, MBE MB ChB, FRCPEd — *Victoria Hospital, Hayfield Road, Kirkcaldy KY2 5AH, UK*

ANTHONY I. TRAUB, MD, FRCOG — *Consultant Obstretrician and Gynaecologist, Royal Maternity Hospital, Grosvenor Road, Belfast BT12 6BA, UK*

F. ANDRÉ VAN ASSCHE, MD, PhD — *Department of Obstetrics and Gynaecology, Universitaire Ziekenhuizen Leuven, Herestraat 49, 3000 Leuven, Belgium*

JOHAN VERHAEGHE, MD, PhD — *Department of Obstetrics and Gynaecology, Universitaire Ziekenhuizen Leuven, Herestraat 49, 3000 Leuven, Belgium*

PAULINE WATT, RN, RM — *Midwife in Charge, Antenatal Clinic, Royal Maternity Hospital, Grosvenor Road, Belfast BT12 6BA, UK*

PETER A.M. WEISS — *Professor of Obstetrics and Gynecology, Director of Maternal Fetal Medicine, University Clinic of Graz, Auenbruggerplatz 14, A-8036 Graz, Austria*

JENNY WOOTTON, RGN — *Jeffrey Kelson Diabetic Centre, Central Middlesex Hospital, Acton Lane, London NW10 7NS, UK*

Preface

This book is intended as a practical guide and introduction to the present state of knowledge regarding diabetes in pregnancy. We have deliberately asked a number of international experts to summarize the world literature as they see it and to provide their own opinion on the best current practice.

We have throughout been conscious of the geographical and ethnic differences in diabetes as a disease, in obstetrical practice, and in medical facilities and expectations. Some chapters are very much state of the art in terms of complex investigations and interpretations, but these will still be relevant to clinical judgement even when facilities are less extensive or therapeutic options less complex. Other chapters are written by nursing, midwifery and dietetic colleagues, drawing on their own practical experience of being part of a multidisciplinary team looking after diabetic women during pregnancy. A chapter is included highlighting the influence social and cultural factors have on the nutritional and medical management of diabetic pregnancies.

The care of a pregnant diabetic woman and her baby involves many members of the health care team. We trust that this book will be useful to all of them: obstetrician, paediatrician both in the neonatal unit and in the later years as the child grows up, and to the diabetes physician and general practitioner who offer adjunctive services at all stages before, during and after the pregnancy.

The thoughts of a diabetic mother herself will serve as a focus for all of us, whatever our particular role in this multifactorial process. The one consistent factor that permeates all chapters is the recognition that a high blood glucose, for whatever reason, in whatever mother, in whatever city or country, will have the same adverse effects on herself and on her baby. The treatment, and ultimately the prevention, of this maternal/fetal interaction remains a challenge to us all.

We have made some editorial decisions on matters of style and spelling which are necessary for a multi-authored volume. The correct spelling is 'fetus' in both Oxford English and American English, but the use of the diphthongs 'ae' and 'oe' in the former but not in the latter (-aemia, emia) is standard practice and we have allowed our American co-authors to retain their language.

More controversial is the tendency for modern medicine to converse in abbreviations; in a multidisciplinary text not all of us will know the codes and for this reason we have tried to eliminate all abbreviations, even some very dear to many of us, such as GDM (gestational diabetes mellitus). The terms IDDM (insulin-dependent diabetes mellitus) and NIDDM (non-insulin-dependent mellitus) may themselves become obsolete and we have also reduced those abbreviations. We trust that those of you who still speak in a technical jargon will allow this move to intelligibility at the expense of a very slight increase in the length of the sentence.

Anne Dornhorst
David R. Hadden

Foreword

The practice of medicine and obstetrics is a continuing evolving process with its foundations in basic science and clinical research, with management adapting to the environmental, cultural and sociological changes of the day. The care of the pregnant diabetic woman highlights these points. Clinical management has evolved into a multi-disciplinary speciality with input from obstetricians, physicians, paediatricians, midwives, dieticians and most importantly the woman herself. This text book, edited by Dr Anne Dornhorst and Professor David Hadden, sets out to discuss the scientific basis on which the management of diabetes in pregnancy is based and to provide useful clinical information for all members of this multi-disciplinary team.

The emphasis on an international approach to the management of women with diabetes in pregnancy and the inclusion of authors from around the world is welcomed, as it acknowledges the influence of geographical and ethnic differences to the clinical presentation and constraints on the management of diabetes in pregnancy. The well publicized improvements in pregnancy outcome associated with diabetes during the last fifty years have been observed predominantly in women with insulin-dependent diabetes living in the Western world. The prevalence, however, of gestational diabetes is uncomfortably high, and essentially untreated, in Third World countries where access to obstetric, medical and public health facilities are often limited. The importance of this condition with respect to fetal wellbeing and the possible damage in utero to the fetal pancreas leading to non-insulin dependent diabetes in later life needs to be established. Improving pregnancy outcome to this important group of women represents a challenge for the next millennium.

The importance of maternal diabetes on the future health of the mother and her child has become an important focus for present day research. The allocation of the final section of the book to this topic is appropriate and timely. The threshold of maternal glucose intolerance which adversely influences the future health of the mother and child needs to be defined. Studies are required to ascertain whether treatment of maternal glycaemia can prevent these changes. If preventative strategies post partum for the mother with previous gestational diabetes are shown to delay the progression to diabetes, the diagnosis and long-term treatment of women with gestational diabetes will become an important public health initiative.

I believe that this text book achieves its objective in laying the scientific basis on which the rationale for the treatment of diabetes in pregnancy should be based. In addition, it provides a body of up-to-date information in this field on which future scientific and clinical research can be based to improve the care of all women with diabetes in pregnancy.

Professor Richard W. Beard, MA, MD, FRCOG
Professor of Obstetrics and Gynaecology
St Mary's Hospital Medical School
London

INTRODUCTION

1

Diabetes in Pregnancy: Past, Present and Future

DAVID R. HADDEN
Royal Victoria Hospital, Belfast, UK

This introductory chapter will focus on two aspects which have been at the centre of interest in the field of diabetes in pregnancy since the early recognition that this was a subject worthy of study by a number of disciplines. The problem of the actual definition and recognition of high blood glucose in a pregnancy, and that of the specific risk to the pregnancy caused by the high glucose, in some ways encapsulate two ways of looking at the same process. In the past, at the present time, and certainly in the future, there has been, is, and will be sufficient interest in what happens during pregnancy in a diabetic mother to justify this book and others which may follow it.

HYPERGLYCAEMIA IN PREGNANCY: NORMAL GLUCOSE LEVELS PRE PREGNANCY

OBSTETRICAL AND EPIDEMIOLOGICAL TERMINOLOGY

There are two different ways of looking at the problem of hyperglycaemia in pregnancy. The traditional obstetrical viewpoint is that the diabetes is a complication of the pregnancy. The alternative epidemiological view is that the pregnancy is in some way superimposed upon the diabetes. There is, of course, truth in both viewpoints and there is also a real difference between the practical requirement of the obstetrician who needs to classify the metabolic condition of the mother so that a treatment programme can be established at that immediate time, and the more contemplative

Diabetes and Pregnancy: An International Approach to Diagnosis and Management.
Edited by A. Dornhorst and D. R. Hadden.
© 1996 John Wiley & Sons Ltd.

retrospective analysis which is a luxury enjoyed by diabetologists and epidemiologists. The very first recorded case of diabetes in pregnancy dates back to 1824, before the medical world became subdivided into specialists of any sort[1]. Dr Bennewitz would have regarded himself as a family physician with broad interests and certainly considered that his case represented diabetes as a complication of the pregnancy, with the implication that it was the pregnancy that caused the metabolic abnormality. He had some justification in that viewpoint as the diabetic symptoms recurred in the subject's fourth, fifth and sixth pregnancies, but disappeared after each. That was long before the days of glucose tolerance tests or even blood glucose measurement in any form. Matthews Duncan in 1882 was an early obstetrician, and had no doubt in his compilation of the very unsatisfactory outcome of 15 pregnancies with diabetes that the situation was one where diabetes was a complication of the pregnancy; although he did admit to a number of problems, including the uncertain prevalence of the condition, the uncertain value of screening all mothers for glycosuria, and whether any special rules of treatment could be laid down[2].

After the discovery of insulin, there was a gradual recognition that improving blood glucose control in pregnancy had a beneficial effect on the outcome. It was in the continued search for perfection in this area that the epidemiological approach developed. The first of these contemplative physicians was Dr Jorgen Pedersen of Copenhagen, who produced the first book on the topic, *The Pregnant Diabetic and her Newborn*, in 1967[3], in which he discussed the terminology and semantics of diabetes. He first used the expression 'gestational diabetes' by which he meant 'chemical diabetes diagnosed for the first time in a pregnant woman with a normal fasting blood sugar and with a non-diabetic curve demonstrated inside the first weeks of the puerperium'. He recognized, therefore, that the final diagnosis could only be made after delivery and he emphasized that no regard be taken of abnormal, borderline or questionable glucose tolerance curves. This strict classification has not found favour as a practical management tool and has proved remarkably difficult to implement, even in epidemiological studies. The obstetrical world found it much easier to adopt the classification suggested by the late Dr Priscilla White, which was based entirely on age of onset and duration of established insulin-dependent diabetes prior to the pregnancy, subsequently adding a number of separate classifications for specific long-term diabetic complications[4]. Dr White did not intend to produce a separate classification for hyperglycaemia diagnosed for the first time in pregnancy, and the apparent simplicity of White's class 'A' (diabetes in pregnancy not treated with insulin) left a legacy of confusion when it was judged necessary to treat even mild hyperglycaemia in pregnancy with insulin. This meant that White class 'A' was an ever-disappearing mirage. Norbert Freinkel recognized this problem in his sub-classification into class 'A1' and 'A2', depending on whether the fasting blood glucose was normal or elevated, and this certainly allowed a more logical approach to treatment and a better understanding of the role of glucose and of other metabolites in the pathological processes[5].

GESTATIONAL DIABETES, OR HYPERGLYCAEMIA RECOGNIZED FOR THE FIRST TIME IN PREGNANCY

Gestational diabetes, as presently recognized, became crystallized in the obstetrical mind following the series of studies initiated in Boston in the late 1950s which eventually established the O'Sullivan criteria[6]. This produced a system which allowed the exact classification of each pregnant woman by the result of a screening 50 g glucose challenge test, followed if indicated by a 100 g glucose tolerance test. The system has proved remarkably resilient and still provides the basis for the obstetrical classification of this problem in many parts of the world. Somewhat later, the World Health Organization (WHO) tried to define gestational diabetes by appointing a committee of epidemiologists who decided, without any fieldwork, to apply non-pregnant criteria for pathological hyperglycaemia to the pregnant state[7]. This led to considerable dissatisfaction from the obstetrical camp. The same committee of the World Health Organization introduced the terminology of 'insulin-dependent' and 'non-insulin-dependent' diabetes mellitus, which has been widely accepted in diabetological medicine but is difficult to apply in the specific context of insulin treatment of hyperglycaemia in pregnancy. Recent studies of the genetic basis of diabetes may throw doubt on the distinction between these two poles of the clinical diabetic condition. The obstetricians have responded to this epidemiological challenge of classification by from time to time dividing the whole world of hyperglycaemia as they see it into either 'gestational' or 'pre-gestational' diabetes, which has a naive simplicity and even manages to ignore the question as to whether the male ever develops a classifiable form of diabetes at all!

The Epidemiological Viewpoint

The epidemiologist would like to take a broad view but sometimes falls into the trap of excessive reliance on minor points of classification and statistical cut-off levels. Soon after the initial WHO classification was promulgated, Jarrett suggested that the whole concept of gestational diabetes might conveniently disappear if the cut-off points for its diagnosis were somewhat raised to those which were considered diagnostic of true diabetes mellitus[8]. This implied a blood glucose of >11.0 mmol/l (200 mg/dl) 2 h after 75 g of glucose, which was a level then accepted by epidemiologists to produce unquestionable long-term complications of the diabetic state. The WHO epidemiological committee also introduced the concept of impaired glucose tolerance to encompass the minor degrees of hyperglycaemia not falling into the major classification. That sub-classification remains controversial and is now recognized to be heterogeneous, because of both the variable distribution of patterns of glucose intolerance in populations and the variability of the test employed to characterize glucose intolerance in individual people. It has even been termed a 'diagnostic rag-bag'[9]. The careful population studies by Harris in the USA have allowed the longer-term viewpoint to be established with some exactitude[10]. It is clear that glucose intolerance and therefore hyperglycaemia is a slowly progressive condition in some individuals in that population, and that this progress occurs in both males and females. If pregnancy supervenes in the female, there will be a short-term effect of the specific insulin resistance of the pregnancy state, but this may not produce any separate long-term effect on the subsequent inexorable progress of the hyperglycaemia in the individual. Harris found just as many cases of impaired glucose tolerance in the male as in the female population which she studied.

The very considerable variation in the diagnosis of gestational diabetes in different countries and in different ethnic groups within the same country has been analysed in detail[11]. The enormous difference between the prevalence of hyperglycaemia in pregnancy amongst the Pima Indian population in the state of Arizona where it is very high, and amongst populations such as rural Tanzania or parts of Chile where it does not appear to occur at all, means that the obstetrical approach in those places will be very different[12]. The equally great ethnic and geographic variation in the prevalence of insulin-dependent diabetes, where the onset is often well before the time of pregnancy, and that of non-insulin-dependent diabetes, where the time of onset is closer to that of the years of pregnancy, produces further epidemiological confusion. There is a marked north/south divide even within Europe, where insulin-dependent diabetes in the Scandinavian countries is relatively much more common than it is in Greece[13]. It is not without reason that the concept of gestational diabetes, defined as diabetes diagnosed for the first time in pregnancy, has found least favour in those northern European countries but is nonetheless judged a severe health problem in Mediterranean areas where non-insulin-dependent diabetes is much more common[14].

The Obstetrical Viewpoint

There is some justification in considering the practical obstetrician as having a narrow viewpoint focused on the individual patient. The persistently increased perinatal mortality and morbidity rates experienced by the known diabetic mother will continue to focus attention on that individual, and there is no case for relaxation of current management guidelines for insulin-dependent diabetic mothers in pregnancy. The association of mild pre-pregnancy hypertension and microalbuminuria with the development of more severe hypertension in pregnancy is diabetes related, although studies in Belfast have shown that pregnancy-induced hypertension or pre-eclampsia is not associated with the increased insulin resistance of the pregnant state (Roberts RN, Henriksen JE, Hadden DR, unpublished). The question, however, is whether a lesser degree of glucose intolerance still conveys a risk of adverse perinatal outcome and whether or not such risk is more associated with other characteristics of the pregnant woman, such as obesity, increasing age, or other medical conditions. From the obstetrical viewpoint the debate is sometimes focused on what is meant by macrosomia and whether that is different from a large-for-dates infant[15]. Associated with that concern is the relationship of macrosomia to the need for operative delivery. There are well-marked differences in the Caesarean section rate between countries, for which the explanation is not entirely based on medical grounds, and these differences have a bearing on the reported Caesarean section rates in pregnancy complicated by hyperglycaemia[16].

In southern California, where gestational diabetes is common among the Latin American population, an alternative diagnostic criterion using ultrasound measurement of fetal abdominal circumference at 30 weeks gestation has been suggested[17]. This direct approach to identifying the pregnancy which is actually producing a macrosomic fetus might be combined with a simple measure of blood glucose: the effect of insulin treatment in reducing the birth weight in these selected macrosomic hyperglycaemic conditions has also been confirmed, even for rather mild hyperglycaemia. There is certainly a need for the obstetrician to have a test which will allow the classification of the pregnancy into a specific high-risk group. There is no doubt that pregnancy in the established diabetic mother is such a high-risk condition and it is very reasonable to assume that there is no exact cut-off for this risk. This leads to the increasing search for lesser degrees of the risk factor[18].

In a northern European non-diabetic population of women attending the Royal Maternity Hospital in Belfast, no relationship has been found between infant birth weight and maternal blood glucose status in the last two months of pregnancy determined by the maternal glycosylated haemoglobin measured on the third postpartum day. This may mean that there is never any such association, but would have to be considered at present as a population-specific finding which might not hold in an ethnic group where unrecognized diabetes was common.

Diagnosis

The obstetrical wish for an exact diagnosis has not been met by a robust epidemiological or individual test. The problem of the distinction between fasting hyperglycaemia and glucose intolerance continues to be debated in the broader field of diabetic medicine. The distinction between sensitivity and specificity of any test is not unique to glucose tolerance, and was discussed in detail by the Reverend Thomas Bayes in his original mathematical theorem which showed that these concepts were entirely related to the frequency of whatever condition was being investigated[19]. If it is a frequent condition, then tests can be both sensitive and specific. If it is rare, neither criterion can be achieved. Thus, if hyperglycaemia in pregnancy is common in a population, useful diagnostic tests can be applied with greater precision. Nevertheless, the problem of reproducibility of either random plasma glucose or of a glucose tolerance test remains as a bar to the exact classification of borderline cases from an obstetrical management point of view. The move towards meal profiles in several centres is a logical development of the wish to classify the carbohydrate tolerance of an individual in relation to the food normally eaten by that person[20]. However, because this moves the challenge to a lower level, the problems of sensitivity and specificity become even greater. Further difficulties in the diagnostic field follow from minor changes in methodology. These have been perhaps unjustifiably held against the original O'Sullivan classification, which was based on the best available technology of 40 years ago, and an entirely satisfactory new population-based diagnostic system has not yet been validated. When such a study is eventually carried out, it will have to address further methodological processes, including that of glycation of haemoglobin or other proteins and, in the longer term, some measure of the genetic or environmental risk of the individual for the diabetic condition. If the identification of hyperglycaemia in pregnancy is to be the ultimate goal, some form of continuous glucose read-out by an implantable glucose sensor may be necessary, and this technology is not impossible.

More complicated diagnostic protocols involving measures of insulin resistance are not likely to find favour from either obstetrical or epidemiological viewpoints, and it has been pointed out that the debate between the role of insulin resistance and that of beta cell failure in the gradual evolution of the diabetic state may itself be a dualistic process, and that insulin resistance can be considered as a 'self-fulfilling prophecy' which depends on the use of a glucose tolerance test for the diagnosis of the hyperglycaemic state[21]. A number of very critical epidemiologically based reviews of the problem of the diagnosis of hyperglycaemia in pregnancy have been produced[22-24]. To some extent these have been specific criticisms of the original Boston criteria, but with recognition of the considerable variability of the glucose tolerance test the conclusion by one group that all such testing should be abolished save as a research tool is understandable[25]. The total confusion which presently exists in obstetrical units throughout the UK justifies this sceptical viewpoint[26]. Nonetheless, there are still mothers who have hyperglycaemia in pregnancy who must be recognized.

Neonatal Outcome

If hyperglycaemia in pregnancy is a clinical entity, there must be demonstrable associated effects on the fetus and newborn baby. That such effects do occur have been best shown in the series of studies of the Pima Indian population, where short-term and long-term effects on the fetal size and on the development of obesity and diabetes in the next generation have been confirmed[27]. Although that population has the highest prevalence of non-insulin-dependent diabetes in the world, there is no reason to suppose that such factors are not also operating in other countries where the risk of non-insulin-dependent diabetes is rapidly rising. There is, however, no evidence that mild hyperglycaemia in pregnancy is of itself associated with any of the long-term complications of established diabetes mellitus, such as retinopathy, nephropathy or neuropathy in the mother, and if those conditions are reported they must presumably represent undiagnosed pre-pregnancy hyperglycaemic states. There is even some evidence that the diagnosis of gestational diabetes is an advantage to pregnancy outcome if it is identified[28], but whether this is due to treatment of the hyperglycaemia or to closer obstetric supervision[29] is not yet clear.

The hypothesis based on epidemiological studies in the UK that small babies have a greater risk of developing diabetes in later life, associated with similar increased risk for coronary heart disease, hypertension and hypertriglyceridaemia, has not been fully confirmed in other countries[30]. The Pima Indian population has been shown to have a U-shaped curve where both small and large babies can be shown to have an increased risk of ultimately developing diabetes themselves[31]. Whether there is a threshold effect of maternal hyperglycaemia on neonatal outcome similar to that which appears to exist for the risk of long-term complications in the adult diabetic is not yet established. If so, the threshold might not be at the same level. There is epidemiological evidence that a sustained postprandial blood glucose of >11.0 mmol/l (200 mg/dl) is necessary to produce long-term microvascular complications. It is possible that a much lesser level of hyperglycaemia throughout the nine months of pregnancy could have a significant programming effect on the developing fetus and its beta cells.

Animal Models

There have been important studies using several different animal models of the risk of hyperglycaemia in pregnancy. To some extent these have focused on more severe hyperglycaemia and therefore are not relevant to the study of mild elevation of blood glucose in pregnancy, and it is clear that the risk of congenital fetal abnormalities in hyperglycaemia diagnosed for the first time in pregnancy is low, although severe experimental hyperglycaemia in the rat model will certainly produce such outcomes[32]. The longer-term follow-up of animal populations exposed to milder degrees of hyperglycaemia *in utero* confirms the importance of the trans-generational passage of diabetes by non-genetic mechanisms[33]. For well-established and well-recognized reasons the diabetic state in experimental animals, particularly in the rat, is not identical to that in human beings[34]. The most relevant studies may be those in the primate models and, in those, a definite relationship has been shown between the growth and development of the fetus and milder degrees of maternal hyperglycaemia[35].

CLASSIFICATION OF HYPERGLYCAEMIA IN PREGNANCY

The above points indicate that the classification of gestational diabetes defined as 'carbohydrate intolerance of variable severity with onset or first recognition during pregnancy' is unsatisfactory for a number of reasons. A number of diabetologists have preferred the term 'hyperglycaemia discovered for the first time in pregnancy'. If this concept is developed, the following scheme of hyperglycaemia in pregnancy can be produced:

Normal glucose levels pre pregnancy

- New insulin-dependent diabetes with onset in pregnancy
- New non-insulin-dependent diabetes with onset in pregnancy
- New impaired glucose tolerance with onset in pregnancy

(All three of these conditions usually improve post partum)

Pre-existing hyperglycaemia (recognized or unrecognized)

- Established insulin-dependent diabetes
- Established non-insulin-dependent diabetes
- Established impaired glucose tolerance

(These conditions are usually permanent and may get worse post partum)

This classification at least avoids the semantic problem of 'pre-gestational diabetes', but does not address the actual definition of hyperglycaemia. The proposed multicentre international study of hyperglycaemia and adverse pregnancy outcome (HAPO) will throw light on this presently confused scene; until then different centres will continue to use their own criteria. The data obtained using the 75 g oral glucose tolerance tests in pregnancy in Southern California will serve as a useful marker towards the adoption of universal standards[36]. The most recent WHO report continues to support this diagnostic tool[37], although thoughtful comparisons between the 2 h post-glucose level and either the fasting glucose or the glycated haemoglobin concentration may point to a much simpler epidemiological diagnosis of hyperglycaemia[38]. These thoughts are developed in more detail by McCance in the next chapter.

The hyperglycaemic state must be severe enough to affect the mother, both in the pregnancy and in later life, and the developing fetus or newborn, *in utero*, at birth, or in later life. To develop these concepts further a study of the value of glycation of haemoglobin as a reliable index of pre-existing hyperglycaemia is needed in a population where this condition is common. In Belfast, where gestational diabetes as usually defined as rare, a study of over 2700 unselected singleton pregnancies not previously known to be diabetic showed no predictive value for either a random plasma glucose, or glycated haemoglobin at the initial booking visit in the first trimester, and subsequent pre-eclampsia, caesarean section or neonatal requirement for special care. However, if the 21 established insulin-dependent diabetic mothers seen during the same time period were included, then a significant prospective association with all of these outcomes could be shown (Roberts, R, unpublished).

PRE-EXISTING HYPERGLYCAEMIA

ESTABLISHED INSULIN-DEPENDENT DIABETES IN PREGNANCY: AN OUTCOME RISK ANALYSIS

When the problem of classification and diagnosis of hyperglycaemia recognized for the first time in pregnancy has been resolved, and appropriate guidelines agreed, there will still be a large number of women who become pregnant *after* the diagnosis of type 1 or insulin-dependent diabetes. This is becoming a more prevalent disease in all parts of the world, and many studies are in progress to address the reasons for this increase. From the pregnancy point of view there is no doubt that it must be considered a high-risk condition, and the risk affects both mother and baby, both now and in their future. The reasons for the metabolic stress and the effects on the mother and the developing fetus are discussed in the three chapters in Part I of this book.

The now discarded White classification attempted to combine estimates of both obstetrical and diabetic risk in a single class: this is now unacceptable, and for any statement of risk to be of use to either doctor or patient it must address a number of points, which are best considered as outcome risks. It is always difficult to construct a memorable list of such items, and previous attempts have perhaps erred too much in the direction of simplicity. This section will discuss the major risks to both mother and baby from both obstetrical and diabetic aspects, in established insulin-dependent diabetic patients.

A systematic review of the importance of the various possible risk factors for the outcome of pregnancy in the diabetic mother, using the principles of the Cochrane Collaboration[39], is not available, although steps are being taken in that direction. In the absence of such a structured protocol, and in the knowledge that relatively few randomized clinical trials have been undertaken in this multidisciplinary field, the pragmatic present-day approach can only try to identify the relevant questions. Whether some of the accepted obstetrical wisdom or diabetic experience will ultimately be proved to be erroneous awaits a future analysis. It is entirely possible that, as for the common general medical interventions used in acute internal medical practice, early pessimism over the extent to which evidence-based obstetrical and diabetic medicine is currently practised will be found to be misplaced[40].

The majority of these risks will be discussed in subsequent chapters in this book. A summary of the major maternal risk factors for a successful pregnancy outcome is shown in Table 1.1. These can be considered as primarily obstetric or primarily diabetic risks, although there is some degree of overlap: there are also more direct fetal risks, both pregnancy and diabetes related.

Table 1.1. Outcome risk factors in diabetic pregnancy

Obstetric	Diabetic
Maternal	
Ethnic/geographic	Insulin-dependent/non-insulin-dependent diabetes mellitus
Age	Onset in pregnancy
Parity	Duration
Weight	Hyperglycaemia/ketoacidosis
Hypertension	Hypoglycaemia
Hydramnios	Hypertension
Miscarriage	Microvascular complications
Multiple pregnancy	Retinopathy
Urinary infection	Nephropathy
Nutrition	Macrovascular complications
Smoking/drug abuse	Cardiac
Late booking	Non-attender
Contraception	Pre-pregnancy counselling
Fetal	
Small-for-dates	Transgenerational programming
Intrauterine death	Large-for-dates
Caesarean section	
Prematurity	
Neonatal	
Breastfeeding	Childhood obesity

Primary Obstetric Risks

Geographical and ethnic maternal outcome risks can to some extent be identified from international tables of perinatal mortality, although this is an unsatisfactory index of total fetal loss. There is of course a very wide range of outcomes within any one population group, and it is difficult to distinguish problems due to deprivation or poverty from those of a purely genetic basis. The same variation exists for the risk of congenital fetal abnormalities, so that outcomes in diabetic pregnancy will be affected by major factors other than the management of the diabetic condition.

Maternal age has to some extent been minimized as a risk factor by the general advice for diabetic mothers to have their family when they are young, before age 30. The increasing secular trend to pregnancy at older ages will also affect the pregnant diabetic woman, and the same constraints will apply. These are not major obstetric reasons for concern, but the likelihood of diabetic complications of all sorts is certainly greater, especially at over age 40 years. Increasing parity is also a possible trend, and with well-controlled diabetes and an efficient mother there should not be a problem; however, the constraints of the present intensive blood glucose monitoring schedules often impose a limit on the desire for more children. Unplanned pregnancy at a very young age has its own obstetric and social problems, and a well-organized educational, family planning and contraceptive advice programme must be available.

Maternal overweight is not usually a risk factor in insulin-dependent diabetic pregnancy, but can be a major problem in non-insulin-dependent diabetes which presents in some populations at age 30 or even younger; these mothers will have to be treated with insulin and there is a major tendency for them to gain even more weight. Maternal underweight due to a pre-existing eating disorder, either anorexia or bulimia nervosa, may produce more difficult problems of adaptation to the physiological fluid balance changes of normal pregnancy, and can be associated with troublesome hyperemesis: when this is superimposed on insulin-dependent diabetes it may be necessary to have a long period of hospital management with nasogastric or intravenous nutrition.

Hypertensive disorders of pregnancy continue to be the leading cause of maternal mortality in the UK. Pre-eclampsia, or proteinuric pregnancy-induced hypertension, is associated with failure of trophoblast invasion of the spiral arterioles of the placenta, but the complete pathophysiological process is still poorly understood. As pregnancy is itself an insulin-resistant state, and insulin resistance is a feature of essential hypertension in non-pregnant individuals, there was a suggestion that pregnancy-induced hypertension was related to insulin resistance. Detailed studies of this situation using the 'minimal model' technique show that as for other forms of secondary hypertension insulin resistance is not involved (Roberts RN, Henriksen JE, Hadden DR, unpublished). Hypertension occurring for the first time in pregnancy can be divided into two distinct groups: pre-eclampsia (or proteinuric pregnancy-induced hypertension), and gestational hypertension. The former is immunologically mediated and most commonly seen in young primigravid women; the latter is not always associated with proteinuria and tends to occur in older multiparous women. This gestational hypertension, in contrast to pre-eclampsia, may still be shown to be associated with insulin resistance.

Proteinuria preceding pregnancy is related to the risk of hypertensive complications, but the exact mechanism is not clear. In one report, a urine protein of more than 190 mg per 24 h before 20 weeks gestation in diabetic women was associated with a 50% risk of pre-eclampsia and preterm delivery[41]. An important point is that angiotensin converting enzyme (ACE) inhibitors are now widely prescribed for diabetic patients with microalbuminuria with or without hypertension. These drugs should not be used during pregnancy because of the potential for adverse effects on fetal renal development and function. Extreme care should be taken to avoid conception in women taking ACE inhibitors.

Optimum blood pressure control for pregnant women with diabetic nephropathy has not been defined, but a figure of less than 130/85 mmHg has been suggested[42]. Drugs which have been proven to be safe during embryogenesis (methyldopa, hydralazine) should be used in early gestation: calcium channel blockers (nifedipine) and α-receptor antagonists (prazosin) may be used at a later stage: β-receptor antagonists may increase the risk of serious hypoglycaemia in insulin-treated patients on very tight metabolic control.

Multiple pregnancy is not an additional risk factor in a diabetic mother although there is a suggestion that hyperglycaemia in pregnancy is more likely, perhaps because of an increased insulin secretory requirement[43]. Hydramnios is difficult to quantify, but may be an indicator for other morbidity, especially a fetal abnormality; it is more frequent in diabetic pregnancy[44], and most series have found an increased perinatal mortality, although whether the hydramnios is of itself a risk is uncertain.

Spontaneous abortion is more common in first trimester diabetic pregnancy, perhaps related to relative maternal insulin deficiency with suboptimal support for early embryo growth[45]. The rate of abortion in mothers with diabetic nephropathy used to be still higher, but more recent studies have not shown this trend[46]. Sudden unexplained fetal death in late pregnancy used to be the major cause of perinatal mortality in diabetic pregnancy, but is now relatively unusual. Coustan has pointed out that the reasons for this decline in the six decades since the discovery of insulin are not entirely clear, and several technological advances such as blood transfusion, safer anaesthesia, fetal monitoring or neonatal intensive care, and ultrasound may all have contributed[47]. Nevertheless, the major contribution of normalization of maternal blood glucose perhaps first shown by Harley and Montgomery in 1965[48] and subsequently widely confirmed, especially with the use of capillary self-monitoring techniques, indicates that maternal hyperglycaemia is a major risk. Sudden unexplained late intrauterine death can still occur, even in very well-controlled diabetic pregnancy: there is no evidence that this is related to maternal hypoglycaemia or undiagnosed ketoacidosis. This risk, although small, continues to promote the concept of not necessarily proceeding to full term delivery in all cases.

Pyelonephritis is considered to be an increased risk in diabetic pregnancy, and to be associated with premature delivery and perinatal mortality; there are no controlled studies to confirm this, nor to suggest that this complication is now less frequent with improved maternal blood glucose levels. Careful monitoring for this condition and appropriate antibiotic therapy, even if asymptomatic, are widely recommended. With better control of blood glucose the amount of glycosuria should be less so that the risk of infection would be less, but the lower renal threshold for glucose in pregnancy means that glycosuria will never be fully eliminated.

Nutrition, smoking, alcohol and drug abuse tend to be linked as risk factors for obstetric outcome, and are all related to social deprivation. Normal nutritional advice should take care of the major changes in food metabolism which occur in normal pregnancy, with a fundamental switch in energy balance to allow a strongly anabolic state with considerable energy storage above the immediate needs of the growing fetus, followed by an overall change in the homeostatic control of almost all nutrients[49]. These concepts have been enshrined in the literature of diabetic pregnancy as 'facilitated anabolism' and 'accelerated starvation', which refer to the early and late adaptations in pregnancy, both of which become more pronounced in a situation where glucose and insulin are present in more than normal concentration[5]. Nutritional guidelines for diabetic pregnancy should not differ greatly from those for normal pregnancy, and excess weight gain should certainly be avoided. No lower limits for a safe level of alcohol or smoking have been established and there is a good case for avoiding both altogether in pregnancy. Dietary supplementation, particularly with folate, iron and free radical scavengers (ascorbic acid, tocopherols), is now widely practised and it may be difficult to obtain actual evidence of benefit. A study of antioxidant status in Belfast in 1995 showed no difference in serum antioxidant concentrations between diabetic and control pregnant women in the first trimester, nor in their intake as assessed by dietetic interview, but animal models point strongly to an association between poor first trimester antioxidant status and congenital fetal malformations[32]. Whether aspartame, now used very widely as an artificial sweetener, will increase the phenylalanine intake to a level which might cause problems in normal or diabetic pregnancy is not entirely clear, but the risk to an unrecognized or poorly controlled phenylketonuric mother must be recognized[50].

A planned pregnancy, with appropriate pre-pregnancy counselling, will give the best chance of addressing all these obstetric risks most effectively. It is well recognized that those who most need the counselling are the least likely to attend in a formal clinical setting, and every effort should be made to reach them by other means. This requires a community and family practice-orientated educational programme for contraception, pregnancy advice and subsequent family support. The role of the obstetrician and internist is to ensure that such facilities exist and are properly used. It has been recognized for many years that the greatest risk to a successful pregnancy outcome for a diabetic woman is non-attendance and non-compliance[51]. That these risks are still a major problem is shown by the results of a literature compilation (1965–1985) comprising the outcome of over 5000 pregnancies in diabetic women: 18% had hypertension (12% pregnancy induced), 9% developed ketoacidosis during the pregnancy, 16% had hydramnios and 4% pyelonephritis. In obstetric management terms, the total caesarean section rate was 41% (27% primary), and 9% went into preterm labour. The maternal mortality was 0.1%[52].

The particular obstetrical risks at delivery, and the possible early neonatal problems in the baby, are considered in detail in Part III of this book.

Primarily Diabetic Risks

The major diabetic risk for pregnancy outcome is maternal hyperglycaemia. The evidence that intensive treatment to correct the high blood glucose as far as possible will reduce maternal morbidity and perinatal mortality is based on a number of long-term reviews of clinical practice in centres with a special interest in this condition. No prospective randomized study has been carried out, nor is one necessary. But there are a number of unanswered questions which still require study, and present-day insulin therapy is far from physiological: the ultimate goal must still be to prevent the development of maternal hyperglycaemia whether identified for the first time in pregnancy or as an aspect of existing insulin-dependent diabetes.

Duration of diabetes is an important risk to pregnancy outcome, but is inextricably linked to both age at pregnancy and age at onset of diabetes. This is one reason why the White classification was unsatisfactory, as a mother aged 25 might have had diabetes for 20 years or for only one year, with widely different risks relating to other complications, and the special categories such as class F for diabetic nephropathy became impossible to assign accurately and again were largely linked to duration of diabetes. It is more satisfactory to note both age and duration of diabetes (or age of onset of diabetes) as separate risks. These measures are also more appropriate in allowing comparisons between countries where the incidence of insulin-dependent and non-insulin-dependent diabetes is widely different.

More important than duration is the degree of control of hyperglycaemia, both in the years preceding pregnancy (where control is linked to long-term complications) and during conception, embryogenesis and subsequent pregnancy (where hyperglycaemia will adversely affect implantation, fetal development and pregnancy outcome). The most striking demonstration of this trend is shown in Figure 1.1, which indicates that at a mean maternal blood glucose of about 5.0 mmol/l (90 mg/dl) the infant mortality falls to the level of the general population. The reasons for this steady fall are of course multifactorial, and not all due to improved blood glucose control.

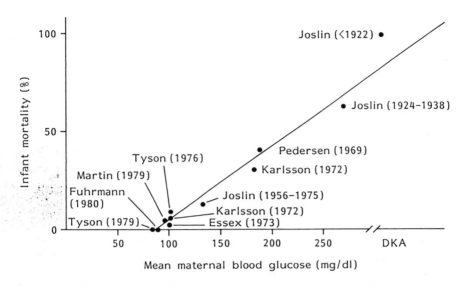

Figure 1.1. Mean maternal blood glucose concentration plotted against reported infant mortality for a number of series of obstetric outcomes in diabetic pregnancy between 1922 (discovery of insulin) and 1980 (introduction of capillary self-monitoring for blood glucose). From Jovanovic L, Peterson CM. Management of the pregnant insulin-dependent diabetic woman. *Diabetes Care* 1980; **3**: 63

Even in centres of excellence it is still not possible to state that the goal of the St Vincent Declaration of 'a pregnancy outcome the same as that of a non-diabetic woman' has been achieved, although for well-motivated and careful diabetic mothers this is likely to be the case. Practical advice in this direction is contained in the chapter by Firth, based on the very extensive experience of the Dublin group (see page 121).

Maternal ketoacidosis has been associated with high perinatal mortality, but this situation is much less common than previously, reflecting the ability of mothers to monitor their own glucose levels and take appropriate action to prevent acute metabolic derangement. Recent reports even suggest that appropriately treated early ketoacidosis does not necessarily carry a high morbidity.

Hyperglycaemia during the pregnancy has a number of consequences. Spontaneous abortion and congenital malformation are both linked to first trimester and periconceptual glucose control, while intrauterine fetal death (stillbirth) and macrosomia and the broader concept of diabetic fetopathy are more related to hyperglycaemia later in the pregnancy. It may be that all these complications have the same basic biochemical mechanism, manifest at different stages of fetal development. There may be abnormalities of placentation because of increased vascular fibrin deposition in early pregnancy, or the early spontaneous abortion may reflect a congenitally malformed conceptus. There are good retrospective and prospective studies linking early pregnancy hyperglycaemia to congenital malformations, although there is still some academic dispute as to whether glucose is the sole teratogen. It is unlikely, in view of the relatively low rate of malformations in human diabetic pregnancy with present-day methods of control of blood glucose, that this question can be answered except in rather artificial animal models, and the very variable background rates and types of malformations in different obstetrical environments mean that it will be difficult to establish the value of any individual change in therapy.

Macrosomia is usually defined as a birth weight greater than the 90th centile when adjusted for gestational age, and occurs in 25–42% of diabetic pregnancies, in contrast to 8–14% in selected control populations[53]. These babies are at a higher risk for unexplained intrauterine death, fetal abnormalities, birth trauma, cardiomyopathy, vascular thrombosis and neonatal hypoglycaemia. There is some evidence that the incidence of macrosomia is less when blood glucose control is very tightly maintained in the second trimester, but that improving control after 30 weeks will not be effective. Nevertheless, even if the risk for fetal weight is normalized, large-for-dates babies (>90th centile) will still be born to about 10% of diabetic mothers who have impeccable blood glucose control and these are presumably genetically rather than metabolically determined. Studies of the other aspects of diabetic fetopathy in this sub-group of 'macrosomic' babies would be of interest.

Maternal hypoglycaemia is an iatrogenic risk, but is a serious problem in tightly controlled first trimester diabetic pregnancy. The major cause is the altered metabolic environment due to the physiological adaptation to pregnancy, with a lower fasting glucose and more rapid swings of plasma glucose relating to meals and exercise. These changes also occur in normal pregnancy, but are more pronounced with insulin-dependent diabetes. Mothers who are determined to achieve normoglycaemia in early pregnancy may find themselves much more prone to severe hypoglycaemia than previously, and they may have less symptomatic warning of rapidly falling glucose levels. This state lasts until about 16 weeks, and then gradually disappears with the onset of insulin resistance in later pregnancy. Careful warning about this risk to the mother, her husband and other close relatives and workmates is necessary and important. Subcutaneous glucagon is often very helpful if available for emergency use by a trained person in the home. Because of this risk, which may very rarely even result in maternal death, the concept of very tight control in early pregnancy to prevent fetal malformation must be tempered with some realism.

Retinal, renal and macrovascular complications of insulin-dependent diabetes all carry their own added risk to the outcome of the pregnancy, which will be discussed in other chapters. The chapters summarizing the experience of the Hammersmith group in London under Kohner on the management of diabetic retinopathy in pregnancy (see page 155), and the detailed update on all aspects of diabetic nephropathy by Kitzmiller (see page 167), will be of great value in actual patient management. With an enthusiastic team approach, a mother with severe microvascular complications may be able to deliver a healthy baby, but the risks are certainly much greater. Severe visual impairment, or renal transplantation, are no longer bars to attempting to become pregnant, but success cannot be guaranteed even if blood glucose control is satisfactory. Macrovascular disease, especially coronary artery disease in an older mother, may produce serious cardiac failure in mid pregnancy. If there is a serious risk to the potential mother's life, or her ability to look after a baby, wise counsel would be to avoid the risk of pregnancy.

From a more optimistic viewpoint, the diabetes-related risks of pregnancy in an insulin-dependent diabetic girl should now be satisfactorily managed by a combined team approach. The chances are good of her producing a normal baby, of normal size, by normal delivery at the usual time. But this outcome will not be achieved without considerable attention to detail and a more supervised pregnancy than that of a non-diabetic mother.

Neonatal considerations still require the availability of intensive care and a cautious approach to possible hypoglycaemia in the infant. The present interest is in transgenerational effects, with 'imprinting' of maternal metabolic events on the fetal metabolism so that subsequent development of hyperglycaemia, hypertension and obesity may be potentially preventable. Curiously, these events have been identified mainly in small babies, and the large baby of the diabetic mother does not seem to have been implicated: this is most probably due to the very small number of successful pregnancies in diabetic mothers 50 years ago, and it is most probable that further prospective studies in this field will confirm the 'U-shaped' distribution already identified in the Pima Indian population[31]. Whether the theories of maternal nutritional deficiency to explain the small babies will be proven, or whether there is a more genetic determination of fetal size awaits the passage of time. But the possibility to extend the knowledge built up by careful observation of the diabetic woman and her baby to the prevention of long-term chronic disease states in the following generation puts a new context into preventive medicine. These concepts are developed in Part IV of this book, with a series of chapters by international experts on the long-term implications of a diabetic pregnancy.

REFERENCES

1 Bennewitz HG. De diabete mellito, graviditatis sympatomate. In: Hadden DR (ed.), The first recorded case of diabetic pregnancy (Bennewitz HG 1824, University of Berlin). *Diabetologia* 1989; **32**: 625.

2 Duncan JM. On puerperal diabetes. *Trans Obstet Soc Lond* 1882; **24**: 256–85.
3 Pedersen J. *The Pregnant Diabetic and her Newborn: Problems and Management.* Munksgaard, Copenhagen, 1967.
4 White P. Pregnancy and diabetes: medical aspects. *Med Clin North Am* 1965; **49**: 1015–30.
5 Freinkel N. Of pregnancy and progeny. *Diabetes* 1980; **27**: 1023–35.
6 O'Sullivan JB, Mahan CM. Criteria for the oral glucose tolerance test in pregnancy. *Diabetes* 1964; **13**: 278–85.
7 WHO. Expert Committee on Diabetes Mellitus, 2nd report. Technical Report Series 646. World Health Organization, Geneva, 1980; 8–14.
8 Jarrett RJ. Reflections on gestational diabetes. *Lancet* 1981; **ii**: 1220–2.
9 Yudkin JS, Alberti KGMM, McLarty DG, Swai ABM. Impaired glucose tolerance: is it a risk factor or a diagnostic ragbag? *Br Med J* 1990; **301**: 397–402.
10 Harris MI. Gestational diabetes may represent discovery of pre-existing glucose intolerance. *Diabetes Care* 1988; **11**: 402–11.
11 Hadden DR. Geographic, ethnic and racial variations in the incidence of gestational diabetes mellitus. *Diabetes* 1985; **34** (Suppl. 2): 8–12.
12 King H, Rewers M. WHO *ad hoc* diabetes reporting group. Global estimates for prevalence of diabetes mellitus and impaired glucose tolerance in adults. *Diabetes Care* 1993; **16**: 157–77.
13 Green A, Gale EAM, Patterson CC, for the Eurodiab ACE Study Group. Incidence of childhood-onset insulin-dependent diabetes mellitus: the Eurodiab Ace Study. *Lancet* 1992; **339**: 905–9.
14 Beard RW, Hoet JJ. Is gestational diabetes a clinical entity? *Diabetologia* 1982; **23**: 307–12.
15 Naeye RL. Infants of diabetic mothers: a quantitative morphologic study. *Pediatrics* 1965; **35**: 980.
16 Drury MI. Management of the pregnant diabetic patient: are the pundits right? *Diabetologia* 1986; **29**: 10–12.
17 Buchanan TA, Kjos SL, Montoro MN *et al.* Use of fetal ultrasound to select metabolic therapy for pregnancies complicated by mild gestational diabetes. *Diabetes Care* 1994; **17**: 275–83.
18 Langer O, Levy J, Brustman L *et al.* Glycaemic control in gestational age versus large for gestational age? *Am J Obstet Gynecol* 1989; **161**: 646–53.
19 Bingley PJ, Bonifacio E, Gale EAM. Perspectives in diabetes: can we really predict IDDM? *Diabetes* 1993; **42**: 213–20.
20 Sutherland HW, Pearson DWM, Lean MWJ, Campbell DM. Breakfast tolerance test in pregnancy. In: Sutherland HW, Stowers JM (eds), *Carbohydrate Metabolism in Pregnancy and the Newborn*. Churchill Livingstone, Edinburgh, 1984; 267–75.
21 O'Rahilly S, Hattersley A, Vaag A, Gray H. Insulin resistance as the major cause of impaired glucose tolerance: a self-fulfilling prophecy? *Lancet* 1994; **344**: 585–9.
22 Ales KL, Santini DL. Should all pregnant women be screened for gestational glucose intolerance? *Lancet* 1989; **ii**: 1187–91.
23 Naylor CD. Diagnosing gestational diabetes mellitus: is the gold standard valid? *Diabetes Care* 1989; **12**: 565–72.
24 Ratner RE. Gestational diabetes mellitus: after three international workshops do we know how to diagnose and manage it yet? *J Clin Endocrinol Metab* 1993; **77**: 1–4.
25 Hunter DJS, Kierse MJNC. Gestational diabetes. In: Chalmers I, Enkin M, Kierse M (eds), *Effective Care in Pregnancy and Childbirth*. Oxford University Press, Oxford, 1989; 403–10.
26 Nelson-Piercy C, Gale EAM. Do we know how to screen for gestational diabetes? Current practice in one Regional Health Authority. *Diabet Med* 1994; **11**: 493–8.
27 Pettitt DJ, Baird HR, Aleck KA *et al.* Excessive obesity in offspring of Pima Indian women with diabetes during pregnancy. *N Engl J Med* 1983; **308**: 242–5.
28 Moses RG, Griffiths RD. Can a diagnosis of gestational diabetes be an advantage to the outcome of pregnancy? *J Soc Gynecol Invest* 1995; **2**: 523–5.
29 Roberts RN, Moohan JM, Foo RLK *et al.* Fetal outcome in mothers with impaired glucose tolerance in pregnancy. *Diabetic Med* 1993; **10**: 438–43.
30 Hales CN, Barker DJP. Type 2 (non-insulin-dependent) diabetes mellitus: the thrifty phenotype hypothesis. *Diabetologia* 1992; **35**: 595–601.
31 McCance DR, Pettitt DJ, Hanson RL *et al.* Birthweight and non-insulin dependent diabetes:

'thrifty genotype', 'thrifty phenotype' or 'surviving small baby genotype'. *Br Med J* 1994; **308**: 942–5.

32 Eriksson UJ. Congenital malformations in diabetic animal models: a review. *Diabetes Res* 1984; **1**: 57–66.

33 Aerts L, Holemans K, van Assche FA. Maternal diabetes during pregnancy: consequences for the offspring. *Diabetes Metab Rev* 1990; **6**: 147–67.

34 Bone AJ, Walker R, Varey A-M *et al.* Effect of cyclosporin on pancreatic events and development of diabetes in BB/Edinburgh rats. *Diabetes* 1990; **39**: 508–14.

35 Chez RA, Mintz DH, Horger EO, Hutchinson DL. Factors affecting the response to insulin in the normal subhuman pregnant primate. *J Clin Invest* 1970; **49**: 1517–27.

36 Sacks DA, Greenspoon JS, Abu-Fadil S *et al.* Towards universal criteria for gestational diabetes: the 75 gram glucose tolerance test in pregnancy. *Am J Obstet Gynecol* 1995; **172**: 607–14.

37 WHO Study Group on Prevention of Diabetes Mellitus. Prevention of diabetes mellitus: report of a WHO study group. WHO Technical Report Series: 844, Geneva, 1994; 32–5.

38 McCance DR, Hanson RL, Charles M-A *et al.* Comparison of tests for glycated haemoglobin and fasting and two-hour plasma glucose concentrations as diagnostic methods for diabetes. *Br Med J* 1994; **308**: 1323–8.

39 Mulrow CD. Rationale for systematic reviews. In: Chalmers I, Altman DG (eds), *Systematic Reviews*. BMJ Publishing Group, London, 1995; 1–8.

40 Ellis J, Mulligan I, Rowe J, Sackett DL. Inpatient general medicine is evidence based. *Lancet* 1995; **346**: 407–10.

41 Combs EA, Rosenn B, Kitzmiller JL *et al.* Early-pregnancy proteinuria in diabetes related to preeclampsia. *Obstet Gynecol* 1993; **82**: 802–7.

42 American Diabetes Association Consensus Statement. Treatment of hypertension in diabetes. *Diabetes Care* 1993; **16**: 1394–7.

43 Dwyer PL, Oats JN, Walstab JE, Beischer NA. Glucose tolerance in twin pregnancy. *Aust NZ J Obstet Gynaecol* 1982; **22**: 131–5.

44 Lufkin G, Nelson R, Hill L. *et al.* An analysis of diabetic pregnancies at Mayo Clinic, 1950–79. *Diabetes Care* 1984; **7**: 539–44.

45 Sutherland HW, Pritchard CW. Increased incidence of spontaneous abortion in pregnancies complicated by diabetes mellitus. *Am J Obstet Gynecol* 1986; **155**: 135–40.

46 Reece EA, Coustan DR, Hyslett JP *et al.* Diabetic nephropathy: pregnancy performance and feto-maternal outcome. *Am J Obstet Gynecol* 1988; **159**: 56–66.

47 Coustan DR. Perinatal morbidity and mortality. In: Reece EA, Coustan DR (eds), *Diabetes Mellitus in Pregnancy: Principles and Practice*. Churchill Livingstone, Edinburgh, 1988; 537–45.

48 Harley JMG, Montgomery DAD. Management of pregnancy complicated by diabetes. *Br Med J* 1965; **i**: 14–16.

49 Hytten FE. Nutritional physiology during pregnancy. In: Campbell DM, Gillmer MDG (eds), *Nutrition in Pregnancy: 10th Study Group*. Royal College of Obstetricians and Gynaecologists, London, 1983; 1–15.

50 Hollingsworth DR, Ney DM. Dietary management of diabetes during pregnancy. In: Reece EA, Coustan DR (eds), *Diabetes Mellitus in Pregnancy: Principles and Practice*. Churchill Livingstone, Edinburgh, 1988; 285–311.

51 Pedersen J, Molsted-Pedersen L. Prognosis of the outcome of pregnancy in diabetics. *Acta Endocrinol* 1965; **50**: 70–8.

52 Cousins L. Obstetric complications. In: Reece EA, Coustan DR (eds), *Diabetes Mellitus in Pregnancy: Principles and Practice*. Churchill Livingstone, Edinburgh, 1988; 455–68.

53 Kitzmiller JL. Macrosomia in infants of diabetic mothers: characteristics, causes, prevention. In: Jovanovic L, Peterson CM, Fuhrmann K (eds), *Diabetes and Pregnancy: Teratology, Toxicology and Treatment*. Praeger, New York, 1986; 85–120.

2

Classification and Diagnosis of Diabetes in Pregnancy

DAVID R. McCANCE

Royal Victoria Hospital, Belfast, UK

There are few other areas of diabetes research which have aroused such confusion and controversy as the classification and diagnosis of diabetes in pregnancy. The diversity of interest in the subject (by epidemiologist, diabetologist, obstetrician, paediatrician, neonatologist, clinical scientist and embryologist alike) is a witness to its perceived importance, but equally has been driven by differing goals and agendas. Respected international bodies[1-3], three international workshops[3-6] and a number of position statements[7-9] have attempted to clarify the situation and offer a uniformity of approach but this is still lacking on a global and even national perspective.

A number of fundamental difficulties exist. The most basic problem is the absence of a threshold separating subjects into low- and high-risk groups for adverse pregnancy outcome. Statistical divisions allow the derivation of sensitivity, specificity and predictive values but these will obviously vary with the choice of diagnostic cutpoint and may be divorced from clinical relevance. A second difficulty concerns the different evolution of diagnostic criteria in the pregnant and non-pregnant states. This has blurred the meaning and understanding of terminology, fostered an entrenchment of attitude and greatly hampered meaningful comparisons among differing populations. A third integrally related problem is the need for a clear definition of the outcome of interest. The maternal–fetal unit is the only relevant consideration and must be rigorously classified and understood by all related disciplines in the field.

Several authors have questioned whether diabetes during pregnancy is a

Diabetes and Pregnancy: An International Approach to Diagnosis and Management.
Edited by A. Dornhorst and D. R. Hadden.
© 1996 John Wiley & Sons Ltd.

disease, or simply a risk factor for disease[10], or glucose intolerance antedating the pregnancy[11] or indeed, whether it is worth diagnosing[12]. A number of provocative reviews have recently challenged established dogma and thinking[13-15].

Against such a background, this chapter does not seek to be didactic or opinionated but rather to offer the reader a balanced overview of the derivation and current usage of nomenclature, classification and diagnostic criteria, highlighting areas of debate and suggesting pertinent questions for further consideration. The subject has an obvious interface with diabetes in the mother and outcome in future generations which are dealt with in other chapters of this book and will only be alluded to here as they relate specifically to diagnosis.

HISTORICAL PERSPECTIVE

The adverse outcome of pregnancy in insulin-dependent diabetes mellitus has been recognized for over a century[16] although in early studies measurements were limited to glycosuria[17]. With the advent of insulin therapy it became possible to contemplate the possibility of successful pregnancy for the diabetic mother. By the 1940s and 1950s an increasing awareness from retrospective analyses that women with overt diabetes often had a history of fetal loss or heavy infants in the years preceding diagnosis led to the concept of a 'prediabetic' state. As many as 58% of diabetic women had given birth to at least one heavy infant during their prediabetic years, compared with 27% of non-diabetic women[18]. Gilbert and Dunlop[19] reported a fetal loss of 50% for the two-year interval before diagnosis. Other authors have cited rates of fetal loss varying between 10% and 35%[20-25] with further emphasis being placed on the significance of blood sugars most proximate to the diagnosis of diabetes.

These observations were consistent with the prevailing belief that early detection of disease and its intensive treatment would postpone or prevent the evolution of the diabetes state or its complications. This necessarily placed a greater importance on diagnosis and raised the possibility that the oral glucose tolerance test (OGTT) (which by then had become widely used) might uncover a defect in glucose metabolism which was not demonstrable in the basal state. An intravenous test[26] had also been developed with good reproducibility and the attraction of bypassing the enterohepatic circulation, but was considered more unphysiological and cumbersome to administer than the OGTT and subsequently was shown to be a poor predictor of fetal outcome[27-29]. Other approaches to diagnosis including stressed OGTT (cortisone GTT and prednisone GTT) were studied in several centres but did not fulfil theoretical expectations[28,30]. All this information posed immediate problems of definition of an abnormal glucose tolerance test, particularly during pregnancy[31].

PHYSIOLOGY

Pathophysiological aspects of the metabolic stress of pregnancy are dealt with elsewhere but a brief mention of the effect of different stages of pregnancy on glucose tolerance is necessary here for a proper understanding of the discussion below. The diabetogenic effect of pregnancy has long been recognized[16] but the exact mechanism remains incompletely understood[32-36]. Various lines of observation including an increase in both fasting and postprandial insulin levels with advancing pregnancy, a blunted response to the intravenous injection of exogenous insulin, the development of abnormal glucose tolerance late in gestation, the need for increasing doses of insulin during pregnancy and resolution of the process after delivery point to pregnancy as inducing a state of insulin resistance. It is generally accepted that fasting glucose values are lower during pregnancy than in non-pregnant individuals[36,37], but are held within a restricted range. The glucose response to a mixed meal or pure glucose challenge is both delayed and increased[38,39]. Fasting glucose levels fall in the first trimester[37,40]. With advancing normal pregnancy, both fasting and postprandial blood glucose levels rise a little although still within the normal non-pregnant range. The practical implication of these observations for diagnosis is that any perceived abnormality of glucose tolerance must be related to a trimester-specific pregnancy reference range. Centile values for each trimester have been established for the 100 g OGTT[41,42] and more recently using a 75 g load[43,44]. Similar trimester-specific data for glycated haemoglobin are also now available[46].

NOMENCLATURE

The exact origin of the term *gestational diabetes* is difficult to ascertain but almost certainly grew from a realization of the relationship between fetal survival, birth weight and hyperglycaemia in pregnancy[19,20,47]. The original concept of gestational diabetes required it to be a temporary state with a return to normal after delivery[48], and was the definition used by Jorgen Pedersen in his pioneering book on the *Pregnant Diabetic and her Newborn*[49]. The present-day situation is more confused. Two slightly different definitions espoused by differing international bodies and reflecting different diagnostic practices have evolved. The American Diabetes Association (ADA)[1,7,9], US National Diabetes Data Group (NDDG) and associated groups define the term as 'carbohydrate intolerance of varying severity with onset or first recognition during pregnancy'. This definition (which has remained unchanged in a subsequent international workshop[6]) applies 'irrespective of whether or not insulin is used for treatment or the condition persists after pregnancy'. By contrast, the World Health Organization (WHO)[2,3] defines diabetes mellitus as 'a state of chronic hyperglycaemia' on the basis of guidelines used for non-pregnant adults and includes an additional category of impaired glucose tolerance (see below). This latter definition is applicable only to women in whom these guidelines are first exceeded during pregnancy.

The meaning of the term 'gestational diabetes' therefore differs depending on which set of diagnostic criteria are used. Both definitions require the fulfilment of criteria after an OGTT but the ADA NDDG defines only two categories – that of normal glucose tolerance and gestational diabetes – while the WHO criteria include categories of normality, impaired glucose tolerance and diabetes.

Few studies have compared the two criteria, but there is some evidence to suggest that 'gestational diabetes' including gestational impaired glucose tolerance, as defined by WHO criteria, will identify two or three times more women than diagnosed by other diagnostic methods[44,50]. This looseness of definition may allow the concept of gestational diabetes to be a useful aetiological risk factor but poses obvious problems from an aetiological and epidemiological point of view.

DIAGNOSIS

The diagnosis of symptomatic insulin-dependent diabetes is usually obvious, being readily confirmed by glycosuria and prompt blood testing. There is international agreement that a random glucose $\geqslant 11.1$ mmol/l (200 mg/dl) or a fasting glucose $\geqslant 7.8$ mmol/l (140 mg/dl) confirms the diabetic state and warrants further investigation[1-3]. The problem relates to those subjects found on screening with few, if any, related symptoms or signs.

Table 2.1 summarizes some of the OGTT criteria for diabetes in pregnancy. In North America the O'Sullivan and Mahan criteria[41], endorsed by the US NDDG[1], are widely used. These were derived from an unselected group of 752 pregnant women recruited on registration in a Boston hospital over a four-month period in the 1950s. On the basis of a 100 g OGTT with fasting and 1, 2 and 3 h samples upper threshold values were created by adding one, two or three standard deviations above the mean result for each time point. For each set of threshold values, the OGTT was positive if blood glucose results for two or more time stages exceeded the corresponding threshold. These criteria were then applied to a second group of 1013 women to determine which set had the best sensitivity and specificity for subsequent diabetes in the non-pregnant state (as defined by US Public Health Criteria) over periods ranging up to eight years. The best set of threshold values were the mean plus two standard deviations for each of the OGTT values, which were rounded off for simplification and later adjusted to modern glucose measurement procedures. Coustan has proposed alternative figures to the O'Sullivan criteria correcting not only for the change from whole blood to plasma but also for the use of glucose

Table 2.1. Oral glucose tolerance test criteria during pregnancy

Author	Sampling times				Load (g)	Comment
	Fasting	1h	2h	3h		
O'Sullivan et al.[52,a]	5.0 (90)	9.2 (165)	8.1 (145)	7.0 (125)	100	2 or more met or exceeded
Gillmer et al.[104]	+	+	+	+	50	>42 area units above baseline
Merkatz et al.[68]	5.8 (105)	10.3 (185)	7.7 (140)	6.9 (125)	75	2 values met or exceeded
Mestman[97]	6.1 (110)	11.1 (200)	8.3 (150)	7.2 (130)	100	2 values met or exceeded
NDDG[1,b]	5.8 (105)	10.6 (190)	9.2 (165)	8.1 (145)	100	2 or more must be met/exceeded
Carpenter and Coustan[51]	5.3 (95)	10.0 (180)	8.7 (155)	7.8 (140)	100	2 values met or exceeded
WHO[2,3] (IGT, G-IGT)	<7.8 (140)		7.8–11.1 (140–199)		75	Both must be met
WHO[2,3] (DM, GDM)	≥7.8		≥200		75	Either fasting or 2h value met or exceeded
Oats and Beischer[55]		9.0 (162)	7.0 (126)		50	Both values met or exceeded

IGT, impaired glucose tolerance; G-IGT, gestational impaired glucose tolerance; DM, diabetes mellitus; GDM, gestational diabetes mellitus.

[a]Measured on whole blood using Somogyi–Nelson method. Figures are rounded to nearest 5 mg/dl. The remaining criteria are based on plasma using glucose oxidase/hexokinase methodology.

[b]Corrects for change from whole blood to plasma or serum glucose and for the use of glucose oxidase or hexokinase methodology. In non-pregnant state a 75 g glucose load is used. IGT is defined as fasting <140, 1 h ≥200, 2 h 140–199 (al. three must be met). Diabetes: fasting ≥140, 1 h ≥200, 2 h ≥200 (either fasting or 1 and 2 h values must be met).

oxidase or hexokinase methodology, which yields values approximately 0.27 mmol/l (5 mg/dl) lower than the Somogi–Nelson method[51].

In the late 1970s and early 1980s several authoritative bodies including the US NDDG and the WHO Expert Committee on Diabetes Mellitus[1-3] reviewed the available evidence and made recommendations about diagnostic standards. There was agreement on the use of a 75 g OGTT, diagnostic cut-off levels and the creation of a new category of impaired glucose tolerance. The groups differed, however, on the application of glycaemic criteria to glucose intolerance in pregnancy, the WHO proposing that the criteria for diabetes in non-pregnant adults should also be applied to pregnant adults, with the proviso that the 'management of impaired glucose tolerance during pregnancy should be the same as for diabetes'[3]. By contrast, the NDDG recommended retention of the procedures and criteria based on those originally proposed by O'Sullivan and Mahan[41,52]. It was hoped by the WHO that this distinction between diabetes and impaired glucose tolerance in pregnancy would allow further elucidation of conflicting reports[13,40,53,54] of the 'effects of minor degrees of glucose intolerance upon maternal and child health'[3].

The WHO criteria are most widely used outside North America and have been further modified by the Diabetes in Pregnancy Study Group of the European Association for the Study of Diabetes[44]. Following realization by this group that conventional WHO criteria identified two or three times more women than did other methods, the upper limit of the 2 h glucose was increased from 8 to 9 mmol/l (144 to 162 mg/dl). Other European criteria have largely been based on various measures of outcome. Oats and Beischer[55] reported a 50 g 3 h OGTT which identified 2.5% of the population whose risk of perinatal mortality was approximately twice the background rate.

DIFFICULTIES IN DIAGNOSIS

DICHOTOMIZING CONTINUOUS VARIABLES

A fundamental problem is the absence of a threshold predicting adverse maternal fetal outcome. The bimodal glucose distribution demonstrated in some non-pregnant populations with a high prevalence of diabetes has not been observed during pregnancy[56]. The glycaemic risk appears to be continuous for both maternal and fetal outcome. Among 249 women who had a 100 g OGTT at 28 weeks gestation, which was not abnormal based on NDDG criteria, higher levels of 2 h glucose were associated with a significant increase in fetal macrosomia, Caesarean section rate and maternal toxaemia[53]. More recently, Sacks *et al.*[57] reported a linear risk with 2 h glucose and fetal birth weight controlled for maternal risk factors. The relevance of glycaemic risk for subsequent maternal diabetes was examined by Metzger *et al.*[58], who showed that among 113 women diagnosed as having gestational diabetes by NDDG criteria, fasting plasma glucose during pregnancy was related to the development of an abnormal OGTT within the first year post partum. Pettitt *et al.*[56] reported that the rate of complications (perinatal mortality, macrosomia, toxaemia, Caesarean section) and the subsequent incidence of diabetes in the mother was continuous through the range of 2 h glucose concentrations studied.

OGTT

Timing of the OGTT During Pregnancy

Variation in fasting and post-load glucose levels during pregnancy dictate the need for comparison with trimester-specific normal ranges and some have criticized the O'Sullivan criteria in this regard[14]. Increased diabetogenic stress with advancing pregnancy is the rationale for the customary diagnostic testing in the third trimester, but the possible benefit of earlier identification of women at risk for adverse maternal–fetal outcome cannot be excluded. There is some evidence that fetal macrosomia is associated with transient abnormalities in maternal glucose metabolism in the second trimester[45]. Conceivably treatment may only be effective if instituted at an early stage.

Reproducibility

Methodological concern over the poor reproducibility of the OGTT applies both to the pregnant and non-pregnant individual. Reproducibility is of the order of 50–70% in non-pregnant subjects[59], but has seldom been examined in pregnancy, with a few exceptions[60,61], and was not considered in the derivation of the O'Sullivan criteria[41]. Patients and controls in various studies frequently differ in the presence or absence of a glucose challenge during an earlier screening procedure. Moreover, the whole category of impaired glucose tolerance introduced by the WHO may be heterogeneous[62].

Glucose Load

The actual amount of glucose ingested (50, 75 or 100 g) varies from centre to centre. A 100 g load is most commonly used in the USA. Some British Commonwealth countries have tended to use a 50 g load mainly because it causes less vomiting. Most European centres have adopted the 75 g OGTT interpreted by WHO criteria. It has been shown, however, that 75 g of glucose gives OGTT values that are virtually identical to those obtained with 100 g glucose[63]. The shorter duration (2 h) removes the opportunity to meet the 3 h O'Sullivan criteria.

SAMPLING AND GLUCOSE ANALYSIS

The O'Sullivan and Mahan criteria were developed using the Somogi–Nelson method of glucose analysis on venous whole blood. This technique measures about 5 mg/100 ml of non-glucose-reducing substances and has now largely been replaced by specific glucose oxidase methods, with a 5% lowering of results. Haemodilution in pregnancy alters the relation between plasma and whole blood concentrations. Plasma contains more glucose than whole blood as after haemolysis there is less glucose inside the red cell; venous blood contains less glucose than arterial blood and capillary glucose approximates more to the arterial level. Fortunately venous plasma (measured in hospital laboratories) and capillary whole blood (measured by an impregnated test strip) are virtually equivalent[64]. These differences may have some importance in pregnancy. There has also been criticism of the attempt to convert the O'Sullivan criteria to current methods of measurement[15,65]. The NDDG criteria were derived by extrapolation of the O'Sullivan data, correcting for the change from venous blood to plasma or sera, and appear to lie outside the 95% confidence intervals of three of the four points chosen[65].

ETHNIC VARIATION

International comparisons of the prevalence of diabetes during pregnancy are made difficult by the use of different methods and cut-off points for diagnosis. The general picture, however, mirrors geographical differences in the prevalence of insulin-dependent and non-insulin-dependent diabetes, being lowest in northernmost parts of Western civilized countries and highest in subtropical and tropical developing countries[66,67]. The contribution of undiagnosed diabetes preceding pregnancy will also vary with location. Using WHO criteria, diabetes during pregnancy was 40 times more prevalent in Pima Indians than in the South Boston population (60% white, 40% non-white) studied by O'Sullivan and 10 times more prevalent than in the Cleveland population (61% white, 39% non-white) studied by Merkatz *et al.*[68]. Adoption of population-specific criteria on a statistical basis will yield greatly differing prevalence rates. It would seem likely that pathological levels of hyperglycaemia are similar for all countries and for all populations[66]. A universal framework of reference has a strong epidemiological appeal.

PREGNANT/NON-PREGNANT DEFINITIONS

The most recent workshop on gestational diabetes acknowledged that glucose intolerance may antedate the pregnancy. No information is usually available before pregnancy but Harris[11] pointed to the similar rates of diabetes and impaired glucose tolerance in pregnant and non-pregnant individuals, together with their association with risk factors for non-insulin-dependent diabetes, and suggested that the condition rather represents the discovery of pre-existing glucose intolerance. This has implications both for diagnosis and the concept and significance of minor degrees of hyperglycaemia.

Postpartum studies of glucose tolerance should be considered an integral part of the diagnostic process but equally suffer from changing practices and differing methodology and criteria for 'normality'. The term gestational diabetes originally implied that the test for abnormal glucose metabolism was repeated in the postpartum period and shown to be normal[49] but this requirement was omitted from both the NDDG and WHO documents. The 'diabetes' predicted by O'Sullivan criteria was defined by US Public Health Criteria and many, if not most of these 'diabetics', would be classified as impaired glucose tolerance by WHO criteria. This disparity makes it difficult to compare estimates of the subsequent development of glucose intolerance. The WHO criteria state that women should be formally retested after pregnancy using a 75 g OGTT and reclassified according to their new non-pregnant results. Unfortunately, for the NDDG criteria, this means that different tests will be used in the same person before and after pregnancy.

MATERNAL RISK FACTORS

The possible confounding by maternal risk factors of the relation of hyperglycaemia and pregnancy outcome continues to be debated[14,69–71] and many reports have failed to control for these factors. Among the early studies, O'Sullivan found an excess perinatal mortality in women who were obese or at least 25 years old[52]. Some consider that the adverse outcome of hyperglycaemia during pregnancy is explicable by these maternal risk factors, while others believe that even minor degrees of hyperglycaemia present an independent risk for adverse pregnancy outcome[53,72]. The situation is further complicated by the fact that some clinical risk factors used to screen subjects (obesity and family history of non-insulin-dependent diabetes) also confer an increased risk of glucose intolerance in the non-pregnant state independent of knowledge of OGTT results during pregnancy[11]. In one study, the 50 g glucose challenge test was significantly associated with fetal macrosomia even when the OGTT was negative[73]. Other recent studies, however, have shown an independent effect of blood glucose for macrosomia and perinatal outcome controlled for maternal risk factors[76].

DETECTION

A survey of clinical obstetric practice clearly reveals that the issue of screening for diabetes during pregnancy is no less confused than that of diagnosis itself[75–79]. Whether all women should be screened and by what method is unclear[13]. It is generally agreed that the simple and traditional documentation of maternal risk factors followed by a full diagnostic test (3 h, 100 g) is only 50–70% sensitive[52,79–81]. In the USA, a 50 g 1 h challenge was first introduced by O'Sullivan in 1973 and has been well validated[52] and endorsed by the ADA. Random sampling of venous[82,83], plasma[84,85] or capillary[86] blood glucose have all been proposed as screening procedures and even as a replacement for the OGTT[14]. Meal tolerance tests are conceptually appealing and have been incorporated into screening paradigms[87,88] but are difficult to standardize.

A universal screening programme of all pregnant women >25 years of age using a 50 g challenge between 24 and 28 weeks of gestation is currently advocated in the USA. The American College of Obstetricians and Gynecologists favour a selective screening policy of women ⩾30 years and younger women with traditional risk factors[8]. By contrast, in other reports[13,44] no convincing evidence of increased fetal or maternal risk was found to justify a universal screening programme other than the increased risk for subsequent diabetes in the mother.

DIAGNOSTIC ENDPOINTS

Central to the diagnosis (and indeed screening) of diabetes during pregnancy is the outcome one wishes to predict (and with treatment to prevent). An inherent weakness and major criticism of the O'Sullivan criteria is their validation by prediction of subsequent maternal diabetes and not fetal outcome[52]. The risk for subsequent retinopathy in the non-pregnant state was the rationale behind the current WHO criteria[2,3] and attention has recently been drawn to the fact that other test variables can only be evaluated in this perspective[89].

In the context of diabetic pregnancy there are immediate and long-term outcomes for both mother and baby. Pregnancy outcome has undoubtedly been affected by improved obstetric practice and neonatal care to the extent that, for perinatal mortality, it may not be possible further to reduce existing rates. Certain endpoints (operative deliveries) may vary as much with traditional practice as with significant metabolic antecedents. Other immediate outcomes suffer from a lack of clear definition and accepted meaning by interrelated disciplines. Several studies have now examined more distant outcomes, but lack of universally agreed diagnostic criteria both during and after pregnancy makes comparisons difficult and almost certainly has contributed to the disparate results obtained. It is conceivable that the glycaemic risk during pregnancy might differ according to the outcome of interest (immediate or long term). There is also the niggling suspicion that any relation of glycaemia to outcome in either parent or child is confounded by maternal risk factors.

OUTCOME

MATERNAL MORBIDITY

The maternal morbidity associated with diabetic pregnancy is well described[90], but few studies have attempted to use morbidity as an outcome variable for diagnosis. Moreover, the very limited evidence of a relation is largely uncontrolled and often retrospective. In one study, prediabetic women had a higher rate of toxaemia (when they may have had glucose intolerance during pregnancy) compared with the general population (14.2% vs 7.0%)[22]. Another (uncontrolled) study reported higher rates of pre-eclampsia and chronic hypertension than would be expected in unaffected populations[91]. Operative delivery was more common in untreated women than in women treated with insulin and diet though the reasons were not discussed[92]. There is also the additional supervision which inevitably attends any possible diagnosis of abnormality[93,94].

MATERNAL DIABETES

It is difficult to compare studies because of the differing diagnostic criteria used in the pregnant and non-pregnant states, differing background prevalence rates of diabetes in the populations studied and the variable time periods elapsed since pregnancy. O'Sullivan reported that 13.5% of index pregnancies showed a 'decompensation of carbohydrate control' (two or more of: postprandial blood glucose >10.0 mmol/l; fasting blood glucose >6.6 mmol/l; and post-glucose peak >16.6 mmol/l) over the next 17–23 years compared with 0.6% mothers with normal glucose tolerance during pregnancy. There is a general agreement[95,96] that overt diabetes may subsequently develop in up to 65% of women with gestational diabetes mellitus[97,98].

FETAL OUTCOME

This is perhaps the most readily appreciated and easily tangible benefit of diagnosis of hyperglycaemia during pregnancy. With increasing standards of obstetric and neonatal care, outcome measures have had to become more sophisticated. Treatment, whether intentional or incidental, has made the question more difficult to answer.

Congenital Abnormalities

There is no evidence for an association between gestational diabetes and this outcome.

Perinatal Mortality

Early studies of O'Sullivan reported an increased perinatal mortality of 6.4% among 187 pregnancies in women with untreated gestational diabetes mellitus compared with 1.5% among 259 randomly selected normal pregnancies[52]. Similarly, Oats and Beischer[55] using a 50 g 3 h OGTT identified 2.5% of the population with a perinatal mortality twice that of the background population. More recent studies almost universally have found no increase in perinatal mortality among pregnancies identified by diagnostic criteria[99–103.]

Neonatal Outcome

Gilmer derived criteria for gestational diabetes on the basis of risk for neonatal hypoglycaemia and reported an increased likelihood of this outcome if the area under a 50 OGTT was >42 area units[104]. A number of studies have shown a direct relationship between the 2 h glucose response and fetal birth weight[55,56,93], controlled for maternal risk factors[93].

OUTCOME IN THE OFFSPRING

If long-term outcomes are to be incorporated into a diagnostic framework, the metabolic fate of the offspring merits as much consideration as the development of maternal diabetes. Several studies have reported an increased risk for both obesity and diabetes in the offspring following diabetes in pregnancy[55,71,105]. In Pima Indians, there was a direct relation between these outcomes and increasing maternal glycaemic response to a 75 g OGTT[106]. Other studies, however, have failed to confirm these findings[101,102]. An association between glucose intolerance and subsequent neurobehavioural development of the offspring requires confirmation[107]. There may well be a difference between the populations of northern Europe, in which the prevalence of diabetes (largely insulin dependent) during pregnancy is low, and other racial groups where the non-pregnant prevalence of non-insulin-dependent diabetes is much higher, often with a strong genetic component to the disease.

UNRESOLVED ISSUES AND FUTURE CONSIDERATIONS

Although the various definitions and methods of diagnosis of diabetes in pregnancy have stimulated much debate and controversy, there is a constant need to keep the critical issues in focus. It may be reasonable to compare the O'Sullivan and WHO criteria for the diagnosis of diabetes, but the fundamental question concerns the best predictor of adverse maternal–fetal outcome. Differences between the various criteria (e.g. WHO and DPSG-EASD (Diabetes Pregnancy Study Group of the European Association for the Study of Diabetes)) reflect the inherent arbitrariness of cutpoints for classifications based on continuously distributed data in the absence of evidence for a threshold predicting adverse outcome on the maternal fetal unit. The choice of exact cutpoints depends on an assessment of the relative costs of diagnosing or failing to diagnose subjects at substantial risk of adverse maternal–fetal outcome. These should be arrived at by organizations making national or international recommendations and clear direction is needed to allow uniform standards of clinical care. The following issues still need consideration:

1. Should the OGTT be recommended as the gold standard for diagnosing diabetes during pregnancy? We have recently challenged the use of the OGTT as the reference standard for diagnosing diabetes in the non-pregnant state[89] and it may well deserve similar scrutiny in the context of pregnancy. A comparison of various test variables can only be judged against their ability to predict adverse pregnancy outcome. Conceptually, there is also the concern that what really affects fetal outcome is not the one-off response to a single challenge with pure glucose but the level of blood glucose which is achieved day after day throughout the nine months of pregnancy.
2. Is it possible that similar information to the OGTT might be obtained by simpler means, such as fasting plasma glucose, or measurement of glycated haemoglobin or glycated proteins? It should be recalled that the categorical division of fasting glucose in early studies arose from its recognized association with adverse pregnancy outcome[4,108]. Of interest is a recent report by Sacks *et al.* which showed that both fasting plasma glucose and 2 h glucose were linearly related to birth weight controlled for maternal risk factors[57]. Several other recent reports have also demonstrated the relevance of fasting glucose to the subsequent development of diabetes in the non-gravid state[109–111]. Glycated proteins have been related to the diagnosis of gestational diabetes but not to pregnancy outcome.
3. What are the relevant clinical endpoints? These must be rigorously defined, clinically robust and universally understood. An additional criterion is the possibility of reversal with treatment. There is the need to differentiate outcome from those improvements which have emerged from the almost uniform increase in obstetric and perinatal care. These may well look beyond perinatal mortality, the reduction in which appears to have reached a plateau[111]. Birth weight (carefully corrected for gestational age) has an obstetric, epidemiological and therapeutic appeal but other important fetal outcomes include fetal hyperinsulinism (assessed by cord blood insulin and C peptide levels), neonatal hypoglycaemia (defined by plasma glucose) and detailed morphological documentation of diabetic fetopathy. The possible long-term risks to

Diabetes and Pregnancy

both mother and baby require confirmation in differing populations and by standardized methodology and criteria for diagnosis.

4. What is the significance of minor degrees of glucose intolerance? This issue is central to the whole concept of 'gestational diabetes' but the evidence remains conflicting. There may well be differences between populations with primarily insulin-dependent and non-insulin-dependent diabetes. With the increased supervision which almost inevitably now follows the diagnosis of glucose intolerance, it is likely that a definitive answer will only be forthcoming in the context of a controlled, multicentre, multicultural clinical trial.

5. What is the significance of the contribution of maternal risk factors to glucose intolerance? These factors must be carefully controlled for in studies seeking to examine the relevance of minor degrees of hyperglycaemia and both must be related to maternal–fetal outcome.

6. What are the benefits of diagnosing hyperglycaemia during pregnancy? As noted above, integral to diagnosis (and detection) of diabetes is a consideration of the relevant costs involved and the assumption that correction of glucose intolerance will have a beneficial effect on maternal–fetal outcome. There are implications here for the optimum timing of diagnosis during pregnancy.

7. Is there a case for the use of similar screening methods in pregnancy as in the non-pregnant individual? Evaluation of a screening test goes beyond prediction of an abnormal test result and must again be related to pregnancy outcome. It should be noted that the same measures (fasting and random plasma glucose levels) customarily are used both for detection and diagnosis in non-pregnant subjects. Fasting values vary little throughout pregnancy, providing a basal index of severity, and were suggested as screening measures in the first GDM International Workshop[4]. More recently they have compared favourably with the post-challenge state[113]. Meal tolerance tests are more difficult to standardize but random glucose values, related to the most recent meal, partially approach this problem and have the added attraction of simplicity, low cost and uniformity with the non-gravid state. Data on both these variables during normal pregnancy are available, and reference ranges for fasting and random glucose levels at varying periods after food have been established. At the very least, a random plasma glucose measurement performed in each trimester of pregnancy allows exclusion of those subjects with unequivocal degrees of hyperglycaemia. Whatever method is adopted, it must be easily applicable to all populations.

CONCLUSIONS

The summary and recommendations of both the Second and Third International Workshop Conference on Gestational Diabetes Mellitus drew attention to the differences in diagnostic practice. Although both recommended continued use of the O'Sullivan and Mahan criteria, the 1985 workshop concluded that 'quantification of the risk for morbidity associated with varying degrees of glucose intolerance at various points of time during pregnancy may provide a more logical basis for refining criteria and nomenclature in the future'. The choice of any test variable is dependent on its ability to predict tightly defined and universally understood clinical endpoints. The only relevant evaluation of various measures of glycaemia is in this perspective.

There is universal agreement on the need to detect clearly abnormal degrees of hyperglycaemia during pregnancy, as defined by both the WHO and the NDDG. The possible adverse consequences of lesser degrees of glucose intolerance (approximating the WHO class of gestational impaired glucose tolerance and contained in the broad NDDG category of gestational diabetes) is much less clear. Particularly in the impaired glucose tolerance range, confounding factors such as maternal age, obesity and parity may play an important role in determining fetal outcome, rather than glucose tolerance alone.

The evidence that glucose intolerance detected in pregnancy is predictive of later maternal non-insulin-dependent diabetes[98] seems reasonably secure although this may simply reflect the predictive power of impaired glucose tolerance for subsequent diabetes mellitus in the non-pregnant state. Increased maternal morbidity with lesser degrees of glycaemia is much less certain. The relation of fetal birth weight and delayed metabolic and behavioural effects on the offspring require clarification.

An internationally agreed document of methods, definitions and outcomes remains the highest priority. The 75 g OGTT has the advantage of allowing a comparison between the pregnant and non-pregnant state. The ultimate clinical challenge is to meet the St Vincent Declaration statement of achieving pregnancy outcome (in the broadest sense of the term) similar to that of the non-pregnant population.

REFERENCES

1 National Diabetes Data Group. Classification and diagnosis of diabetes mellitus and other categories of glucose intolerance. *Diabetes* 1979; **28**: 1039–57.
2 World Health Organization Expert Committee on Diabetes Mellitus. Second Report. Technical Report Series 646. WHO, Geneva, 1980.
3 World Health Organization Study Group on Diabetes Mellitus. Technical Report Series 727. WHO, Geneva, 1985.
4 Freinkel N, Josimovich J. Summary and Recommendations of American Diabetic Association Workshop Conference on Gestational Diabetes. *Dabetes Care* 1980; **3**: 499–501.
5 Summary and Recommendations of the Second International Workshop Conference on Gestational Diabetes Mellitus. *Diabetes* 1985; **34** (Suppl. 2): 123–6.
6 Metzger BE. Summary and Recommendations of the Second International Workshop Conference on Gestational Diabetes Mellitus. *Diabetes* 1991; **40** (Suppl. 2): 197–201.

7 American Diabetes Association. Position statement: gestational diabetes mellitus. *Diabetes Care* 1986; **9**: 430–1.
8 American College of Obstetricians and Gynaecologists. Management of diabetes in pregnancy. *ACGO Tech Bull* 1986; **92**: 1–5.
9 American Diabetes Association Inc. Position statement on gestational diabetes mellitus. *Diabetes Care* 1991; **14**: 5–6.
10 Coustan DR. Diagnosis of gestational diabetes: what are our objectives? *Diabetes* 1991; **40** (Suppl. 2): 14–17.
11 Harris MI. Gestational diabetes may represent discovery of preexisting glucose tolerance. *Diabetes Care* 1988; **11**: 402–11.
12 Jarrett RJ. Gestational diabetes: a non-entity? *Br Med J* 1993; **306**: 37–8.
13 Ales KL, Santini DL. Should all pregnant women be screened for gestational glucose intolerance? *Lancet* 1989; **i**: 1187–91.
14 Hunter DJS, Kierse MJNC. Gestational diabetes. In: Chalmers I, Enkin M, Keirse MJNC (eds), *Effective Care in Pregnancy and Childbirth*, Vol. 1. Oxford University Press, Oxford, 1989; 403–10.
15 Naylor CD. Diagnosing gestational diabetes mellitus: is the gold standard valid? *Diabetes Care* 1989; **12**: 565–72.
16 Matthews Duncan J. On puerperal diabetes. *Trans Obstet Soc Lond* 1882; **24**: 256–85.
17 Williams JW. The clinical significance of glycosuria in pregnant women. *Am J Med Sci* 1909; **137**: 1–26.
18 Kriss JP, Futcher PH. The relation between infant birth weight and subsequent develoment of maternal diabetes mellitus. *J Clin Endocrinol* 1948; **8**: 380–9.
19 Gilbert JAL, Dunlop DM. Diabetic fertility, maternal mortality and foetal loss. *Br Med J* 1949; **i**: 48–51.
20 Miller HC, Hurwitz D, Kuder K. Fetal and neonatal mortality in pregnancies complicated by diabetes mellitus. *JAMA* 1944; **124**: 271–5.
21 Barnes HHF, Morgans ME. Prediabetic pregnancy. *J Obstet Gynaecol Br Empire* 1948; **55**: 449–54.
22 Moss JM, Mulholland JB. Diabetes and pregnancy with special reference to the prediabetic state. *Ann Intern Med* 1951; **34**: 678–91.
23 Pedowitz P, Shlevin EL. Perinatal mortality in the unsuspected diabetic. *Obstet Gynecol* 1957; **9**: 524–32.
24 Malins JM, Fitzgerald MG. Childbearing prior to the recognition of diabetes recollected birth weights and stillbirth rate in babies born to parents who developed diabetes. *Diabetes* 1965; **14**: 175–8.
25 Jackson WPU, Woolf N. Maternal prediabetes as a cause of the unexplained stillbirth. *Diabetes* 1958; **7**: 446–8.
26 Silverstone FA, Solomons E, Rubricus J. The rapid intravenous glucose tolerance test in pregnancy. *J Clin Invest* 1961; **140**: 2180–9.
27 O'Sullivan JB, Synder PJ, Sporer AC *et al*. Intravenous glucose tolerance test and its modification by pregnancy. *J Clin Endocrinol Metab* 1970; **31**: 33–7.
28 Hadden DR, Harley JMG, Kajtar TJ, Montgomery DAD. A prospective study of three tests of glucose tolerance in pregnant women selected for potential diabetes with reference to the fetal outcome. *Diabetologia* 1971; **7**: 87–93.
29 Farmer G, Russell G, Hamilton-Nichol DR *et al*. The influence of maternal glucose metabolism on fetal growth and morbidity in 917 singleton pregnancies in nondiabetic women. *Diabetologia* 1988; **31**: 134–41.
30 Billis A, Rastogi GK. Studies in methods of investigating carbohydrate metabolism in pregnancy. *Diabetologia* 1966; **2**: 169–77.
31 West KM. Substantial differences in the diagnostic criteria used by diabetes experts. *Diabetes* 1975; **24**: 641–4.
32 Kuhl C. Glucose metabolism during and after pregnancy in normal and gestational diabetic women: influence of normal pregnancy on serum glucose and insulin concentration during basal fasting conditions and after a challenge with glucose. *Acta Endocrinol* 1975; **79**: 709–19.
33 Kuhl C, Andersen O. Pathophysiological background for gestational diabetes. In: Weiss

PAM, Coustan DR (eds), *Gestational Diabetes*. Springer-Verlag, Vienna, 1988; 67–71.

34 Kuhl C. Insulin secretion and insulin resistance in pregnancy and GDM: implications for diagnosis and management. *Diabetes* 1991; **40**: (Suppl. 2): 18–24.

35 Cousins L. Insulin sensitivity in pregnancy. *Diabetes* 1991; **40**: (Suppl. 2): 39–44.

36 Felig P, Lynch V. Starvation in human pregnancy: hypoglycemia, hypoinsulinemia and hyperketonemia. *Science* 1970; **124**: 900–2.

37 Lind T, Belewicz WZ, Brown G. A serial study of changes occurring in the glucose tolerance test during pregnancy. *J Obstet Gynecol Br Commonw* 1973; **80**: 1033–9.

38 Hagen A. Blood sugar findings during normal and possible prediabetics. *Diabetes* 1961; **10**: 438–44.

39 Phelps RL, Metzger BE, Freinkel N. Carbohydrate metabolism in pregnancy. XVII. diurnal profiles of plasma glucose, insulin, free fatty acids, triglycerides, cholesterol and individual fatty acids. *Am J Obsetet Gynecol* 1981; **140**: 730–6.

40 Freinkel N. The Banting Lecture 1980. Of pregnancy and progeny. *Diabetes* 1980; **29**: 1023–35.

41 O'Sullivan JB, Mahan CM. Criteria for the oral glucose tolerance test in pregnancy. *Diabetes* 1964; **13**: 278–85.

42 Forest JC, Garrido-Russo M, Lemay A *et al*. Reference values for the oral glucose tolerance test at each trimester of pregnancy. *Am J Clin Pathol* 1983; **80**: 828–31.

43 Hatem M, Anthony F, Hogston P *et al*. Reference valus for the 75 g oral glucose tolerance test in pregnancy. *Br Med J* 1988; **296**: 676–8.

44 Diabetes Pregnancy Study Group. A prospective multicentre study to determine the influence of pregnancy upon the 75 g oral glucose tolerance test (OGTT). In: Sutherland HN, Stowers JM, Pearson DWM (eds), *Carbohydrate Metabolism in Pregnancy and the Newborn IV*. Springer-Verlag, London 1989; 209–26.

45 Morris MA, Grandis AS, Litton JC. Glycosylated hemoglobin concentration in early gestation associated with neonatal outcome. *Am J Obstet Gynecol* 1985; **153**: 651–4.

46 Phelps RL, Honig G, Green D *et al*. Biphasic changes in hemoglobin AIC concentrations during normal human pregnancy. *Am J Obstet Gynecol* 1983; **147**: 651–3.

47 Jackson WPV. Studies in prediabetes. *Br Med J* 1952; **ii**: 690.

48 Bennewitz HG. De diabete mellito, graviditatis symptomate. MD dissertation, Berlin, 1824.

49 Pedersen J. *The Pregnant Diabetic and her Newborn*, 2nd edn., Munksgaard, Copenhagen, 1977.

50 O'Sullivan JB. The Boston gestational diabetes studies: review and perspectives. In: Sutherland HW, Stowers JM, Pearson DWM (eds). *Carbohydrate Metabolism in Pregnancy and the Newborn IV*. Springer-Verlag, London, 1989; 287–94.

51 Carpenter MW, Coustan DR. Criteria for screening tests for gestational diabetes. *Am J Obstet Gynecol* 1982; **159**: 768–73.

52 O'Sullivan JB, Mahan CM, Charles D, Dandrow RV. Screening criteria for high-risk gestational diabetic patients. *Am J Obstet Gynecol* 1973; **116**: 895–900.

53 Tallarigo L, Gianpetro O, Penno G *et al*. Relation of glucose tolerance to complications of pregnancy in nondiabetic women. *N Engl J Med* 1986; **315**: 989–92.

54 Jarrett RJ. Reflections on gestational diabetes mellitus. *Lancet* 1989; **ii**: 1220–2.

55 Oats JN, Beischer NA. Gestational diabetes. *Aust NZ J Obstet Gynecol* 1986; **26**: 2–10.

56 Pettitt DJ, Knowler WC, Baird HR, Bennett PH. Gestational diabetes: infant and maternal complications of pregnancy in relation to third trimester glucose tolerance in the Pima Indians. *Diabetes Care* 1980; **3**: 458–64.

57 Sacks DA, Greenspoon JS, Salim AF *et al*. Toward universal criteria for gestational diabetes: the 75-gram glucose tolerance test in pregnancy. *Am J Obstet Gynecol* 1995; **172**: 607–14.

58 Metzger BE, Bybee DE, Freinkel N *et al*. Gestational diabetes mellitus: correlation between the phenotypic and genotypic characteristics of the mother and abnormal glucose tolerance during the first year postpartum. *Diabetes* 1985; **34** (Suppl. 2): 111–15.

59 McDonald GWM, Fisher GF, Burham C. Reproducibility of the oral glucose tolerance test. *Diabetes* 1965; **14**: 473–80.

60 Furhman GI, Steinberg MC. Diabetes screening during pregnancy. *Diabetes* 1987; **36** (Suppl. 1): 90–4.

61 Neiger R, Coustan DR. The role of repeat glucose tolerance tests in the diagnosis of gestational diabetes. *Am J Obstet Gynecol* 1991; **165**: 787–90.

62 Yudkin JS, Alberti KGMM, McLarty DG *et al*. Impaired glucose tolerance: is it a fact or a diagnostic ragbag? *Br Med J* 1990; **301**: 397–402.

63 Leonards JR, McCullagh EP, Christopher TC. A new carbohydrate solution for testing glucose tolerance. *Diabetes* 1965; **14**: 96–9.

64 Neely RDG, Kiwanuka JB, Hadden DR. Influence of sample type on the interpretation of the oral glucose test for gestational diabetes mellitus. *Diabetic Med* 1991; **8**: 129–34.

65 Sacks DA, Abu-Fadil S, Greenspoon JS, Fotheringham N. Do the current standards for glucose tolerance in pregnancy represent a valid conversion of O'Sulivan's original criteria? *Am J Obstet Gynecol* 1989; **161**: 638–41.

66 Hadden DR. Geographic, ethnic, and racial variations in the incidence of gestational diabetes mellitus. *Diabetes* 1985; **34** (Suppl. 2): 8–12.

67 Green JR, Pawson JG, Schumacher LB *et al*. Glucose tolerance in pregnancy: ethnic variation and influence of body habitus. *Am J Obstat Gynecol* 1990; **163**: 86–92.

68 Merkatz IR, Duchon MA. Yamashita TS, Houser HB. A pilot community based program for gestational diabetes. *Diabetes Care* 1980; **3**: 453–7.

69 Jarrett RJ. REflections on gestational diabetes mellitus. *Lancet* 1981; **i**: 1220–1.

70 Metzger BR, Bybee DR, Freinkel N *et al*. Gestational diabetes mellitus: correlations between the phenotypic and genotypic characteristics of the mother and abnormal glucose tolerance during the first year postpartum. *Diabetes* 1985; **34** (Suppl. 2): 111–15.

71 Coustan DR, Nelson C, Carpenter MW *et al*. Maternal age and screening for gestational diabetes: a population-based study. *Obstet Gynecol* 1989; **73**: 557–61.

72 Langer O, Brustman L, Anyaegbunam A, Mazze R. The significance of one abnormal glucose tolerance test value on adverse outcome in pregnancy. *Am J. Obstet Gynecol* 1987; **159**: 1478–83.

73 Leiken EL, Jenkins JH, Pomerantz GA, Klein L. Abnormal glucose screening tests in pregnancy: a risk factor for fetal macrosomia. *Obstet Gynecol* 1987; **69**: 570–3.

74 Weeks, JW, Major CA, de Veciana M, Morgan MA. Gestational diabetes: does the presence of risk factors influence perinatal outcome? *Am J Obstet Gynecol* 1994; **171**: 1003–7.

75 Mazze RS, Krogh CL. Gestational diabetes mellitus: now is the time for detection and treatment. *Mayo Clin Proc* 1992; **67**: 995–1002.

76 Hunter A, Doery JC, Miranda V. Diagnosis of gestational diabetes in Australia: a national survey of current practice. *Med J Aust* 1990; **153**: 290–2.

77 Burnett L. An audit of glucose tolerance test requests. *Med J Aust* 1990; **152**: 607–8.

78 Nelson-Piercy C, Gale EAM. Do we know how to screen for gestational diabetes? Current practice in one regional health authority. *Diabetic Med* 1994; **11**: 493–8.

79 Landon MB, Gabbe SG, Sachs L. Management of diabetes mellitus and pregnancy: a survey of obstetricians and materno-fetal specialists. *Obstet Gynecol* 1990; **75**: 635–40.

80 Coustan DR, Nelson C, Carpenter MW *et al*. Maternal age and screening for gestational diabetes: a population-based study. *Obstet Gynecol* 1989; **73**: 557–61.

81 Lavin JP. Screening of high-risk and general populations for gestational diabetes. *Diabetes* 1985; **34** (Suppl. 2): 24–41.

82 Lind T, Anderson T. Does random blood glucose sampling outdate testing for glycosuria in the detection of glycosuria during pregnancy. *Br Med J* 1984; **289**: 1569–71.

83 Lind T. Antenatal screening for diabetes mellitus. *Br J Obstet Gynecol* 1984; **91**: 833–4.

84 Hadden DR. Random plasma glucose as a screening tool for hyperglycaemia in pregnancy. In: Sutherland HW, Stowers JW (eds), *Carbohydrate Metabolism in Pregnancy and the Newborn*. Churchill Livingstone, Edinburgh, 1984; 203–5.

85 Hatem M, Dennis KJ. A random plasma glucose method for screening for abnormal glucose tolerance in pregnancy. *Br J Obstet Gynaecol* 1987; **94**: 213–16.

86 Stangenberg M, Persson B, Norlander E. Random capillary blood glucose and conventional selection criteria for glucose tolerance testing during pregnancy. *Diabetes Res* 1985; **2**: 29–33.

87 Hadden DR. Medical management of diabetes in pregnancy. *Bailliere's Clin Obstet Gynaecol* 1991; **5**: 369–94.

88 Sutherland HW, Pearson DWM, Lean MEJ *et al*. Breakfast tolerance test in pregnancy. In: Sutherland HW, Stowers JM, Person DWM (eds), *Carbohydrate Metabolism in Pregnancy and the Newborn IV*. Springer-Verlag, London, 1989; 267–75.

89 McCance DR, Hanson RL, Charles MA *et al*. Comparison of tests for glycated haemoglobin and fasting and two hour plasma glucose concentrations as diagnostic methods for diabetes. *Br Med J* 1994; **308**: 1323–8.

90 Coustan DR. Hyperglycaemia–hyperinsulinaemia: effect on the infant of the diabetic mother. In: Jovanovic L, Peterson CM, Fuhrman K (eds), *Diabetes and Pregnancy: Teratology, Toxicity and Treatment*. Praeger, New York, 1986; 291–320.

91 Du Muylder X. Perinatal complications of gestational diabetes: the influence of the timing of the diagnosis. *Eur J Obstet Reprod Biol* 1984; **18**: 35–42.

92 Coustan DR, Imarah J. Prophylactic insulin treatment of gestational diabetes reduces the incidence of macrosomia, operative delivery and birth trauma. *Am J Obstet Gynecol* 1984; **150**: 836–42.

93 Widness JA, Cowett RM, Coustan DR *et al*. Neonatal morbidities in infants of mothers with glucose intolerance in pregnancy. *Diabetes* 1985; **34** (Suppl. 2): 61–5.

94 Cousins L. Pregnancy complications among diabetic women: review 1965–1985. *Obstet Gynecol Surv* 1987; **42**: 140–9.

95 O'Sullivan JB, Charles D,l Dandrow RV. Treatment of verified prediabetics in pregnancy. *J Reprod Med* 1971; **7**: 21–4.

96 O'Sullivan JB. Gestational diabetes: factors influencing the rates of subsequent diabetes. In: Sutherland HW, Stowers JM (eds), *Carbohydrate Metabolism in Pregnancy and the Newborn*. Springer-Verlag, New York, 1979; 425–35.

97 Mestman JH. Follow-up studies in women with gestational diabetes mellitus: the experience at Los Angeles County University of Southern California Medical Centre. In: Weiss PA, Coustan DR (eds), *Gestational Diabetes*. Springer-Verlag, New York, 1988; 191–8.

98 Oats JN, Beischer NA, Grand PT. The emergence of diabetes and impaired glucose tolerance in women who had gestational diabetes. In: Weiss PA, Coustan DR (eds), *Gestational Diabetes*. Springer-Verlag, New York, 1988; 199–207.

99 Gyves MT, Rodman HM, Little AB *et al*. A modern approach to management of pregnant diabetics: a two-year analysis of perinatal outcomes. *Am J Obstet Gynecol* 1977; **128**: 606–16.

100 Lavin JP, Lovelace DR, Miodovnik M. *et al*. Clinical experience with one hundred and seven diabetic pregnancies. *Am J Obstet Gynecol* 1983; **147**: 742–52.

101 Hadden DR. Screening for abnormalities of carbohydrate metabolism in pregnancy 1966–1977. The Belfast Experience. *Diabetes Care* 1980; **3**: 440–6.

102 Roberts RN, Moohan JM, Foorl K *et al*. Fetal outcome in mothers with impaired glucose tolerance in pregnancy. *Diabetic Med* 1993; **10**: 438–3.

103 Philipson EH, Kalhan SC, Rosen MG *et al*. Gestational diabetes mellitus: is further improvement necessary? *Diabetes* 1985; **34** (Suppl. 2): 55–60.

104 Gillmer MDG, Beard RW, Brooke FM, Oakley NW. Carbohydrate metabolism in pregnancy. *Br Med J* 1975; **3**: 399–404.

105 Pettitt DJ, Baird HR, Aleck KA *et al*. Excessive obesity in offspring of Pima Indian women with diabetes during pregnancy. *N Engl J Med* 1983; **308**: 242–5.

106 Pettitt DR, Bennett PH, Saad MF *et al*. Abnormal glucose tolerance during pregnancy in Pima Indian women. Long-term effects on offspring. *Diabetes* 1991; **40** (Suppl. 2): 126–30.

107 Rizzo T, Metzger BE, Burns WJ, Burns K. Correlations between antepartum maternal metabolism and inteligence of offspring. *N Engl J Med* 1991; **325**: 911–16.

108 American Diabetes Association. International Workshop Conference on Gestational Diabetes, Chicago 1979. *Diabetes Care* 1980; **3**: 399–501.

109 Aufmann RC, Schleyhahn FT, Huffman DG, Amankwah KS. Gestational diabetes diagnostic criteria: long term maternal follow up. *Am J Obstet Gynecol* 1995; **172**: 621–5.

110 Coustan DR, Carpenter MD, Ivan PS, Carr SR. Gestational diabetes: predictors of subsequent disordered glucose metabolism. *Am J Obstet Gynecol* 1993; **168**: 1139–45.

111 Kjos SL, Buchanan TA, Greenspoon JS *et al*. Gestational diabetes mellitus: the prevalence of glucose intolerance and diabetes mellitus in the first two months post partum. *Am J*

Obstet Gynecol 1990; **163**: 93–8.

112 Gregory R, Scott AR, Mohajer M, Tattersall RB. Diabetic pregnancy 1977–1990: have we reached a plateau? *J R Coll Phys Lond* 1992; **26**: 162–6.

113 Fuhrmann K. Targets in oral glucose tolerance. In: Sutherland HN, Stowers JM, Pearson DWM (eds), *Carbohydrate Metabolism in Pregnancy and the Newborn IV*. Springer-Verlag, London, 1989; 227–37.

Part I

PATHOPHYSIOLOGY

3

The Metabolic Stress of Pregnancy

THOMAS A. BUCHANAN[1] and ANNE DORNHORST[2]

[1]University of Southern California School of Medicine, Los Angeles, USA and
[2]Royal Postgraduate Medical School, London, UK

INTRODUCTION

A successful pregnancy requires a high degree of maternal physiological adaptation which draws on maternal reserves not fully utilized outside pregnancy. Metabolic changes occur which help optimize fetal growth over a wide range of nutritional circumstances[1]. The added energy cost of pregnancy has to be met through a combination of increased energy intake, utilization of endogenous energy stores and energy conservation. An important metabolic change in pregnancy is the associated decrease in insulin sensitivity[2]. The fall in insulin sensitivity throughout pregnancy helps optimize metabolic efficiency. A variety of placental hormones modify insulin action, facilitating maternal fat disposition in the fed state. During fasting human placental lactogen increases lipolysis, providing an early maternal energy source while sparing carbohydrate nutrients for the fetus[3]. Optimal fetal growth is dependent on this delicate balance between maternal anabolism and catabolism. As maternal insulin sensitivity falls in pregnancy insulin secretion needs to increase to maintain maternal glucose tolerance[2,4]. Although most women have the necessary beta cell reserves to meet the extra demands of pregnancy, a minority of women do not and develop glucose intolerance that is detected for the first time when pregnant. Maternal diabetes, either predating or arising for the first time during the pregnancy, has the potential to upset this delicate balance between enhanced maternal anabolism and accelerated catabolism.

Diabetes and Pregnancy: An International Approach to Diagnosis and Management.
Edited by A. Dornhorst and D. R. Hadden.

Untreated diabetes can lead to an uncontrolled supply of fetal nutrients and an increased risk of maternal ketosis, both highly detrimental to pregnancy outcome.

This chapter looks at the maternal changes that occur in normal pregnancy, and examines the effects on maternal insulin sensitivity and insulin secretion, and subsequent changes in glucose, lipid and protein metabolism. The added effects of maternal diabetes (both established and that arising in pregnancy) on these metabolic changes are subsequently discussed.

INSULIN SENSITIVITY

Decreased insulin sensitivity is a universal feature of normal pregnancy. Fasting insulin concentration and the insulin response to ingested glucose both increase as a direct consequence of this fall in insulin sensitivity[5,6]. Pregnancy is usually associated with a decrease in maternal glucose tolerance. The reduced effect of exogenous insulin on lowering plasma glucose in pregnant women was first described by Burt in the 1950s[7]. More recently, whole body insulin sensitivity has been assessed using the euglycaemic clamp technique[4,7] and computerized modelling of the intravenous glucose tolerance test[2,8,9]. These newer techniques have shown that by late pregnancy an individual's insulin sensitivity falls by 45–70%, achieving values similar to those associated with non-insulin-dependent diabetes[10,11]. With the proviso that there is adequate maternal beta cell function, this fall in insulin sensitivity is advantageous, facilitating the diversion of glucose to the fetus in the postprandial state, while providing a metabolic milieu that favours maternal fat deposition which can then be utilized as an energy source during fasting. Theoretically, decreased insulin sensitivity may further improve metabolic efficiency by reducing postprandial thermogenesis, thereby optimizing anabolic usage of undigested calories[12].

The decrease in insulin sensitivity during pregnancy parallels the growth of the fetoplacental unit[11,13] and reverses abruptly following the delivery of the placenta[14,15]. The metabolic effects of the fetoplacental unit are likely to account for most of the fall in insulin sensitivity[3,16]; however, other maternal contributory factors will include increased food intake, increased adiposity and decreased activity. The fetoplacental hormones, human placental lactogen[17,18] and progesterone[19], as well as the maternal hormones raised in pregnancy, prolactin and cortisol[20], all reduce insulin sensitivity *in vivo*. Studies *in vitro* on adipocytes[21,22] and skeletal muscle[23] have shown that these fetoplacental hormones both individually and synergistically decrease insulin-mediated glucose uptake. In addition, human placental lactogen through its lipolytic action is likely further to decrease insulin sensitivity[24], as circulating free fatty acids are known to decrease insulin sensitivity outside pregnancy[25]. In animal studies suppression of maternal lipolysis in late pregnancy improves insulin sensitivity[26], implying that circulating free fatty acids contribute to this change.

In pregnancy the major site of the decreased insulin sensitivity is skeletal muscle, and by full term insulin-mediated glucose uptake into this tissue will have fallen by >40%[27]. Animal work has also shown that insulin-mediated glucose uptake by cardiac muscle[28] and fat cells[23,29,30] is reduced. In addition to decreased peripheral insulin sensitivity, decreased hepatic insulin sensitivity has been described in pregnant rats[31,32] and rabbits[26,32]. Whether a decrease in hepatic insulin sensitivity in human pregnancy accounts for the increase in hepatic glucose output in late pregnancy is unclear. Glucose has a suppressive effect on hepatic glucose output which is itself synergistic with insulin[33,34], and the increase in hepatic glucose output in pregnancy could result simply from a lowering of the maternal plasma glucose concentration. However, a reduction in hepatic insulin sensitivity from mid to late pregnancy despite similar ambient plasma glucose concentrations has been reported in animals[35]. A possible effect of circulating free fatty acid in decreasing hepatic insulin sensitivity in late pregnancy is suggested by work in rabbits[36]. Nevertheless, studies in non-obese human pregnancies have failed to demonstrate a decreased hepatic sensitivity to insulin with increasing gestation, but these workers used relatively high doses of insulin[4] and subtle differences in insulin sensitivity may have been missed.

The cellular mechanisms that underlie the decreased insulin sensitivity of pregnancy have not been fully identified. While insulin binding to adipocytes is decreased in pregnancy[37-39], that to hepatocytes[40,41] and to skeletal muscle[42,43] is unaffected. As insulin sensitivity is influenced most by insulin-mediated glucose disposal in muscle it is most likely that the decrease in insulin sensitivity in muscle is due to post-receptor binding events affecting some aspect of cell signalling[41-45].

INCREASED INSULIN SECRETION

A normal consequence of the pregnancy-related fall in insulin sensitivity is an increase in maternal insulin secretion. The hyperinsulinaemia of pregnancy results from increased synthesis and release of insulin as opposed to decreased insulin clearance[46,47]. This hyperinsulinaemia represents intact insulin rather than increases in proinsulin or other immunoreactive but less biologically active precursor molecules. Fasting insulin concentrations rise throughout pregnancy as does glucose-stimulated insulin secretion[5,48,49]. In glucose-tolerant women by the last trimester the first- and second-phase insulin responses to oral and intravenous glucose will have increased approximately three-fold[2]. The increase in insulin secretion is associated with morphological pancreatic changes, including beta cell hypertrophy and hyperplasia[50]. The 10–15% estimated increase in beta cell mass[50] may help explain the fasting hyperinsulinaemia in late pregnancy which occurs in the presence of normal or low plasma glucose values[2,4]. Postprandial hyperinsulinaemia, which may be two to three times non-pregnant levels, is more likely to be explained by an enhanced beta-cell sensitivity to secretogogues, and both progesterone and human placental lactogen increase insulin secretory responses of isolated rat islets to known secretogogues[51-54]. The protein kinase activity of rat islets increases in pregnancy, which suggests a possible cellular mechanism for this enhanced insulin secretion[55,56].

CARBOHYDRATE METABOLISM

By the eighth week of pregnancy fasting plasma glucose falls[48]. This physiological fall in fasting glucose precedes any changes in insulin production and sensitivity. An increase in the renal clearance of glucose[57], and a decrease in the availability of gluconeogenic precursors, notably alanine, are thought to contribute to this early fall in fasting glucose[58,59]. By the second trimester a 72 h fast results in plasma glucose values significantly lower than in non-pregnant women[60]. By the third trimester following a 10 h fast plasma glucose values are 0.5–1 mmol/l lower than for non-pregnant women[2-4,6,16,26], and glucose values fall further in the pregnant woman over the subsequent 4 h[62].

Fasting hypoglycaemia during pregnancy cannot be explained by a decrease in hepatic glucose production, which increases in pregnancy[4,61,64]. The volume of distribution for glucose in late pregnancy is markedly increased[61] and by the third trimester the fasting endogenous glucose production is unable to keep up with the increase in glucose clearance following a 14–18 h fast. The reduced availability of alanine as a gluconeogenic substrate in pregnancy[58,59,65] will also contribute to the lower fasting glucose values.

LIPID METABOLISM

Throughout pregnancy fasting lipolysis and ketogenesis are increased[66]. The placental hormone human placental lactogen directly stimulates free fatty acid release from adipose tissue which contributes to fasting lipolysis. In the postprandial state the exaggerated hyperinsulinaemia that occurs following food ingestion suppresses free fatty acid concentrations[67], but as circulating insulin concentrations fall in the postabsorptive period the lipolytic actions of placental hormones are unmasked, and circulating free fatty acid concentrations rise again. As in the non-pregnant state free fatty acids are a primary energy source, being utilized by both skeletal and cardiac muscle. Free fatty acids also provide the substrate for the production of hepatic ketone which can be metabolized directly by the central nervous system as an energy source, thereby reducing maternal obligatory glucose requirements. By the third trimester accelerated ketone production occurs after relatively short periods of starvation (14–16 h)[60–63], which helps to optimize the supply of fetal nutrients during periods of fasting[62].

Normal pregnancy is associated with hypertriglyceridaemia[68]. Serum triglycerides begin to rise in the first trimester, increasing two-fold by the third[67]. Fasting and postprandial hepatic triglyceride synthesis is increased in pregnancy, due to a direct effect of oestrogens on hepatic triglyceride synthesis[69] and to increased substrate availability secondary to the increase in circulating free fatty acids[70,71]. Postprandial hypertriglyceridaemia is further exaggerated by decreased peripheral triglyceride clearance, due to reduced adipose tissue lipoprotein lipase activity as a result of decreased insulin sensitivity[72]. Increased maternal food consumption further increases circulating triglyceride concentrations due to the production of chylomicrons by the gut.

PROTEIN METABOLISM

Hypoaminoacidaemia is a metabolic feature of pregnancy, when most circulating concentrations of amino acids fall[73]. Placental hormones and insulin inhibit amino acid release from skeletal muscle under fasting conditions[74,75]. Maternal hyperinsulinaemia contributes to the postprandial hypoaminoacidaemia by accelerating amino acid uptake. The expanding volume of distribution during pregnancy further decreases circulating amino acid concentrations. Theoretically, increased fetal amino acid utilization in late pregnancy could contribute to hypoaminoacidaemia but in humans, as opposed to polytocous species, this does not appear to be an important factor.

INTERMEDIARY METABOLISM

In pregnancy the changes between carbohydrate, fat and protein metabolism that usually occur during the transition from feeding to fasting are exaggerated, with more rapid swings observed between the anabolic state of feeding and the catabolic state of fasting. Decreased insulin sensitivity results in a more rapid rise and fall in plasma glucose and insulin levels following feeding. While postprandial hyperinsulinaemia is sufficient to minimize hyperglycaemia, plasma glucose values 1 h after a mixed meal are consistently higher in pregnant than non-pregnant subjects[57]. Postprandial hyperinsulinaemia also accounts for the rapid fall of glycerol and free fatty acids following food ingestion. Between meals, glucose levels fall more rapidly and to lower levels in pregnant compared to non-pregnant women. The accompanying fall in circulating insulin concentrations leaves the lipolytic effects of placental hormones unopposed, causing free fatty acid and ketone concentrations to rise earlier than in non-pregnant women. Other metabolites including circulating triglycerides and amino acids fluctuate less in late pregnancy, even though their mean plasma concentrations may change.

The exaggerated postprandial excursions of maternal carbohydrate and lipid metabolites promote transplacental passage of nutrients to the fetus[76]. During feeding, nutrients are preferentially diverted to maternal fat synthesis due to the less marked decrease in insulin sensitivity in adipose tissue compared to skeletal muscle[22,29,77]. The accelerated fat catabolism and hypoglycaemia that occur with fasting allow the mother to switch quickly from utilizing carbohydrate to fat as her predominant energy source. This rapid switch from carbohydrate to fat metabolism underlies Freinkel's concept of 'accelerated starvation'[78] and all these metabolic adaptations can be seen as advantageous to the developing fetus.

IMPLICATIONS FOR DIABETES IN PREGNANCY

The ability of the pancreatic beta cell to increase its secretory function two- to three-fold is essential for normal glucose tolerance in pregnancy. Women who lack this beta cell reserve, either due to an absolute deficiency as in insulin-dependent diabetes or to a relative deficiency as in non-insulin-dependent diabetes, display abnormalities of carbohydrate, lipid and protein metabolism. These are abnormalities which if uncorrected can adversely affect both fetal development and maternal well-being. The decrease in insulin sensitivity and accelerated fat catabolism which are found in normal pregnancy also occur in pregnancies complicated by diabetes. Insulin requirements similarly increase in diabetic pregnant women and increasing doses of exogenous insulin need to be given[15]. Anticipating the insulin requirements in diabetic pregnancies is imperative if maternal hyperglycaemia and ketoacidosis, with their ensuing complications, are to be prevented[79].

INSULIN REQUIREMENTS IN INSULIN-DEPENDENT AND NON-INSULIN-DEPENDENT DIABETES

Insulin deficiency, be it absolute or relative, results in elevated plasma concentrations of glucose, triglycerides and many amino acids. To achieve normoglycaemia during pregnancy women with insulin-dependent diabetes always require exogenous insulin, which needs to be given in increasing amounts to counteract the increasing fall in insulin sensitivity. It is not unusual for the insulin requirements of an insulin-dependent diabetic woman to increase three-fold by the end of the third trimester[14,15]. Women with non-insulin-dependent diabetes also require exogenous insulin in pregnancy to maintain normoglycaemia and insulin treatment is often started for the first time in these women during a pregnancy. Women with previously diet-controlled diabetes inevitably become too hyperglycaemic in early pregnancy to continue to be controlled by diet alone. Those with non-insulin-dependent diabetes previously treated with oral hypoglycaemic agents are usually switched to insulin therapy before pregnancy. As decreased insulin sensitivity is a universal finding in non-insulin-dependent diabetes and as many of these women are obese and physically inactive before pregnancy, their insulin requirements are frequently higher than for women with insulin-dependent diabetes[15,80]. Following delivery, insulin requirements fall rapidly to pre-pregnancy levels or less in both types of diabetic women[14,15], and those previously controlled on diet only are usually able to stop insulin treatment altogether.

ACCELERATED FAT CATABOLISM

The normal physiological adaptation of increased fat catabolism in pregnancy puts women with insulin-dependent diabetes at particular risk for ketoacidosis. The development of ketoacidosis in these pregnancies can occur at lower plasma glucose levels and after shorter periods of insulin deficiency than in non-pregnant diabetic women[81]. The need for sufficient and continual insulin treatment throughout pregnancies must be stressed to all insulin-dependent diabetic women and their carers. Potential precipitating factors for ketoacidosis include nausea and anorexia in early pregnancy, and urinary tract infections in later pregnancy[82]. At term the use of β-sympathomimetic and other tocolytic agents used to inhibit preterm labour[83] and the administration of high-dose steroids given for fetal lung maturation can all precipitate ketoacidosis if the necessary adjustments to insulin dosage are not made[79]. Ketoacidosis should be preventable by the continual prediction and adjustment of insulin dosage throughout pregnancy. However, if this condition develops, rapid treatment with intravenous insulin is imperative as severe maternal ketoacidosis is associated with a high fetal mortality (between 30% and 90%), especially when the mother presents in coma[81,84]. The mechanism of fetal death associated with maternal ketoacidosis is attributed to fetal acidosis. Studies involving cordocentesis in the third trimester have shown that the fetus of a diabetic compared to a non-diabetic woman is more susceptible to acidosis and hyperlacticaemia[85-87]. Acidosis results when fetal oxygen requirements exceed the delivery of oxygen to the fetal tissues. In diabetic pregnancies fetal hyperglycaemia and hyperinsulinaemia cause an enhancement of fetal substrate metabolism which increases fetal oxygen requirement which is often not met by any increase in placental oxygen transfer[88]. In maternal ketoacidosis the associated acidosis, hypovolaemia and high circulating catecholamines all act to reduce uterine blood flow, thereby further compromising the balance between oxygen delivery and oxygen requirement in fetal tissues.

Pregnant women with non-insulin-dependent diabetes rarely develop diabetic ketoacidosis. However, the accelerated fat catabolism of pregnancy can be further exaggerated if excessive dietary restriction is enforced in the management of non-insulin-dependent diabetes[62,89,90]. While the magnitude of the fasting ketosis is not sufficient to cause changes in maternal acid–base status, concern exists on the effect of maternal ketonuria[91,92] and ketonaemia[93] on motor and intellectual development of the offspring.

THE INFLUENCE OF ESTABLISHED DIABETES ON CARBOHYDRATE, LIPID AND PROTEIN METABOLISM IN PREGNANCY

The extent of the derangement of carbohydrate, lipid and protein metabolism in pregnant women with established diabetes is highly dependent on the degree of maternal glycaemic control. Intensive insulin therapy resulting in normal plasma glucose control can also normalize the concentrations of circulating triglyceride, free fatty acid, ketone and amino acids[80,94–97]. Even when the mean concentrations of circulating metabolites are normal, the fluctuations in the concentrations of glucose and ketones are more marked than in non-diabetic pregnancies[80,95,97]. With poor glycaemic control ketone, free fatty acid, triglyceride and amino acid concentrations all increase, resulting in an abnormal metabolic environment for the developing embryo and fetus.

GESTATIONAL DIABETES

Gestational diabetes mellitus is glucose intolerance first recognized in pregnancy[98]. Metabolically it is a heterogeneous disorder[99]. The degree of glucose intolerance encountered ranges from the frankly diabetic to that which forms a continuum with the glucose tolerance changes observed in normal pregnancy, and the extent of the metabolic derangements in carbohydrate, lipid and protein metabolism reflects the degree of glucose intolerance.

The diagnosis of gestational diabetes has implications affecting the pregnancy and the future health of the mother[100] and her child[101]. The exact degree of glucose intolerance that adversely affects pregnancy outcome remains to be defined, and may be higher than that which is associated with an increased predisposition to non-insulin-dependent diabetes in later life. The degree of maternal glucose intolerance required to affect the fetal pancreas adversely and therefore predispose the infant to later diabetes is also unknown.

Women who develop gestational diabetes form a heterogeneous group[99]. Many develop glucose intolerance as a direct consequence of the pregnancy, with glucose tolerance deteriorating in the second trimester, coinciding with the fall in insulin sensitivity[11]. Other women, also classified as having gestational diabetes, have previously undiagnosed diabetes or impaired glucose tolerance. The metabolic abnormalities encountered in these women are more severe, present earlier in pregnancy, and persist post partum. By contrast, women who develop glucose intolerance for the first time in pregnancy usually become glucose tolerant again post partum. However, these women have a high likelihood of gestational diabetes recurring at progressively earlier gestation in subsequent pregnancies, and of diabetes developing in later life[102]. A few of these women (about 5% in most ethnic groups) are in the early phases of developing insulin-dependent diabetes with evidence of an active autoimmune destruction of their beta cells[103–105]. The increased demands on beta cell function in pregnancy result in the earlier manifestation of this usually silent phase of insulin-dependent diabetes[106].

BETA CELL FUNCTION IN GESTATIONAL DIABETES

The metabolic characteristic of women with gestational diabetes is insufficient insulin secretion to counteract the pregnancy related fall in insulin sensitivity[2,4]. A degree of beta cell dysfunction appears to be a common finding in these women even when the diagnosis is made using the less stringent criteria of the World Health Organization (120 min plasma glucose >7.8 mmol/l following a 75 g oral glucose tolerance test)[107]. Women with a history of previous gestational diabetes, even when glucose tolerant, have evidence of persistent beta cell dysfunction[108,109], and the degree of this beta cell dysfunction appears to be influenced by ethnicity[109]. During a pregnancy complicated by gestational diabetes there is an impaired, delayed and attenuated insulin response to oral and intravenous glucose. During a 75 g oral glucose tolerance test there is an inverse correlation between the 30 min insulin response and the 120 min plasma glucose value[107] and evidence of beta cell dysfunction is further provided by the increased levels of circulating proinsulin[110]. Indeed, increased circulating proinsulin levels early in pregnancy are predictive for the subsequent need for insulin treatment in later pregnancy[111].

The exact nature of the beta cell defects in gestational diabetes is unclear. A minority of women have mutations in the glucokinase gene which cause abnormalities in the glucose sensor of the beta cell[112], and another small group have evidence of cell and humoral immunity directed against their own pancreatic islets[99,113]. One of the more intriguing scenarios that has been proposed to contribute to the beta cell defect in gestational diabetes is that the beta cell mass of the woman was adversely influenced during her own fetal development, as a result of hyperglycaemia in her own mother, a hypothesis which implies that diabetes can beget diabetes through environmental mechanisms that bypass Mendelian genetics. The association between intrauterine growth retardation and an increased later susceptibility for diabetes has also been used to support the hypothesis that the intrauterine environment can adversely influence beta cell mass and function in later life[114,115].

INSULIN SENSITIVITY IN GESTATIONAL DIABETES

The two most important risk factors for the development of gestational diabetes also influence insulin sensitivity, namely obesity and ethnicity[116,117]. Similarly, the progression to diabetes following a gestational diabetes pregnancy is highly influenced by obesity and weight gain which lowers insulin sensitivity. Both the incidence of gestational diabetes and the progression to diabetes post partum is highest in those ethnic groups characterized by low levels of insulin sensitivity, women from the Indian subcontinent[118], native American women[119] and women of Hispanic origin[120] being examples of this phenomenon. Decreased insulin sensitivity also occurs in individuals with a family history of non-insulin-dependent diabetes[121], and in the presence of increasing obesity, especially abdominal obesity[122,123], which is another important risk factor for gestational diabetes. Women whose gestational diabetes is diagnosed early in pregnancy[4,11] may therefore have other factors than pregnancy contributing to their lower insulin sensitivity[124,125]. The persistence of reduced insulin sensitivity in these women post partum in combination with their inherent beta cell dysfunction is likely to explain the much higher rate of progression from impaired glucose tolerance to non-insulin-dependent diabetes than in the background population[120,126]. For these reasons many women with previous gestational diabetes will have had low insulin sensitivities preceding and following the pregnancy[127]. What has been more difficult to ascertain is whether the fall in insulin sensitivity that occurs in a normal pregnancy is greater in a pregnancy complicated by gestational diabetes. To examine this question insulin sensitivity must be measured in women with and without gestational diabetes who are otherwise matched for ethnicity, degree of obesity, age and gestational week.

Studies on insulin sensitivity in late pregnancy in women with mild or moderate gestational diabetes[2,4,107] have consistently shown that by late pregnancy the insulin sensitivity has fallen to values similar to those seen in women with normal glucose tolerance[127]. Although by late pregnancy there is no difference in insulin-mediated glucose disposal between women with and without gestational diabetes, the suppression of hepatic glucose output by insulin infusion is reduced in women with the latter[127], despite similar increases in glucose production[127].

The mechanisms for the decreased insulin sensitivity both early in pregnancy and after pregnancy in women who develop gestational diabetes is likely to be multifactorial, and different among various ethnic groups and family kindred. Abnormalities of $GLUT_4$ content and subcellular trafficking have been reported in adipocytes of women with gestational diabetes by Garvey *et al.*[128]; however, the same group found similar $GLUT_4$ content of rectus abdominis muscles obtained at term in women with and without gestational diabetes[44]. Ethnic differences in the frequencies for restriction fragment length polymorphisms in the region of the insulin receptor gene and the IGF-II gene have been reported in women with gestational diabetes compared with ethnically matched non-diabetic controls[129].

ACCELERATED FAT CATABOLISM IN GESTATIONAL DIABETES

The major implication of accelerated fat catabolism for women with gestational diabetes is the risk of fasting ketosis. In the case of overweight patients this risk has been shown to be no greater than for non-diabetic pregnant women[89]. Most overweight patients with gestational diabetes tolerate mild caloric restriction (~25 kcal/kg actual body weight each day during the latter half of gestation) without significant ketonuria[90]. However, more severe caloric restriction may cause fasting ketosis with the potential for long-term developmental problems in offspring[91–93].

INTERMEDIARY METABOLISM IN GESTATIONAL DIABETES

As is true for established diabetes in pregnancy, the imbalance between insulin resistance and pancreatic beta cell function that characterizes gestational diabetes results in abnormal concentrations of carbohydrate, lipid and protein nutrients. Metzger *et al.*[130] reported that concentrations of glucose, free fatty acids, triglycerides and several branched-chain amino acids were increased in the circulation of women with gestational diabetes compared to glucose-tolerant women in the third trimester. The extent of the elevation of these metabolites reflects the degree of hyperglycaemia and normalization of maternal hyperglycaemia normalizes circulating free fatty acid and triglyceride concentrations[131]. Reduced suppression of serum glycerol and free fatty acids following food ingestion is seen in gestational diabetes, which probably reflects the poor postprandial insulin response in these women, and similar abnormalities have been reported to persist after delivery[132].

METABOLIC PREDICTORS FOR FUTURE DIABETES

The most important factors influencing the progression to diabetes following gestational diabetes are ethnicity and the background incidence of impaired glucose tolerance and non-insulin-dependent diabetes. The requirement for insulin in pregnancy, obesity and further weight gain post partum are also associated with an increased risk of future diabetes, mostly non-insulin-dependent diabetes[102,110,126]. A maternal family history of non-insulin-dependent diabetes and a relatively insulinopenic response to oral glucose are further predictors of early progression[126]. A further pregnancy following a pregnancy complicated by gestational diabetes has been reported to increase the annual incidence of developing non-insulin-dependent diabetes post partum three-fold in Hispanic women[102]. An important subgroup (approximately 5%) of women with gestational diabetes develop insulin-dependent diabetes[104,110]. Recently maternal antibodies to glutamic acid decarboxylase, a beta cell enzyme, have been shown to be a good predictor for future insulin-dependent diabetes, which can develop 10 years or more following the pregnancy[103,105].

SUMMARY

In summary, a number of maternal metabolic changes occur early in pregnancy and continue throughout pregnancy which help optimize the transfer of nutrients to the fetus. These changes include a decrease in insulin sensitivity, an increase in fasting lipolysis and an increase in fat disposition following food ingestion. For glucose tolerance to be maintained in pregnancy it is necessary for maternal insulin secretion to increase sufficiently to counteract the fall in insulin sensitivity. Women with insufficient pancreatic beta cell reserve can develop diabetes for the first time in pregnancy. Women with established diabetes need to increase their exogenous insulin therapy to counteract the decrease in insulin sensitivity. Normalization of all metabolic parameters in the pregnant diabetic woman is important for optimal fetal growth and development; it is therefore important that all physicians who look after these women have an understanding of the metabolic changes that occur at this time.

REFERENCES

1   Poppitt SD, Prentice AM, Goldberg GR, Whithead RG. Energy-sparing strategies to protect human fetal growth. *Am J Obstet Gynecol* 1994; **171**: 118–25.
2   Buchanan TA, Metzger BE, Freinkel N, Bergman RN. Insulin sensitivity and beta-cell responsiveness to glucose during late pregnancy in lean and moderately obese women with normal glucose tolerance or mild gestational diabetes. *Am J Obstet Gynecol* 1990; **162**: 1008–114.

3   Handwerger S. Clinical counterpoint: the physiology of placental lactogen in human pregnancy. *Endocr Rev* 1991; **12**: 329–36.

4   Catalano PM, Tyzbir ED, Wolfe RR *et al*. Longitudinal changes in basal hepatic glucose production and suppression during insulin infusion in normal pregnant women. *Am J Obset Gynecol* 1992; **167**: 913–19.

5   Spellacy WN, Goetz FC. Plasma insulin in normal late pregnancy. *N Engl J Med* 1963; **268**: 988–91.

6   Bleicher SJ, O'Sullivan JB, Freinkel N. Carbohydrate metabolism in pregnancy V. The interrelations of glucose, insulin and free fatty acids in later pregnancy and postpartum. *N Engl J Med* 1964; **271**: 866–72.

7   Burt RL. Peripheral utilization of glucose in pregnancy. III. Insulin tolerance. *Obstet Gynecol* 1956; **2**: 558–664.

8   Bergman RN, Phillips LS, Cobeli C. Physiological evaluation of factors controlling glucose tolerance in man: measurement of insulin sensitivity and beta-cell sensitivity from the response to intravenous glucose. *J Clin Invest* 1981; **68**: 1456–67.

9   Cousins L. Insulin sensitivity in pregnancy. *Diabetes* 1991; **40** (Suppl. 2): 39–43.

10 Bergman RN, Finegood DT, Ader M. Assessment of insulin sensitivity *in vivo*. *Endocr Rev* 1985; **6**(1): 45–86.

11 Kühl C. Insulin secretion and insulin resistance in pregnancy and gestational diabetes. Implications for diagnosis and management. *Diabetes* 1991; **40** (Suppl. 2): 18–24.

12 Robinson SR, Johnson DJ. Advantage of diabetes? *Nature* 1995; **375** (letter): 640.

13 Ryan EA, O'Sullivan MJ, Skyler JS. Insulin action during pregnancy: studies with the euglycemic glucose clamp technique. *Diabetes* 1985; **34**: 380–9.

14 Jovanovic L, Peterson CM. Optimal insulin delivery for the pregnant diabetic patient. *Diabetes Care* 1982; **5** (Suppl. 1): 24–37.

15 Langer O, Anyaegbunam A, Brustman L *et al*. Pregestational diabetes: insulin requirements throughout pregnancy. *Am J Obstet Gynecol* 1988; **159**: 616–21.

16 Langhoff-Roos J, Wibell L, Gebre-Medhin M, Lindmark G. Placental hormones and maternal glucose tolerance: a study of fetal growth in normal pregnancy. *Br J Obstet Gynaecol* 1989; **96**: 320–6.

17 Samaan N, Yen SCC, Gonzalaez D. Metabolic effects of placental lactogen in man. *J Clin Endocrinol Metab* 1968; **28**: 485–91.

18 Kalkhoff RK, Richardson BL, Beck P. Relative effects of pregnancy human placental lactogen and prednisolone on carbohydrate tolerance in normal and subclinical diabetic subjects. *Diabetes* 1969; **18**: 153–75.

19 Kalkhoff RK, Jacobson M, Lemper D. Progesterone, pregnancy and the augmented plasma insulin response. *J Clin Endocrinol* 1970; **31**: 24–8.

20 Taylor R. Insulin action. *Clin Endocrinol* 1991; **34**: 159–71.

21 Martin JW, Friesen HG. Effect of human placental lactogen on the isolated islets of Langerhans. *Endocrinology* 1969; **84**: 619–22.

22 Ryan EA, Enns L. Role of gestational hormones in the induction of insulin resistance. *J Clin Endrocinol Metab* 1988; **67**: 341–7.

23 Leturque A, Hauguel S, Sutter-Dub MT, Girard J. Effects of placental lactogen and progesterone on insulin stimulated glucose metabolism in rat muscles in vitro. *Diabete Metab* 1989; **15**: 176–81.

24 Randle PJ, Garland PB, Hales CN, Newsholme EA. The glucose fatty acid cycle: its role in insulin sensitivity and the metabolic disturbances of diabetes mellitus. *Lancet* 1963; **i**: 785–9.

25 Bonadonna RC, Groop LC, Simonson DC, Defronzo RA. Free fatty acid and glucose metabolism in human ageing: evidence for operation of the Randle cycle. *Am J Physiol* 1994; **266**: 501–9.

26 Gilbert M, Basile S, Buadelin A, Pere MC. Lowering plasma free fatty acid levels improves insulin action in conscious pregnant rabbits. *Am J Physiol* 1993; **264**: E576–82.

27 DeFronzo RA. Lilly Lecture 1987. The triumvirate: beta-cell, muscle, liver: a collusion responsible for non insulin dependent diabetes. *Diabetes* 1988; **37**: 667–87.

28 Hauguel S, Leturque A, Gilbert M, Girard J. Effects of pregnancy and fasting on muscle glucose utilization in the rabbit. *Am J Obstet Gynecol* 1988; **158**: 1215–18.

29 Leturque A, Ferre P, Burnol AF *et al*. Glucose utilization rates and insulin sensitivity in vivo in tissues of virgin and pregnant rats. *Diabetes* 1986; **35**: 172–7.

30 Toyoda N, Murata K, Sugiyama Y. Insulin binding, glucose oxidation and methylglucose transport in isolated adipocytes and pregnant rats near term. *Endocrinology* 1985; **116**: 998–1002.

31 Leturque A, Burnol AF, Ferre P, Girard J. Pregnancy-induced resistance in the rat: assessment by glucose clamp technique. *Am J Physiol* 1984; **246**: E25–31.

32 Rossi G, Sherwin RS, Penzias AS *et al*. Temporal changes in resistance and secretion in 24 hr-fasted conscious pregnant rats. *Am J Physiol* 1993; **265**: E845–51.

33 Ader M, Bergan RN. Glucose synergies insulin suppression of hepatic glucose output: mechanism to avoid hyperglycemia. Abstract. *Diabetes* 1988; **37** (Suppl. 1): 77A.

34 Liu Z, Gardner LB, Barrett EJ. Insulin and glucose suppress hepatic glucose glycogenolysis by distinct enzymatic mechanisms. *Metabolism* 1993; **42**: 1546–51.

35 Hauguel S, Gilbert M, Girard J. Pregnancy-induced insulin resistance in liver and skeletal muscle of the conscious rabbit. *Am J Physiol* 1987; **252**: E165–9.

36 Gilbert M, Basile S, Buadelin A, Pere MC. Lowering plasma free fatty acid levels improves insulin action in conscious pregnant rabbits. *Am J Physiol* 1993; **263**: E576–82.

37 Pagano G, Cassader M, Massobrio M *et al*. Insulin binding to human adipocytes during late pregnancy in healthy, obese and diabetic state. *Horm Metab Res* 1980; **12**: 177–81.

38 Hjolland E, Pedersen O, Espersen T, Klebe JG. Impaired insulin receptor binding and postbinding defects of adipocytes from normal and diabetic women. *Diabetes* 1986; **35**: 598–603.

39 Ciraldi TP, Kettel M, El-Roeiy A *et al*. Mechanisms of cellular insulin resistance in human pregnancy. *Am J Obstet Gynecol* 1994; **170**: 635–41.

40 Davidson M. Insulin resistance of late pregnancy does not include the liver. *Metabolism* 1984; **33**: 532–7.

41 Martinez C, Ruiz P, Andres A *et al*. Tyrosine kinase activity of the liver insulin receptor is inhibited in rats at term gestation. *Biochem J* 1989; **263**: 267–72.

42 Damm P, Handberg A, Kühl C *et al*. Insulin receptor binding and tyrosine kinase activity in skeletal muscle from normal pregnant women and women with gestational diabetes. *Obstet Gynecol* 1993; **82**: 251–9.

43 Toyada N, Deguchi T, Murata K *et al*. Postbinding insulin resistance around parturition in the isolated rat epitrochlearis. *Am J Obstet Gynecol* 1991; **165**: 1475–80.

44 Garvey WT, Maianu L, Hancock JA *et al*. Gene expression of GLUT$_4$ in skeletal muscle from insulin resistant patients with obesity, IGT, GDM, and NIDDM. *Diabetes* 1992; **41**: 465–75.

45 Okuno S, Maeda Y, Yamamguchi Y *et al*. Expression of GLUT$_4$ glucose transporter mRNA and protein in skeletal muscle and adipose tissue from rats in late pregnancy. *Biochem Biophys Res Commun* 1993; **191**: 405–12.

46 Burt RL, Davidson IWF. Insulin half-life and utilization in normal pregnancy. *Obstet Gynecol* 1974; **43**: 161–70.

47 Bellman O, Hartman E. Influence of pregnancy on the kinetics of insulin. *Am J Obstet Gynecol* 1975; **122**: 829–33.

48 Lind T, Billewicz WZ, Brown G. A serial study of changes occurring in the oral glucose tolerance test during pregnancy. *J Obstet Gynaecol Br Commonw* 1973; **80**: 1033–9.

49 Cousins L, Rigg L, Hollingsworth D *et al*. The 24-hour excursion and diurnal rhythm of glucose, insulin, and C-peptide in normal pregnancy. *Am J Obstet Gynecol* 1980; **136**: 483–8.

50 Van Assche FA, Aerts L, De Prins F. A morphological study of the endocrine pancreas in human pregnancy. *Br J Obstet Gynaecol* 1978; **85**: 818–20.

51 Costrini NV, Kalkhoff RK. Relative effects of pregnancy, estradiol and progesterone on plasma insulin and pancreatic islet insulin secretion. *J Clin Invest* 1971; **50**: 992–9.

52 Malaisse WJ, Malaisse-Lagae F, Picard C, Flament-Durand J. Effects of pregnancy and chronic growth hormone upon insulin secretion. *Endocrinology* 1969; **84**: 41–4.

53 Hager D, Georg RH, Leitner JW, Beck P. Insulin secretion and content in isolated rat pancreatic islets following treatment with gestational hormones. *Endocrinology* 1972; **91**: 977–81.

54 Kalkhoff RK. Effects of pregnancy on insulin and glucagon secretion by perifused rat pancreatic islets. *Endocrinology* 1978; **102**: 623–31.
55 Hubinot CJ, Duframe SP, Malaisse WJ. Effect of pregnancy on protein kinase A and C in rat pancreatic islets. *Horm Metab Res* 1985; **17**: 104–109.
56 Tanigawa K. Tsuchiyama S, Kato Y. Differential sensitivity of pancreatic β-cells to phorbol ester TPA and C-kinase inhibitor H-7 in nonpregnant and pregnant rats. *Endocrinol Jpn* 1990; **37**: 883–91.
57 Lind T. Metabolic changes in pregnancy relevant to diabetes mellitus. *Postgrad Med J* 1979; **55**: 353–7.
58 Felig P, Kim YJ, Lynch V, Hendler R. Amino acid metabolism during starvation in human pregnancy. *J Clin Invest* 1972; **51**: 1195–202.
59 Metzger BE, Agnoli FS, Hare JW, Freinkel N. Carbohydrate metabolism in pregnancy. X. Metabolic disposition of alanine by the perfused liver of the fasting pregnant rat. *Diabetes* 1973; **22**: 601–12.
60 Felig P, Lynch V. Starvation in human pregnancy: hypoglycemia, hypoinsulinemia and hyperketonemia. *Science* 1970; **170**: 990–2.
61 Kalhan SC, D'Angelo LJ, Savin SM, Adam PAJ. Glucose production in pregnant women at term gestation. *J Clin Invest* 1979; **63**: 388–94.
62 Metzger BE, Ravnikar V, Vilesis R, Freinkel N. Accelerated starvation and the skipped breakfast in late normal pregnancy. *Lancet* 1982; **i**: 588–92.
63 Metzger BE, Freinkel N. Accelerated starvation in pregnancy: implications for dietary treatment of obesity and gestational diabetes mellitus. *Biol Neonate* 1987; **51**: 78–85.
64 Cowett RM. Hepatic and peripheral responsiveness to a glucose infusion in pregnancy. *Am J Obstet Gynecol* 1985; **153**: 272–9.
65 Kalhan SC, Gilfillian CA, Tserng KY, Savin SM. Glucose–alanine relationship in normal human pregnancy. *Metabolism* 1988; **37**: 152–8.
66 Turtle JR, Kipnis DM. The lipolytic action of human placental lactogen in isolated fat cells. *Biophys Acta* 1967; **144**: 583–93.
67 Phelps RL, Metzger BE, Freinkel N. Diurnal profiles of glucose, insulin free fatty acids, triglycerides, cholesterol, and individual amino acids in late normal pregnancy. *Am J Obstet Gynecol* 1981; **140**: 730–6.
68 Potter JM, Nestel PJ. The hyperlipidemia of pregnancy in normal and complicated pregnancy. *Am J Obstet Gynecol* 1979; **64**: 704–12.
69 Glueck CJ, Fallat RW, Sheel D. Effect of estrogenic compounds on triglyceride kinetics. *Metabolism* 1975; **24**: 537–45.
70 Merrera E, Gomez-Coronado D, Lasuncion MA. Lipid metabolism in pregnancy. *Biol Neonate* 1987; **51**: 70–7.
71 Topping DL, Mayes PA. The immediate effect of insulin and fructose on the metabolism of perfused liver. *Biochem J* 1972; **126**: 295–311.
72 Herrera E, Lasuncion MA, Gomez-Coronado D *et al.* Role of lipoprotein lipase activity on lipoprotein metabolism and the fate of circulating triglycerides in pregnancy. *Am J Obstet Gynecol* 1988; **158**: 1575–83.
73 Bruschetta H, Buchanan TA, Steil GM *et al.* Reduced glucose production accounts for the fall in plasma glucose during brief extension of an overnight fast in women with gestational diabetes. Abstract. *Clin Res* 1994; **42**: 27A.
74 Morrow PG, Marshall WP, Kim H-J, Kalkoff RK. Metabolic response to starvation I. Relative effects of pregnancy and sex steroid administration in the rat. *Metabolism* 1981; **30**: 268–73.
75 Morrow PG, Marshall WP, Kim H-J, Kalkoff RK. Metabolic response to starvation II. Effects of sex steroid administration to pre- and post-menopausal women. *Metabolism* 1981; **30**: 274–8.
76 Freinkel N. Of pregnancy and progeny. *Diabetes* 1980; **29**: 1023–35.
77 Andersen O, Kühl C. Adipocyte insulin receptor binding and lipogenesis at term in normal pregnancy. *Eur J Clin Invest* 1988; **18**: 575–81.
78 Freinkel N. Effects of the conceptus on maternal metabolism during pregnancy. In: Leibel BS, Wrenshall GA (eds), *On the Nature and Treatment of Diabetes.* Excerpta Medica, Amsterdam, 1965; 679–91.

79 Hagay ZJ. Diabetic ketoacidosis in pregnancy: etiology, pathophysiology and management. *Clin Obstet Gynecol* 1994; **37**: 39–49.

80 Rigg L, Cousins L, Hollingsworth D *et al*. Effects of exogenous insulin on excursions and diurnal rhythm of plasma glucose in pregnant patients with and without residual β-cell function. *Am J Obstet Gynecol* 1980; **136**: 537–44.

81 Montoro MN, Myers VP, Mestman JH *et al*. Outcome of pregnancy in diabetic ketoacidosis. *Am J Perinatol* 1993; **10**: 17–20.

82 Kilvert JA, Nicholson HO, Wright AD. Ketoacidosis in diabetic pregnancy. *Diabetes Med* 1993; **10**: 278–81.

83 Tibaldi JM, Lorber DL, Nerenberg A. Diabetic ketoacidosis and insulin resistance with subcutaneous terbutelin infusion: a case report. *Am J Obstet Gynecol* 1990; **163**: 509–10.

84 Miodovnik M, Peros N, Holroyde JC, Siddiqi TA. Treatment of premature labor in insulin-dependent diabetic women. *Obstet Gynecol* 1985; **65**: 621–7.

85 Myers RE. Brain damage due to asphyxia: mechanism of causation. *J Perinat Med* 1981; **9**: 78–86.

86 Philips AF, Dubin JW, Matty PJ, Raye JR. Arterial hypoxemia and hyperinsulinemia in the chronically hyperglycemia fetal lamb. *Pediatr Res* 1982; **16**: 653–8.

87 Bradley RJ, Brudenell JM, Nicolaides KH. Fetal acidosis and hyperlacticaemia diagnosed by cordocentesis in pregnancies complicated by maternal diabetes mellitus. *Diabetic Med* 1991; **8**: 464–8.

88 Milley JR, Papacostas JS. Effect of insulin on metabolism of fetal sheep hindquarters. *Diabetes* 1989; **38**: 597–603.

89 Buchanan TA, Metzger BE, Freinkel N. Accelerated starvation in late pregnancy: a comparison between obese normal pregnant women and women with gestational diabetes. *Am J Obstet Gynecol* 1990; **162**: 1015–20.

90 Knopp RH, Hagee MS, Raisys V, Benedetti T. Metabolic effects of hypocaloric diets in management of gestational diabetes. *Diabetes* 1991; **40** (Suppl. 2): 165–71.

91 Churchill JA, Berendez HW, Nemore J. Neuropsychological deficits in children of diabetic mothers. *Am J Obstet Gynecol* 1966; **105**: 257–68.

92 Stehbens JA, Baker GL, Kitchell M. Outcome at ages 1, 3 and 5 years of children born to diabetic women. *Am J Obstet Gynecol* 1977; **127**: 408–13.

93 Rizzo T, Metzger BE, Burns WJ, Burns K. Correlation between antepartum maternal metabolism and intelligence of offspring. *N Engl J Med* 1991; **325**: 408–13.

94 Reece EA, Coustan DR, Sherwin RS *et al*. Does intensive glycaemic control in diabetic pregnancies result in normalization of other metabolic fuels? *Am J Obstet Gynecol* 1991; **165**: 126–30.

95 Potter JM, Reckless JPD, Cullen DR. The effect of continuous subcutaneous insulin infusion and conventional insulin regimes on 24-hour variation of blood glucose and intermediary metabolites in the third trimester of diabetic pregnancy. *Diabetologia* 1981; **21**: 534–9.

96 Hertz RH, King KC, Kalhan SC. Management of third trimester pregnancies with the use of continuous subcutaneous insulin infusion therapy: a pilot study. *Am J Obstet Gynecol* 1984; **149**: 256–60.

97 Jervell J, Stokke KT, Moe N *et al*. Metabolic profiles in closely controlled diabetic pregnancies during the third trimester. *Diabetologia* 1979; **16**: 229–33.

98 Metzger BE. Summary and recommendations of the Third International Workshop Conference on Gestational Diabetes Mellitus. *Diabetes* 1991; **40** (Suppl. 2): 197–201.

99 Freinkel N, Metzger BE, Phelps RL *et al*. Gestational diabetes mellitus: heterogeneity of maternal age, weight, insulin secretion, HLA antigens, and islet cell antibodies and the impact of maternal metabolism on pancratic β-cell function and somatic growth in the offspring. *Diabetes* 1985; **34** (Suppl. 2): 1–7.

100 Dornhorst A, Beard RW. Implications of gestational diabetes for the health of the mother. *Br J Obstet Gynaecol* 1994; **101**: 286–90.

101 Pettitt D, Aleck K, Baird H *et al*. Congenital susceptibility to non insulin dependent diabetes: role of intrauterine environment. *Diabetes* 1988; **37**: 622–8.

102 Peters RK, Kjos SL, Xiang A, Buchanan TA. Long-term diabetogenic effect of single pregnancy in women with previous gestational diabetes mellitus. *Lancet* 1996; **347**:

227–30.

103 Tuomilehto J, Zimmet P, Mackay IR *et al.* Antibodies to glutamic acid decarboxylase as predictors of insulin-dependent diabetes mellitus before clinical onset of the disease. *Lancet* 1994; **343**: 1383–5.

104 Damm P, Kuhl C, Buschard K *et al.* Prevalance and predictive value of islet cell antibodies in women with gestational diabetes. *Diabetic Med* 1994; **11**: 558–63.

105 Beischer NA, Wein P, Sheedy MT *et al.* Prevalence of antibodies to glutamic acid decarboxylase in women who have had gestational diabetes. *Am J Obstet Gynecol* 1995 (in press).

106 Buschard K, Buch I, Molsted-Pedersen L *et al.* Increased incidence of true type I diabetes acquired during pregnancy. *Br Med J* 1987; **294**: 275–9.

107 Nicholls JSD, Chan SP, Ali K *et al.* Insulin secretion and sensitivity in women fulfilling WHO criteria for gestational diabetes. *Diabetic Med* 1995; **12**: 56–60.

108 Dornhorst A, Bailey PC, Anyaoku V *et al.* Abnormalities of glucose tolerance following gestational diabetes. *Q J Med* 1990; **284** (New Series 77): 1219–28.

109 Dornhorst A, Chan SP, Gelding SV *et al.* Ethnic differences in insulin secretion in women at risk of future diabetes. *Diabetic Med* 1992; **9**: 258–62.

110 Dornhorst A, Davies M. Anyakou V *et al.* Abnormalities in fasting proinsulin concentrations in mild gestational diabetes. *Clin Endocrinol* 1991; **34**: 211–13.

111 Nicholls JSD, Ali K, Gray IP *et al.* Increased maternal fasting proinsulin as a predictor of insulin requirements in women with gestational diabetes. *Diabetic Med* 1994; **11**: 57–61.

112 Stoffel M, Bell KL, Blackburn CL *et al.* Identification of glucokinase mutations in subjects with gestational diabetes mellitus. *Diabetes* 1993; **42**: 937–40.

113 Catalano PM, Tyzbir ED, Sims EA. Incidence and significance of islet cell antibodies in women with previous gestational diabetes. *Diabetes Care* 1990; **13**: 478–83.

114 Swenne I. Pancreatic beta-cell growth and diabetes mellitus. *Diabetologia* 1992; **35**: 193–201.

115 Swenne I, Borg LA, Crace CJ, Schnell Landström A. Persistent reduction in pancreatic beta-cell mass after limited period of protein-energy malnutrition in the young rat. *Diabetologia* 1992; **35**: 932–45.

116 Dornhorst A, Paterson CM, Nicholls JSD *et al.* High prevalence of gestational diabetes in women from ethnic minority groups. *Diabetic Med* 1992; **9**: 820–5.

117 Dooley SL, Metzger BE, Cho NH. Gestational diabetes mellitus: influence of race on disease prevalence and perinatal outcome in a U.S. population. *Diabetes* 1991; **40** (Suppl. 2): 25–9.

118 Motala AA, Omar MAK, Gouws E. High risk of progression to non insulin dependent diabetes in South-African Indians with impaired glucose tolerance. *Diabetes* 1993; **42**: 556–63.

119 Benjamin E, Winters D, Mayfield J, Gohdes D. Diabetes in pregnancy in Zuni Indian women: prevalence and subsequent development of clinical diabetes after gestational diabetes. *Diabetes Care* 1993; **16**: 1231–5.

120 Kjos SL, Peters RK, Xiang A *et al.* Predicting future diabetes in Latino women with gestational diabetes. *Diabetes* 1995; **44**: 586–91.

121 Eriksson J, Franssila K, Allunki A *et al.* Early metabolic defects in persons at increased risk for non-insulin-dependent diabetes mellitus. *N Engl J Med* 1989; **231**: 337–43.

122 Haffner SM, Stern MP, Mitchell BD *et al.* Incidence of type II diabetes in Mexican Americans predicted by fasting insulin and glucose levels, obesity and body fat distribution. *Diabetes* 1990; **39**: 283–8.

123 Martin BC, Warram JH, Krolweski AS *et al.* Role of glucose and insulin resistance in the development of type 2 diabetes mellitus: results of a 25 year follow-up study. *Lancet* 1992; **340**: 925–9.

124 Ward WK, Johnston CL, Beard JC *et al.* Abnormalities of islet β-cell function, insulin action and fat distribution in women with a history of gestational diabetes: relation to obesity. *J Clin Endocrinol Metab* 1985; **61**: 1039–45.

125 Ward WK, Johnston CL, Beard JC *et al.* Insulin resistance and impaired insulin secretion in subjects with histories of gestational diabetes. *Diabetes* 1985; **34**: 861–9.

126 Metzger BE, Cho NH, Roston SM, Radvany R. Prepregnancy weight and antepartum

insulin secretion predict glucose tolerance five years after gestational diabetes mellitus. *Diabetes Care* 1993; **16**: 1598–605.

127 Catalano PM, Tyzbir ED, Wolfe RR *et al*. Carbohydrate metabolism during pregnancy in control subjects and women with gestational diabetes. *Am J Physiol* 1993; **264** (Endocrinol. Metab.): E60–7.

128 Garvey WT, Maianu L, Zhu J-H *et al*. Multiple defects in the adipocyte glucose transport system cause cellular insulin resistance in gestational diabetes. *Diabetes* 1993; **42**: 1773–85.

129 Ober C, Xiang KS, Thisted RA *et al*. Increased risk of gestational diabetes associated with insulin receptor and insulin-like growth factor II restriction fragment polymorphisms. *Gen Epidemiol* 1989; **6**: 559–69.

130 Metzger BE, Phelps RL, Frienkel N, Navickas IA. Effects of gestational diabetes on diurnal profiles of plasma glucose, lipids and individual amino acids. *Diabetes Care* 1980; **3**: 402–9.

131 Cowett RM, Carr SR, Ogburn PL. Lipid tolerance testing in pregnancy. *Diabetes Care* 1993; **16**: 51–6.

132 Chan SP, Gelding SV, McManus RJ *et al*. Abnormalities of intermediate metabolism following a gestational diabetic pregnancy. *Clin Endocrinol* 1992; **36**: 417–20.

4

Embryo Development in Diabetic Pregnancy

ULF J. ERIKSSON
University of Uppsala, Uppsala, Sweden

Maternal diabetes affects embryonic development in several ways, leading to increased morbidity and mortality in the offspring[1]. During the embryonic period in particular two types of disturbance in the embryonic development have been noted. These are retarded growth, denoted as early growth delay[2], and increased incidence of congenital malformations[3]. In this chapter we will review the clinical and experimental findings of these disturbances in embryonic development in diabetic pregnancy, and some of the current theoretical concepts suggested to explain these processes.

EARLY GROWTH DELAY

This phenomenon was first described by Pedersen and Mølsted-Pedersen[2], who performed serial ultrasound measurements in early normal and diabetic pregnancy. They reported an early growth retardation among the embryos of diabetic mothers. This early growth disturbance amounted to a mean delay of five to six days, although considerable individual variation was noted[2]. Growth retardation was also found to be associated with an increased risk for congenital malformations[4], as well as postnatal psychological and motor dysfunction[5]. These studies suggested a coupling between early growth disturbance and teratogenic susceptibility in diabetic pregnancy.

However, several authors have been unable to confirm an early growth delay in diabetic pregnancy[6,7], others have reported a growth retardation

Diabetes and Pregnancy: An International Approach to Diagnosis and Management.
Edited by A. Dornhorst and D. R. Hadden.
© 1996 John Wiley & Sons Ltd.

but no coupling to congenital malformations[8], and other investigators failed to demonstrate any long-term psychomotor or psychological effects on the infants of the diabetic mother[9,10].

Several experimental studies have reported detrimental effects on early embryonic development exerted by a diabetic or a diabetes-like environment. Thus, in pre-implantation embryos of diabetic animals pronounced retardation of growth and development have been described. This effect is found in embryos of experimentally diabetic rodents[11–13] and in blastocysts of spontaneously diabetic NOD mice[14]. In addition, it has been shown that an increased ambient concentration of glucose[15–17] or ketone bodies[18,19] during *in vitro* culture of pre-implantation rodent embryos causes growth retardation. The growth and development of the embryoblast (the inner cell mass) of the rodent conceptus appear to be particularly sensitive to a diabetic environment[17,20].

There are several indices of the importance of adequate levels of insulin for normal pre-implantation embryonic development. Insulin treatment of the diabetic pregnant rodent mother normalizes somatic growth in pre-implanted embryos[13,16], presumably by stimulating DNA and RNA synthesis[21]. Insulin also stimulates glucose metabolism (increased glucose consumption and anaerobic lactate production) in chick embryos during the gastrula and neural stages[22], and has also been shown to stimulate protein synthesis in pre-implantation mouse embryos *in vivo*[23], as well as to influence their glucose metabolism *in vitro*[24] and to stimulate cellular proliferation in culture[25,26], leading to an improved implantation rate following transfer into recipient females[27].

In conclusion, there seems to be clinical and experimental support for an early growth-retarding effect in embryos exerted by a (maternal) diabetic environment. This effect is associated with increased ambient levels of glucose and ketone bodies, as well as with a decrease in insulin concentration.

CONGENITAL MALFORMATION

In general the risk of giving birth to a malformed child appears to be increased two to four times in diabetic pregnancy[1,3,28–32] although the incidence may vary between different clinical centres and time periods[33–39]. The congenital malformations are induced early in gestation, according to Mills and collaborators[40], who designated the embryonic period up to the seventh gestational week as the teratologically susceptible time period, based on theoretical considerations. Strong indirect support for this notion was also obtained from studies where early pre-conception counselling and treatment of the mothers yielded markedly reduced malformation rates[41,42]. The problem of the timing of the teratological induction has been studied experimentally. The outcome of pregnancy in animals with either spontaneous diabetes (BB rat), or chemically (streptozotocin) induced diabetes has been analysed. The pregnant diabetic rats were either given streptozotocin on gestational day 6, or treated with insulin – a treatment which was interrupted for two to four days, thus exposing their offspring to a manifest maternal diabetic state during a limited period of the gestation. The findings in these studies implicate the post-conception days 6–10 in the rat (which correspond to human post-conception weeks 2–4) as the teratogenic period for skeletal malformations[43-45].

The exact nature of the teratological insult in diabetic pregnancy, and the cell biological details of the induced disturbances, are not known. In recent years, however, a number of clinical reports and experimental findings have addressed this question. Thus, the effects on embryogenesis exerted by the diabetic state seem to be different if the major developmental disturbance occurs in early, middle, or late pregnancy[11,20,31,40,43-45]. The teratologic insult is clearly related to the degree of maternal metabolic imbalance. It has been shown that elevated HbA_{1c} levels in early pregnancy, indicative of impaired metabolic control during the immediate post-implantation period, are associated with an increased risk for fetal maldevelopment[46-49]. The impaired control of the maternal diabetic state involves alterations of several metabolites, of which excess glucose concentration has been suggested as the major teratogenic agent. In addition, several other alterations in maternal and fetal physiology have been implicated in diabetic teratogenesis; some of these are discussed in Tables 4.1 and 4.2.

Table 4.1. Suggested teratological agents of a diabetic environment

Teratological agent	References
Excess glucose	15,17,50–57,61,63–67,69,71–74,78,93,107,108, 115,120,122,123
Deficiency of glucose	79–82
Excess β-hydroxybutyrate	19,53,56,72–74,77,88–93
Excess branched-chain amino acids (α-ketoisocaproic acid)	74,93
Excess somatomedin inhibitor(s)	72,73,96
Excess triglycerides	74
Multifactorial	73,74,77,78,93
Genetic predisposition	53,56,104

Table 4.2. Metabolic consequences of a diabetic environment in embryos

Teratological effect	References
Accumulation of sorbitol	58–61
Deficiency of *myo*-inositol	58,60,65–70
Deficiency of zinc	99,100
Altered prostaglandin metabolism	67,71
Excess free oxygen radicals	93,104,107–109,120,123,131

HYPERGLYCAEMIA

An increased ambient glucose level has been suggested as the primary teratogen in diabetic pregnancy. This notion is based upon the covariation between HbA_{1c} concentration and malformation rate, as discussed above, as well as ample experimental evidence, most of which emanates from *in vitro* studies of rodent embryos. It has been repeatedly demonstrated that increased concentration of glucose in the culture medium in a dose–response manner increases the degree of dysmorphogenesis and growth retardation in post-implantation embryos[50-53]. Retarded development is found in pre-implanted embryos[15-17,54] as well as in cranial neural crest cells[55] and embryonic (pre)chondrocytes from the mandibular and limb bud regions[56,57].

Several biochemical consequences of increased ambient glucose concentration have been suggested to play a role in disturbed embryogenesis, such as hyperaccumulation of sorbitol[58-62], arachidonic acid depletion[63,64] and deficiency of *myo*-inositol[58,60,62,65-70]. However, when the embryonic sorbitol accumulation was blocked by aldose reductase inhibitors there was no effect on the dysmorphogenesis of the conceptus[59-62]. In contrast, *myo*-inositol and arachidonic acid supplementation have been shown to alleviate the glucose-induced embryonic malformations *in vitro* to a significant extent[60,62,63,66-68]. Also addition of some prostaglandins to the culture medium has decreased the malformation rate in embryos subjected to high glucose levels[67,71].

The notion of excess glucose as the single teratogenic agent in diabetic pregnancy has in recent years been replaced by the view of a multifactorial aetiology of congenital malformations[72-74]. There is now both clinical[75,76] and experimental[74,77,78] support for the existence of teratogens other than an increased maternal glucose level in diabetic pregnancy.

HYPOGLYCAEMIA

Decreased glucose concentration in the culture medium may induce embryonic malformations *in vitro*[79-81] and severe hypoglycaemia in pregnant rats *in vivo* also leads to fetal dysmorphogenesis[82]. Extremely low glucose levels may result from the intensive insulin treatment advocated in pregnant diabetic women, and there has been widespread concern that hypoglycaemia may be teratogenic in human diabetic pregnancy. There is one report of a four-fold increase in heart disease in insulin-dependent diabetic mothers when the pregnancy was complicated by hypoglycaemia[83], but in contrast to these findings Mølsted-Pedersen and collaborators reported that only eight of 65 diabetic mothers with malformed infants had insulin-related hypoglycaemic reactions during the first trimester of pregnancy[84] – findings that are supported by several recent clinical trials which have failed to demonstrate an increase in the incidence of congenital anomalies in diabetic pregnancy despite severe and frequent maternal hypoglycaemia[85-87]. Furthermore, there is an *ad hoc* argument against a possible teratogenic effect of hypoglycaemia. Frequent hypoglycaemic episodes occur rather commonly with tight glucose control, and since this stringent metabolic control is clearly associated with a decreased malformation rate, hypoglycaemia is not likely to be a major contributor to the genesis of congenital anomalies.

HYPERKETONAEMIA

Increased ketone body concentration is a teratogen *in vitro*[18,19,72,73,88-92] and may act together with high glucose concentration *in vivo*[74]. Free oxygen radical scavenging diminishes the *in vitro* dysmorphogenesis induced by excess β-hydroxybutyrate[93].

ALTERATION OF OTHER SUBSTANCES

Increased triglyceride levels, as well as increased levels of branched-chain amino acids, have been suggested to exert teratologic influence on the developing embryo, based on experimental studies[44,74,93].

SOMATOMEDIN INHIBITOR(S)

A serum fraction from severely diabetic rats, which reduces the growth-promoting activity of somatomedins in costal cartilage *in vitro*[94,95], has been identified as teratogenic. This serum fraction causes growth retardation and malformations both in mouse[96] and rat embryos[72], a teratogenic effect that is additive to those of high glucose and β-hydroxybutyrate concentrations[96]. The exact biochemical identity of the active compound(s) in this serum fraction has not been determined, and its role in the teratogenic process is not clear at present.

ZINC DEFICIENCY

Deficiency of trace metals, in particular zinc, is a recognized animal teratogen[97,98]. In rat diabetic pregnancy, a zinc deficiency has been demonstrated in the fetuses[99,100]. This decrease in the fetal content of zinc amounts to 25%, a decrease which is refractory to supplementation of extra zinc via the drinking water[99]. Trace metal disturbances, leading to zinc deficiency, have been implicated in a few clinical studies of diabetic pregnancies[101,102]. A lowered serum concentration of zinc in early human diabetic pregnancy could induce zinc deficiency in the embryo resulting in fetal malformation[101,102].

GENETIC BACKGROUND

The importance of both the maternal and fetal genomes for the induction of congenital malformations was studied in two closely related rat strains (U and H) which display markedly different malformation patterns in experimental diabetic pregnancy[53]. The cross-breeding of normal males with manifestly diabetic female rats (U, H or the F_1 hybrid H/U) showed that if there was 50% or more of the U genome on the maternal side, 3–5% malformations and 16–21% resorptions resulted. If the U proportion of the fetal genome was increased from 50% to 75–100%, the malformation and resorption rates increased further[53]. These findings suggested a mixed genetic–environmental pathogenesis of the congenital malformations. A subsequent study of biochemical markers, in accordance with Bender *et al*.[103], revealed a polymorphism of the catalase locus, denoted Cs-1. In the H strain and in the inbred U substrain B, which showed almost no malformations, the allele Cs-1[b] was found to be predominant. In contrast, in the outbred U strain, as well as in the two inbred U substrains A and C where malformations were present, the allele Cs-1[a] was predominant. This suggests that the Cs-1[a] allele cosegregates with the susceptibility for skeletal malformations[104]. This finding may either implicate the isoenzyme of catalase in the teratological process, by its role in the defence against free oxygen radicals (see below), or indicate an alteration in a chromosomal area which – by way of analogy with the mouse genome – may be close to genes coding for abnormal skeletal development[104]. There are a few published reports on a possible teratological predisposition in human diabetic pregnancy where the authors have compared the rates of malformations among offspring of diabetic and non-diabetic fathers[28,105,106]. There were no significant differences in the malformation rates in any of these studies, thereby demonstrating that the genes predisposing for diabetes mellitus in the father do not at the same time induce an increased risk of congenital malformations in the offspring[28,105,106].

EMBRYONIC EXCESS OF FREE OXYGEN RADICALS

Based upon experimental findings *in vitro* of blocked embryonic dysmorphogenesis by increased oxygen radical scavenging activity, the concept of embryonic excess of free oxygen radicals was proposed[93,107] as an integral component in the teratogenic process of diabetic pregnancy. Recently, transgenic mouse embryos, with an increased activity of the scavenging enzyme superoxide dismutase, have displayed resistance toward the teratogenic effect of a diabetic environment, both *in vitro*[108] and *in vivo*[109].

The notion of excess oxygen radicals in embryos may serve as a metabolic common denominator for the teratogenic processes reviewed above. A substantial interrelationship between all of these processes is evident. For instance, one effect of excess free oxygen radicals would be an enhanced intra- and extracellular lipid peroxidation. This constitutes a link to prostaglandin metabolism since hydroperoxides are strong stimulants of prostaglandin biosynthesis and also inhibit the production of prostacyclin[110] – an imbalance which may have profound effects on embryonic development. The beneficial effects of arachidonic acid[63,64] or *myo*-inositol[62,67] supplementation to embryos in a diabetic environment may thus be the result of a normalized prostaglandin metabolism. The latter compound (*myo*-inositol) normalizes phospholipase A_2 activity[111] by restoring decreased cellular levels of phosphatidylinositol and *myo*-inositol[65]. Recent observations of a beneficial effect on glucose-induced malformations by addition of various prostaglandins to the culture medium support the notion of prostaglandin imbalance *in vitro*[67,71].

Another possible effect of increased oxygen radical activity is DNA damage[112,113]. Results in favour of DNA damage being present in the offspring of diabetic pregnancy have been published[114,115].

The concept of free oxygen radicals causing embryonic maldevelopment is supported by the finding of dysmorphogenesis in embryos subjected to buthionine sulphoximine[116,117], a compound which decreases the concentration of reduced glutathione, one of the primary cellular antioxidants. Disturbed glutathione metabolism may also constitute a bridging pathway between free oxygen radical-induced damage and disturbed prostaglandin biosynthesis in embryos subjected to a diabetic environment[118,119]. This concept was supported by the recent demonstration of diminished glucose-induced dysmorphogenesis in embryos cultured in 0.5–1 mM *N*-acetylcysteine[120], a glutathione supplementing agent which has shown beneficial effects in several tissues exposed to oxidative damage[121].

The nature of an excess of free oxygen radicals could be of two types: either increased generation of the radicals or decreased defence against the radicals. Both of these mechanisms have gained experimental support. The generation concept is indirectly supported by the demonstration of mitochondrial swelling in the neuroepithelial tissues of embryos of diabetic rats[122], and by the finding that the pyruvate transport inhibitor CHC (cyano-hydroxy-cinnamic acid) was able to block glucose- and pyruvate-induced teratogenesis *in vitro*[93]. In contrast, Trocino and collaborators recently reported that high-glucose cultured embryos displayed decreased γGCS (gamma-glutamylcysteine synthetase) activity and diminished glutathione levels, thereby suggesting decreased antioxidant defence in these embryos[123].

FUTURE INTERVENTION STRATEGIES

The interrelationship between increased oxidative stress, excess of free oxygen radicals, prostaglandin biosynthesis and embryogenesis in a metabolically altered environment awaits further studies[124-126]. In this line of work a direct interaction between oxygen radical excess and gene expression, as suggested by recent reports[127,128], should be investigated. Understanding the cellular relationships between maternal diabetes and disturbed embryonic development should enable us to develop new strategies for blocking the teratogenic process of diabetic pregnancy. In this context antioxidant therapy may be a logical step, as implied by the encouraging results *in vitro*[93,107,120,123]. I concur with recent studies reporting diminished neurological complications in diabetic animals following administration of antioxidant compounds[129,130]; there are emerging data from *in vivo* administration of butylated hydroxytoluene and vitamin E to pregnant diabetic rats which indicate lower malformation rates and improved somatic growth of the offspring[131,132].

CONCLUDING REMARKS

As evident from the discussion above, a unifying concept for the mechanism of diabetic teratogenesis may be embryonic excess of free oxygen radicals. The biochemical consequences of this notion should be found in several metabolic compartments within and outside the embryonic cells, and the challenge of future research in this field will be to discover the interrelationships between the many processes found to be altered in these embryos. Thus, the relations between excess oxygen radicals, glutathione metabolism, reduced *myo*-inositol level, alterations in arachidonic acid and prostaglandin metabolism, all need elucidation. When this is achieved, we will have a better understanding of the cellular events linking the abnormal metabolic milieu to altered growth and differentiation, and access to new therapeutic intervention strategies, perhaps with implications also for other types of pregnancies when the maternal metabolism is compromised.

ACKNOWLEDGEMENTS

The author gratefully acknowledges the support from the Swedish Medical Research Council (grants no. 12X-7475 and 12X-109), the Family Ernfors Fund, the Novo Nordisk Foundation, the Swedish Diabetes Association, the Juvenile Diabetes Foundation International, and the Bank of Sweden Tercentenary Foundation.

REFERENCES

1 Pederson J. *The Pregnant Diabetic and her Newborn: Problems and Management* 1977; (2nd edn). Munksgaard, Copenhagen.
2 Pedersen JF, Mølsted-Pedersen L. Early growth retardation in diabetic pregnancy. *Br Med J* 1979; i: 18–19.
3 Kucera J. Rate and type of congenital anomalies among offspring of diabetic women. *J Reprod Med* 1971; 7: 61–70.
4 Pedersen JF, Mølsted-Pederson L. Early growth delay detected by ultrasound marks increased risk for congenital malformation in diabetic pregnancy. *Br Med J* 1981; 283: 269–71.
5 Petersen MB, Pedersen SA, Greisen G *et al.* Early growth delay in diabetic pregnancy: relation to psychomotor development at age 4. *Br Med J* 1988; 296: 598–600.
6 Harper MA, Morrow RJ. Early growth delay in diabetic pregnancy. *Br Med J* 1988; 296: 1005–6.
7 Heita-Heikurainen H, Teramo K. Comparison of menstrual history and basal body temperature with early fetal growth by ultrasound in diabetic pregnancy. *Acta Obstet Gynecol Scand* 1989; 68: 457–9.
8 Brown ZA, Mills JL, Metzger BE *et al.* Early sonographic evaluation for fetal growth delay and congenital malformations in pregnancies complicated by insulin-requiring diabetes. *Diabetes Care* 1992; 15: 613–19.
9 Hadden DR, Byrne E, Trotter I *et al.* Physical and psychological health of children of type 1 (insulin-dependent) diabetic mothers. *Diabetologia* 1984; 26: 250–4.
10 Persson B. Longterm morbidity in infants of diabetic mothers. *Acta Endocrinol* 1986; (Suppl. 277): 156–8.
11 Diamond MP, Moley KH, Pellicer A *et al.* Effects of streptozotocin- and alloxan-induced diabetes mellitus on mouse follicular and early embryo development. *J Reprod Fertil* 1989; 86: 1–10.
12 Vercheval M, De Hertogh R, Pampfer S *et al.* Experimental diabetes impairs rat embryo development during the preimplantation period. *Diabetologia* 1990; 33: 187–91.
13 Beebe LFS, Kaye PL. Maternal diabetes and retarded preimplantation development of mice. *Diabetes* 1991; 40: 457–61.
14 Moley KH, Vaughn WK, DeCherney AH, Diamond MP. Effect of diabetes mellitus on mouse pre-implantation embryo development. *J Reprod Fertil* 1991; 93: 325–32.
15 Zusman I, Ornoy A, Yaffe P, Shafrir E. Effects of glucose and serum from streptozotocin-diabetic and non-diabetic rats on the *in vitro* development of preimplantation mouse embryos. *Isr J Med Sci* 1985; 21: 359–65.
16 Diamond MP, Harvert-Moley K, Logan J *et al.* Manifestation of diabetes mellitus on mouse follicular and pre-embryo development: Effects of hyperglycemia per se. *Metabolism* 1990; 39: 220–4.
17 De Hertogh R, Vanderheyden I, Pampfer S *et al.* Stimulatory and inhibitory effects of glucose and insulin on rat blastocyst development *in vitro*. *Diabetes* 1991; 40: 641–7.
18 Zusman I, Yaffe P, Ornoy A. Effects of metabolic factors in the diabetic state on the *in vitro* development of preimplantation mouse embryos. *Teratology* 1987; 35: 77–85.
19 Moley KH, Vaughn WK, Diamond MP. Manifestations of diabetes mellitus on mouse preimplantation development: effect of elevated concentration of metabolic intermediates. *Hum Reprod* 1994; 9: 113–21.
20 Pampfer S, De Hertogh R, Vanderheyden I *et al.* Decreased inner cell mass proportion in blastocysts from diabetic rats. *Diabetes* 1990; 39: 471–6.
21 Rao LV, Wikarczuk ML, Heyner S. Functional roles of insulin and insulin like growth factors in preimplantation mouse embryo development. *In Vitro Cell Dev Biol* 1990; 26: 1043–8.
22 Baroffio A, Raddatz E, Markert M, Kucera P. Transient stimulation of glucose metabolism by insulin in the 1-day chick embryo. *J Cell Physiol* 1986; 127. 288–92.
23 Harvey MB, Kaye PL. Insulin stimulates protein synthesis in compacted mouse embryos. *Endocrinology* 1988; 122: 1182–4.
24 Wales RG, Khurana NK, Edirisinghe WR, Pike IL. Metabolism of glucose by

preimplantation mouse embryos in the presence of glucagon, insulin, epinephrine, cAMP, theophylline and caffeine. *Aust J Biol Sci* 1985; **38**: 421–8.

25 Caro CM, Trounson A. The effect of protein on preimplantation mouse development in vitro. *J In Vitro Fertil Embryo Transf* 1984; **1**: 183–7.

26 Gardner DK, Kaye PL. Insulin increases cell number and morphological development in mouse preimplantation embryos in vitro. *Reprod Fertil Dev* 1991; **3**: 79–91.

27 Zhang X, Armstrong DT. Presence of amino acids and insulin in a chemically defined medium improves development of 8-cell rat embryos *in vitro* and subsequent implantation *in vivo*. *Biol Reprod* 1990; **15**: 662–8.

28 Chung CS, Myrianthopoulos NC. Factors affecting risks of congenital malformations. II. Effect of maternal diabetes on congenital malformations. *Birth Defects* 1975; **11**: 23–38.

29 Kitzmiller JL, Cloherty JP, Younger MD *et al*. Diabetic pregnancy and perinatal morbidity. *Am J Obstet Gynecol* 1978; **131**: 560–80.

30 Mills JL. Malformations in infants of diabetic mothers. *Teratology* 1982; **25**: 385–94.

31 Hadden DR. Diabetes in pregnancy 1985: clinical controversy. *Diabetologia* 1986; **29**: 1–9.

32 Freinkel N. Diabetic embryopathy and fuel-mediated organ teratogenesis: lessons from animal models. *Horm Metab Res* 1988; **20**: 463–75.

33 Duncan JM. On puerperal diabetes. *Trans Obstet Soc Lond* 1882; **24**: 256–85.

34 Drury MI, Green AT, Stronge JM. Pregnancy complicated by clinical diabetes mellitus: a study of 600 pregnancies. *Am J Obstet Gynecol* 1977; **49**: 519–22.

35 Simpson JL, Elias S, Martin AO *et al*. Diabetes in pregnancy, Northwestern University series (1977–1981). I. Prospective study of anomalies in offspring of mothers with diabetes mellitus. *Am J Obstet Gynecol* 1983; **146**: 263–70.

36 Mølsted-Pedersen L, Kühl C. Obstetrical management in diabetic pregnancy: the Copenhagen experience. *Diabetologia* 1986; **29**: 13–16.

37 Becerra JE, Khoury MJ, Cordero JF, Erickson JD. Diabetes mellitus during pregnancy and the risks for specific birth defects: a population-based case–control study. *Pediatrics* 1990; **85**: 1–9.

38 Hanson U, Persson B, Thunell S. Relationship between haemoglobin A1c in early type 1 (insulin-dependent) diabetic pregnancy and the occurrence of spontaneous abortion and fetal malformation in Sweden. *Diabetologia* 1990; **33**: 100–4.

39 Kitzmiller JL, Gavin LA, Gin GD *et al*. Preconception care of diabetes: glycemia control prevents congenital anomalies. *JAMA* 1991; **265**: 731–6.

40 Mills J, Baker L, Goldman AS. Malformations in infants of diabetic mothers occur before the seventh gestational week. *Diabetes* 1979; **28**: 292–3.

41 Mølsted-Pedersen L. Pregnancy and diabetes, a survey. *Acta Endocrinol* 1980; **94** (Suppl. 238): 13–19.

42 Fuhrmann K, Reiher H, Semmler K, Glöckner E. The effect of intensified conventional insulin therapy before and during pregnancy on the malformation rate in offspring of diabetic mothers. *Exp Clin Endocrinol* 1984; **83**: 173–7.

43 Baker L, Egler JM, Klein SM, Goldman AS. Meticulous control of diabetes during organogenesis prevents congenital lumbosacral defects in rats. *Diabetes* 1981; **30**: 955–9.

44 Eriksson RSM, Thunberg L, Eriksson UJ. Effects of interrupted insulin treatment on fetal outcome of pregnant diabetic rats. *Diabetes* 1989; **38**: 764–72.

45 Eriksson UJ, Bone AJ, Turnbull DM, Baird JD. Timed interruption of insulin therapy in diabetic BB/E rat pregnancy: effects on maternal metabolism and fetal outcome. *Acta Endocrinol* 1989; **120**: 800–10.

46 Leslie RDG, Pyke DA, John PN, White JM. Hemoglobin A1 in diabetic pregnancy. *Lancet* 1978; **ii**: 958–9.

47 Miller E, Hare JW, Cloherty JP *et al*. Elevated maternal hemoglobin A1c in early pregnancy and major congenital anomalies in infants of diabetic mothers. *N Engl J Med* 1981; **304**: 1331–4.

48 Ylinen K, Aula P, Stenman U-H *et al*. Risk of minor and major fetal malformations in diabetics with high hemoglobin A1c values in early pregnancy. *Br Med J* 1984; **289**: 345–6.

49 Greene MF, Hare JW, Cloherty JP *et al*. First-trimester hemoglobin A1 and risk for major malformation and spontaneous abortion in diabetic pregnancy. *Teratology* 1989; **39**: 225–31.

50 Cockroft DL, Coppola PT. Teratogenic effects of excess glucose on head-fold rat embryos in culture. *Teratology* 1977; **16**: 141–6.
51 Sadler TW. Effects of maternal diabetes on early embryogenesis II: Hyperglycemia-induced exencephaly. *Teratology* 1980; **21**: 349–56.
52 Garnham EA, Beck F, Clarke CA, Stanisstreet M. Effects of glucose on rat embryos in culture. *Diabetologia* 1983; **25**: 291–5.
53 Eriksson UJ. Importance of genetic predisposition and maternal environment for the occurrence of congenital malformations in offspring of diabetic rats. *Teratology* 1988; **37**: 365–74.
54 Diamond MP, Pettway ZY, Logan J *et al.* Dose–response effects of glucose, insulin and glucagon on mouse pre-embryo development. *Metabolism* 1991; **40**: 566–70.
55 Suzuki N, Svensson K, Eriksson UJ. High glucose concentration inhibits migration of rat cranial neural crest cells *in vitro*. *Diabetologia* 1996; (in press).
56 Styrud J, Eriksson UJ. Effects of D-glucose and β-hydroxybutyric acid on the *in vitro* development of (pre)chondrocytes from embryos of normal and diabetic rats. *Acta Endocrinol* 1990; **122**: 487–98.
57 Styrud J, Eriksson UJ. *In vitro* effects of glucose and growth factors on limb bud and mandibular arch chondrocytes maintained at various serum concentrations. *Teratology* 1991; **44**: 65–75.
58 Sussman I, Matschinsky FM. Diabetes affects sorbitol and *myo*-inositol levels of neuroectodermal tissue during embryogenesis in rat. *Diabetes* 1988; **37**: 974–81.
59 Eriksson UJ, Naeser P, Brolin S. Increased accumulation of sorbitol in embryos of manifest diabetic rats. *Diabetes* 1986; **35**: 1356–63.
60 Hod M, Star S, Passonneau JV *et al.* Effect of hyperglycemia on sorbitol and myo-inositol content of cultured rat conceptus: failure of aldose reductase inhibitors to modify myo-inositol depletion and dysmorphogenesis. *Biochem Biophys Res Commun* 1986; **140**: 974–80.
61 Eriksson UJ, Naeser P, Brolin SE. Influence of sorbitol accumulation on growth and development of embryos cultured in elevated levels of glucose and fructose. *Diabetes Res* 1989; **11**: 27–32.
62 Hashimoto M, Akazawa S, Akazawa M *et al.* Effects of hyperglycemia on sorbitol and myo-inositol contents of cultured embryos: treatment with aldose reductase inhibitor and myo-inositol supplementation. *Diabetologia* 1990; **33**: 597–602.
63 Goldman AS, Baker L, Piddington R *et al.* Hyperglycemia-induced teratogenesis is mediated by a functional deficiency of arachidonic acid. *Proc Natl Acad Sci USA* 1985; **82**: 8227–31.
64 Pinter E, Reece EA, Leranth CS *et al.* Arachidonic acid prevents hyperglycemia-associated yolk sac damage and embryopathy. *Am J Obstet Gynecol* 1986; **155**: 691–702.
65 Weigensberg MJ, Garcia-Palmer FJ, Freinkel N. Uptake of *myo*-inositol by early-somite rat conceptus: transport kinetics and effects of hyperglycemia. *Diabetes* 1990; **39**: 575–82.
66 Hod M, Star S, Passonneau JV *et al.* Glucose-induced dysmorphogenesis in the cultured rat conceptus: prevention by supplementation with myo-inositol. *Isr J Med Sci* 1990; **26**: 541–4.
67 Baker L, Piddington R, Goldman A *et al.* Myo-inositol and prostaglandins reverse the glucose inhibition of neural tube fusion in cultured mouse embryos. *Diabetologia* 1990; **33**: 593–6.
68 Akashi M, Akazawa S, Akazawa M *et al.* Effects of insulin and myo-inositol on embryo growth and development during early organogenesis in streptozotocin-induced diabetic rats. *Diabetes* 1991; **40**: 1574–9.
69 Strieleman PJ, Connors MA, Metzger BE. Phosphoinositide metabolism in the developing conceptus: effects of hyperglycemia and scyllo-inositol in rat embryo culture. *Diabetes* 1992; **41**: 989–97.
70 Strieleman PJ, Metzger BE. Glucose and scyllo-inositol impair phosphoinositide hydrolysis in the 10.5 day cultured rat conceptus: a role in dysmorphogenesis? *Teratology* 1993; **48**: 267–78.
71 Goto MP, Goldman AS, Uhing MR. PGE2 prevents anomalies induced by hyperglycemia or diabetic serum in mouse embryos. *Diabetes* 1992; **41**: 1644–50.
72 Freinkel N, Cockroft DL, Lewis NJ *et al.* Fuel-mediated teratogenesis during early

organogenesis: the effects of incrased concentrations of glucose, ketones, or somatomedin inhibitor during rat embryo culture. *Am J Clin Nutr* 1986; **44**: 986–95.

73 Sadler TW, Hunter III ES, Wynn RE, Phillips LS. Evidence for multifactorial origin of diabetes-induced embryopathies. *Diabetes* 1989; **38**: 70–4.

74 Styrud J, Thunberg L, Nybacka O, Eriksson UJ. Correlations between maternal metabolism and deranged development in the offspring of normal and diabetic rats. *Pediatr Res* 1995; **37**: 343–53.

75 Mills JL, Knopp RH, Simpson JL *et al.* Lack of relation of increased malformation rates in infants of diabetic mothers to glycemic control during organogenesis. *New Engl J Med* 1988; **318**: 671–6.

76 Mills J, Simpson J, Driscol SG *et al.* Incidence of spontaneous abortion among normal women and insulin dependent diabetic women whose pregnancies were identified within 21 days of conception. *N Engl J Med* 1988; **319**: 1617–23.

77 Buchanan TA, Denno DM, Sipos GF, Sadler TW. Diabetic teratogenesis: *in vitro* evidence for a multifactorial etiology with little contribution from glucose *per se*. *Diabetes* 1994; **43**: 656–60.

78 Wentzel P, Eriksson UJ. Insulin treatment fails to abolish the teratogenic potential of serum from diabetic rats. *Eur J Endocrinol* 1996; (in press).

79 Akazawa S, Akazawa M, Hashimoto M *et al.* Effects of hypoglycaemia on early embryogenesis in rat embryo organ culture. *Diabetologia* 1987; **30**: 791–6.

80 Ellinton SKL. *In vivo* and *in vitro* studies of the effects of maternal fasting during embryonic organogenesis in the rat. *Reprod Fertil* 1980; **60**: 383–8.

81 Sadler TW, Horton WE Jr. Effects of maternal diabetes on early embryogenesis: the role of insulin and insulin therapy. *Diabetes* 1983; **32**: 1070–4.

82 Buchanan TA, Schemmer JK, Freinkel N. Embryotoxic effects of brief maternal insulin-hypoglycemia during organogenesis in the rat. *J Clin Invest* 1986; **78**: 643–9.

83 Rowland TW, Hubbell JP, Nadas AS. Congenital heart disease in infants of diabetic mothers. *J Pediatr* 1973; **83**: 815–20.

84 Mølsted-Pedersen L, Tygstrups I, Pedersen J. Congenital malformations in newborn infants of diabetic women: correlation with maternal diabetic vascular complications. *Lancet* 1964; **i**: 1124–6.

85 Bergman M, Seaton TB, Auerhahn CC *et al.* The incidence of gestational hypoglycemia in insulin-dependent and non-insulin-dependent diabetic women. *NY State J Med* 1986; **86**: 174–7.

86 Rayburn W, Piehl E, Joacober S *et al.* Severe hypoglycemia during pregnancy: its frequency and predisposing factors in diabetic women. *Int J Gynaecol Obstet* 1986; **24**: 263–8.

87 Kimmerle R, Heinemann L, Delecki A, Berger M. Severe hypoglycemia incidence and predisposing factors in 85 pregnancies of type I diabetic women. *Diabetes Care* 1992; **15**: 1034–7.

88 Horton WE, Sadler TW. Effects of maternal diabetes on early embryogenesis: alterations in morphogenesis produced by the ketone body β-hydroxybutyrate. *Diabetes* 1983; **32**: 610–16.

89 Horton WE, Sadler TW, Hunter ES. Effects of hyperketonemia on mouse embryonic and fetal glucose metabolism *in vitro*. *Teratology* 1985; **31**: 227–33.

90 Sheehan EA, Beck F, Clarke CA, Stanisstreet M. Effects of β-hydroxybutyrate on rat embryos grown in culture. *Experientia* 1985; **41**: 273–5.

91 Hunter ES, Sadler TW, Wynn RE. A potential mechanism of DL-β-hydroxybutyrate-induced malformations in mouse embryos. *Am J Physiol* 1987; **253**: E72–80.

92 Moore DCP, Stanisstreet M, Clarke CA. Morphological and physiological effects of β-hydroxybutyrate on rat embryos grown in vitro at different stages. *Teratology* 1989; **40**: 237–51.

93 Eriksson UJ, Borg LAH. Diabetes and embryonic malformations: role of substrate-induced free-oxygen radical production for dysmorphogenesis in cultured rat embryos. *Diabetes* 1993; **42**: 411–19.

94 Philips LS, Belosky DC, Young HS, Reichard LA. Nutrition and somatomedin. VI. Somatomedin activity and somatomedin inhibitory activity in sera from normal and

diabetic rats. *Endocrinology* 1979; **104**: 1519–24.
95 Phillips LS, Bajaj VR, Fusco AC, Matheson CK. Nutrition and somatomedin. XI. Studies of somatomedin inhibitors in rats with streptozotocin-induced diabetes. *Diabetes* 1983; **32**: 1117–25.
96 Sadler TW, Phillips LS, Balkan W, Goldstein S. Somatomedin inhibitors from diabetic rat serum alter growth and development of mouse embryos in culture. *Diabetes* 1986; **35**: 861–5.
97 Hurley LS, Swenerton H. Congenital malformations resulting from zinc deficiency in rat. *Proc Soc Exp Biol Med* 1966; **123**: 692–7.
98 Styrud J, Dahlström VE, Eriksson UJ. Induction of skeletal malformations in the offspring of rats fed a zinc-deficient diet. *Ups J Med Sci* 1986; **91**: 29–36.
99 Eriksson UJ. Diabetes in pregnancy: retarded fetal growth, congenital malformations and feto-maternal concentrations of zinc, copper and manganese in the rat. *J Nutr* 1984; **114**: 477–86.
100 Uriu-Hare JY, Stern JS, Reaven GM, Keen CL. The effect of maternal diabetes on trace element status and fetal development in the rat. *Diabetes* 1985; **34**: 1031–40.
101 Jameson S. Effects of zinc deficiency in human reproduction. Thesis. *Acta Med Scand* 1976; (Suppl. 593): 1–89.
102 Breskin MW, Worthinton-Roberts BS, Knopp RH *et al.* First trimester serum zinc concentrations in human pregnancy. *Am J Clin Nutr* 1983; **38**: 943–53.
103 Bender K, Adams M, Baverstock PR *et al.* Biochemical markers in inbred strains of the rat (*Rattus norvegicus*). *Immunogenetics* 1984; **19**: 257–66.
104 Eriksson UJ, den Bieman M, Prins JB, van Zutphen LFM. Differences in susceptibility for diabetes induced malformations in separated rat colonies of common origin. In: *Proc 4th FELASA Symp*, Lyon, France, 1990; 53–7.
105 Comess LJ, Bennett PH, Burch TA, Miler M. Congenital anomalies and diabetes in the Pima Indians of Arizona. *Diabetes* 1969; **18**: 471–7.
106 Neave C. Congenital malformations in offspring of diabetics. *Perspect Pediatr Pathol* 1984; **8**: 213–22.
107 Eriksson UJ, Borg LAH. Protection by free oxygen radical scavenging enzymes against glucose-induced embryonic malformations in vitro. *Diabetologia* 1991; **34**: 325–31.
108 Eriksson UJ, Borg LAH, Hagay Z, Groner Y. Increased superoxide dismutase (SOD) activity in embryos of transgenic mice protects from the teratogenic effects of a diabetic environment. *Diabetes* 1993; **42** (Suppl. 1): 85A.
109 Hagay ZJ, Weiss Y, Zusman I *et al.* Prevention of hyperglycemia-associated embryopathy by embryonic overexpression of the free radical scavenger copper zinc superoxide dismutase gene. *Am J Obstet Gynecol* 1995; **173**: 1036–41.
110 Warso MA, Lands WEM. Lipid peroxidation in relation to prostacyclin and thromboxane physiology and pathophysiology. *Br Med Bull* 1983; **39**: 277–80.
111 Lapetina EG. Regulation of arachidonic acid production: role of phospholipases C and A2. *Trends Pharmacol Sci* 1982; **3**: 115–18.
112 Bucala R, Model P, Cerami A. Modification of DNA by reducing sugars: a possible mechanism for nucleic acid ageing and age-related dysfunction in gene expression. *Proc Natl Acad Sci USA* 1984; **81**: 105–9.
113 Morita J, Ueda K, Nanjo S, Komano T. Sequence specific damage of DNA induced by reducing sugars. *Nucleic Acid Res* 1985; **13**: 449–58.
114 Lee AT, Plump A, DeSimone C *et al.* A role for DNA mutations in diabetes-associated teratogenesis in transgenic embryos. *Diabetes* 1995; **44**: 20–4.
115 Lee AT, Eriksson UJ. Embryos exposed to high glucose *in vitro* show congenital malformations and increased frequency of DNA mutations. *Diabetologia* 1995; **38** (Suppl. 1): A281.
116 Hales BF, Brown H. The effect of *in vivo* glutathione depletion with buthionine sulfoximine on rat embryo development. *Teratology* 1991; **44**: 251–7.
117 Stark KL, Harris C, Juchau MR. Influence of electrophilic character and glutathione depletion on chemical dysmorphogenesis in cultured rat embryos. *Biochem Pharmacol* 1989; **38**: 2685–92.
118 Kashiwagi A, Asahina T, Ikebuchi M *et al.* Abnormal glutathione metabolism and

increased cytotoxicity caused by H_2O_2 in human umbilical vein endothelial cells cultured in high glucose medium. *Diabetologia* 1994; **37**: 264–9.

119 Hempel SL, Wessels DA. Prostaglandin E2 synthesis after oxidant stress is dependent on cell glutathione content. *Am J Physiol* 1994; **266** (Cell Physiol. 35): C1392–9.

120 Eriksson UJ. Rat embryos exposed to a teratogenic diabetic environment *in vitro* are protected by the antioxidant N-acetylcysteine. *Eur J Endocrinol* 1994; **130** (Suppl. 1): 20.

121 Hoffer E, Avidor I. Benjaminov O *et al*. N-Acetylcysteine delays the infiltration of inflammatory cells into the lungs of paraquat-intoxicated rats. *Toxicol Appl Pharmacol* 1993; **120**: 8–12.

122 Yang X, Borg LAH, Eriksson UJ. Altered mitochondrial morphology of rat embryos in diabetic pregnancy. *Anat Rec* 1995; **241**: 255–67.

123 Trocino RA, Akazawa S, Ishibashi M *et al*. Significance of glutathione depletion and oxidative stress in early embryogenesis in glucose-induced rat embryo culture. *Diabetes* 1995; **44**: 992–8.

124 Hunt JV, Dean RT, Wolff SP. Hydroxyl radical production and autooxidative glycosylation. *Biochem J* 1988; **256**: 205–12.

125 Gillery P, Monboisse J-C, Maquart F-X, Borel J-P. Does oxygen free radical increased formation explain long term complications of diabetes mellitus? *Med Hypotheses* 1989; **29**: 47–50.

126 Wolff SP. Diabetes mellitus and free radicals: free radicals, transition metals and oxidative stress in the aetiology of diabetes mellitus and complications. *Br Med Bull* 1993; **49**: 642–52.

127 Kashihara N, Watanabe Y, Makino H *et al*. Selective decreased de novo synthesis of glomerular proteoglycans under the influence of reactive oxygen species. *Proc Natl Acad Sci USA* 1992; **89**: 6309–13.

128 Schreck R, Rieber P, Baeuerle PA. Reactive oxygen intermediates as apparently widely used messengers in the activation of the NF-αB transcription factor and HIV-1. *EMBO J* 1991; **10**: 2247–58.

129 Bravenboer B, Kappelle AC, Hamers FPT *et al*. Potential use of glutathione for the prevention and treatment of diabetic neuropathy in the streptozotocin-induced diabetic rat. *Diabetologia* 1992; **35**: 813–17.

130 Cameron NE, Cotter MA, Archibald V *et al*. Anti-oxidant and pro-oxidant effects on nerve conduction velocity, endoneurial blood flow and oxygen tension in non-diabetic and streptozotocin-diabetic rats. *Diabetologia* 1994; **37**: 449–59.

131 Simán CM, Eriksson UJ. Protection from malformations in fetuses of diabetic rats treated with the antioxidant butylated hydroxytoluene (BHT). *Eur J Endocrinol* 1995; **132** (Suppl. 1): 26.

132 Bonet B, Viana M, Herrera E. Teratogenic effects of diabetes: protection by vitamin E. *Proc 2nd Int Symp Diab Pregn in the 90's* 1995; 131.

5

Fetal Growth and Development

LEONA AERTS, ROBERT PIJNENBORG, JOHAN VERHAEGHE,
KATHLEEN HOLEMANS and F. ANDRÉ VAN ASSCHE
Universitaire Ziekenhuizen Leuven, Leuven, Belgium

Fetal growth and development are primarily determined by the fetal genome, but the genetic regulation of fetal growth is influenced by different factors, which can exert a stimulatory or an inhibitory effect. On one hand fetal growth is determined by the capacity of the mother to supply nutrients and by the capacity of the placenta to transport these nutrients to the fetus. On the other hand the fetus has its own factors which influence growth and differentiation, the fetal growth factors. Specific cells of the fetus have to produce these factors in appropriate amounts, and other cells have to respond to their stimulus. Both processes can be influenced by endogenous factors (hormones or central nervous system).

Normal growth demands an equilibrium in the interaction between these different compartments and between the stimulatory and inhibitory factors affecting each of these steps. Disturbance of this equilibrium at either stage can result in intrauterine growth retardation and microsomia, or in fetal overgrowth and macrosomia.

The main substrate for fetal development is glucose, which is completely derived from the maternal circulation, since it cannot be synthesized by the fetus itself. Glucose is supplied from mother to fetus by facilitated diffusion through the placenta, and is mainly determined by the maternal plasma glucose levels. The maternal metabolic condition therefore is the first important determinant of fetal growth. Malnutrition of the mother resulting in maternal and fetal hypoglycaemia interferes with normal fetal growth; maternal metabolic disorders of glucohomeostasis, such as diabetes,

Diabetes and Pregnancy: An International Approach to Diagnosis and Management.
Edited by A. Dornhorst and D. R. Hadden.
© 1996 John Wiley & Sons Ltd.

provide the fetus with an abundance of glucose and force it to adapt its own metabolism. These two maternal conditions therefore can affect placental and fetal development within an abnormal intrauterine milieu.

PLACENTAL NUTRIENT TRANSPORT

NORMAL DEVELOPMENT

Adequate maternal and fetal blood flow is important for placental function. In species with haemochorial placentation, such as the rat and the human, substantial adaptive changes occur within the placental bed spiral arteries that deliver maternal blood to the placenta. It is well known that trophoblast invasion of the spiral arteries in the placental bed plays an essential role in that process[1,2]. As far as transport function within the placental tissue is concerned, the availability of an adequate surface area for physiological exchange is important. Apart from direct nutrient transfer to the fetus, consumption or conversion of the nutrients within the placental tissue must also be taken into account. Not only do they have obvious effects on placental growth and weight, but also a significant impact on nutrient transfer and pregnancy maintenance. At the cellular level glucose transfer through the placenta is effected by facilitated diffusion, mediated by glucose transporters (GLUT). In the rat, $GLUT_1$ and $GLUT_3$ have been demonstrated in the placenta within different placental layers[3-5], but only $GLUT_3$ is exclusively expressed within the labyrinth, which is the zone of physiological exchange between maternal and fetal circulations. It has been suggested therefore that $GLUT_1$ is responsible for supplying glucose as a placental fuel and that $GLUT_3$ is important for glucose transfer to the fetus[6]. In the human, $GLUT_1$ is abundant in both syncytiotrophoblast and cytotrophoblast and fetal endothelial cells in placental villi at term. Controversies still exist whether $GLUT_3$ is also expressed in the human placenta[3,7]. As far as possible regulatory factors are concerned, it has been found that insulin has no effect on glucose uptake and metabolism in a perfused *in vitro* system[8], only the maternal glucose concentration has been shown to direct its own uptake[9].

DIABETIC PREGNANCY

Abnormal maternal blood supply to the placenta may be one of the crucial defects in diabetic pregnancy. Although in the rat functional data are available illustrating impaired maternal blood flow to the placenta[10], no histological studies have been published to illustrate a lack of adaptive changes within the uteroplacental arteries, which is normally effected by invading trophoblast. Also in the human few data exist about the placental bed in diabetic women. Although occasional thickening of the arterial wall and artherosclerotic lesions in spiral arteries have been reported[11,12], other studies have failed to reveal pathological lesions[13,14]. Furthermore, recent Doppler studies have failed to detect any obvious aberration in uteroplacental blood flow in diabetic patients[15,16].

Diabetic placentae are heavier than normal, both in the human[17-19] and in the rat, at least when maternal diabetes is severe and associated with fetal microsomia[20]. It is not yet clear which factors determine the increased placental growth in this situation or whether it influences transplacental flow and nutrient transport. In the rat, the overgrowth of the diabetic placenta is associated with increased glycogen content[17-20]. The placental glycogen is stored primarily within the glycogen cells—a subpopulation of specialized trophoblastic cells within the trophospongium[21], which undergo gradual lysis near term. In severe diabetic rats huge cystic structures are formed within the trophospongium[22], which are probably derived by lysis of extensive areas of glycogen cells. In the human, the placentae of diabetic women also show increased glycogen concentration. This material is stored within the syncytiotrophoblast as well as along the fetal blood vessels of the villous stroma[23]. Changes in expression of insulin receptors on trophoblast cell membranes in diabetic women may play a role[24], although it has been shown that trophoblast isolated from normal placentae does not show increased glycogen accumulation after treatment with glucose or insulin *in vitro*[25]. In diabetic rats $GLUT_3$ mRNA and protein increase up to five-fold, while the expression of $GLUT_1$ remains unaltered. The same effect could be obtained in pregnant normal rats that were made hyperglycaemic, but not in hyperinsulinaemic animals[5].

It is important to evaluate the effect of placental adaptations on the maternal–fetal transfer. Does the increased placental tissue mass in diabetes also reflect an increased transport capacity or does it induce pathological defects that may compromise placental function? Apart from the development of trophospongial cysts in the diabetic rats, no obvious abnormality could be found within the labyrinth[22]. However, proper evaluation would require detailed morphometric analysis of surface areas of physiological exchange, which has not yet been reported. In the human, numerous histological and ultrastructural studies have been performed on placentae of diabetics, but there is no agreement on any typical pathological feature[26]. However, among the numerous observations published, the occurrence of focal necrosis of villous syncytiotrophoblast and compensatory proliferation of cytotrophoblast is regularly reported, as well as villous fibrinoid necrosis, oedema or fibrosis of the villous stroma, and increased syncytial sprout formation, which may all compromise placental function. An increased villous surface area has been reported in diabetes[27,28] but these findings were not confirmed in a more recent study[29], although an increased fetal capillary surface area was observed within the villous stroma. It is important to notice that in these morphometric studies the possible existence of areas of focal necrosis within the syncytiotrophoblastic covering of the villi was not taken into account.

MATERNAL MALNUTRITION

Maternal malnutrition during pregnancy obviously leads to intrauterine growth retardation and microsomia in the human as well as in experimental animals. The decreased availability of nutrients for transplacental transport and a decreased placental blood flow[30] must result in a decreased nutrient supply to the fetus. No studies are available concerning effects of malnutrition on uteroplacental vascular adaptations within the placental bed development. In the rat, malnutrition leads to decreased placental weights[31] with reduction in glucose transfer and glycogen content[32]. No histological studies have been performed so far in this species. In the human, lower placental weights were reported, but no significant change in glycogen content was noted[32,33]. A variety of histopathological defects are increased, including infarction, fibronoid necrosis of the villi, syncytial knotting and proliferation of the cytotrophoblastic cells within the villi[34], which may all compromise placental transport functions.

INSULIN AS A FETAL GROWTH FACTOR

The major factor for fetal growth throughout late gestation is insulin. Withdrawal of fetal insulin by pancreatectomy reduces fetal growth rate by 50%, which can be completely corrected by insulin replacement[35]. For normal insulin-dependent fetal growth two related effects are needed. On one hand insulin must be produced by the fetal pancreatic beta cells in an appropriate quality and quantity, and on the other hand insulin must effect appropriately the uptake of glucose by the fetal tissues, which must be equipped to do so.

NORMAL DEVELOPMENT

Insulin Production

In the rat the initial formation of the pancreatic diverticulum from the gut epithelium occurs at 10 days of gestation. During the early period of formation the primitive organ comprises cords of cells with little structural organization[36]. From day 12, insulin immunoreactivity is observed in small clusters of cells, sometimes together with glucagon. However, 'islet-like' formations, composed mainly of insulin-containing cells, are clearly present only from day 18; these cells already co-express $GLUT_2$, the typical glucose transporter of the beta cells[37]. Within a few days an explosive development of these clusters occurs: their number and size increase considerably, partly by neogenesis of endocrine cells from primordial stem cells, partly by replication of existing differentiated cells[38]. By day 20 they appear organized into real 'mantle-islets' with a core of insulin-producing beta cells, surrounded by a mantle of glucagon (A), somatostatin (D) and pancreatic polypeptide (PP)-containing cells[39]. At the ultrastructural level these cell types are clearly recognizable by their secretory granules. They all appear as mature, synthesizing and secreting cells. In the beta cells granulation increases with fetal age, parallel to the increase in pancreatic insulin content, while emeiocytotic images increase in parallel with the rise in fetal plasma insulin[40]. In term fetuses, at day 22 of gestation, beta cells appear as mature adult cells.

From day 20 of gestational age, the fetal rat pancreas responds to glucose stimulation by a clear insulin response, *in vivo* and *in vitro*[41-43]. The magnitude of this response increases with age and becomes clearly biphasic by the end of gestation[42]. In the human, stimulated insulin release, although monophasic, is already present as early as 14 weeks of gestation[44] and matures into a biphasic response before the end of the pregnancy, as demonstrated in preterm babies at birth[45]. The sensitivity of the fetal beta cell to glucose is significantly enhanced by the presence of amino acids which circulate at high levels in the fetal blood. This allows modulation of the insulin secretion by small changes in blood glucose and provides the basis for the growth-promoting action of insulin during fetal life[42].

The response of beta cells to glucose stimulation is initiated by glucose transport into the beta cells, followed by glycolysis. This assumes the presence of the glucose transporter $GLUT_2$ in the fetal beta cells, and the glycolytic enzymes, mainly glucokinase. Although little is known about the development of these steps in the fetal pancreas, it has been shown that the $GLUT_2$ protein is present in rat fetal pancreatic beta cells from day 18 of gestation[37]. However, at day 20 it only reaches 50% of its amount in neonatal beta cells[46]. In the human fetus, $GLUT_2$ and glucokinase mRNA expression in the beta cells remain very low up to 24 weeks of gestation, when glucose sensitivity is still immature[47]. No data are available concerning late gestation. Also glucose metabolism is quantitatively lower in fetal than in neonatal islets and the immature secretory response observed in fetal islets, at least up to day 20 of rat gestation, may be a consequence of reduced glucose transport into the pancreatic beta cells and the resulting reduction in glycolytic flux[46]. We may conclude that in the last days of fetal life an explosive development of the fetal beta cell mass coincides with progressive maturation of beta cell function and response, and with increasing insulin levels in the fetal plasma. In fact, plasma insulin levels in the term fetus are much higher than at any other period in life and are associated with an exceptional increase in body weight.

Insulin Action

High circulating insulin levels during late fetal life coincide with the spectacular increase in body weight, suggesting an important role for insulin in the anabolic processes. In order to profit from the abundance of insulin, the fetal tissues must be equipped to capture the insulin (insulin receptors), to internalize and degrade it (post-receptor mechanisms), and to initiate glucose entry (GLUT) and metabolism (glucokinase) in their cells.

Insulin receptors are present from day 17 of gestation in the fetal lungs, gastrointestinal tract and heart, but most abundantly in the fetal liver, where their number increases with fetal age[48,49]. Internalization of the hormone occurs in the hepatocytes from day 17 up to term, and the rate at which this mechanism proceeds increases with the degree of liver maturation. Considering the whole body receptor compartment, it appears that its size in one-day preterm fetuses is similar to that in the adult rat, but that the events subsequent to insulin binding to its receptors are slower in young fetuses and mature with fetal age[48]. Thus by the end of gestation the fetal tissues show an abundance of insulin receptors, an adult capacity to bind insulin and a progressive maturation of the post-receptor processes. This allows the fetus to profit maximally from the circulating nutrients for its growth and development.

Little is known, however, about the mechanism by which insulin affects the glucose uptake by the fetal tissues. The glucose transporter regulating insulin-dependent glucose uptake is known to be $GLUT_4$. However in the rat, $GLUT_4$ mRNA expression and protein are at the limit of detection during fetal and early postnatal life, and are enhanced only at the time of weaning, when the pups switch from a low to a high carbohydrate diet[50]. Also hepatic glucokinase first appears at the time of weaning, concomitant with the progressive change of nutrient[51]. In embryonic and fetal tissues the main glucose transporter is $GLUT_1$[52,53]. Since its activity is not insulin dependent, at least in adult tissues, the role of insulin in fetal glucose uptake remains unclear.

MATERNAL DIABETES AND FETAL HYPERINSULINAEMIA

Diabetes in the mother during pregnancy involves an abnormal intrauterine milieu for the developing fetus. The abundant fuel supply from mother to fetus induces alteration in both fetal insulin production and insulin action, and thereby influences fetal growth and development.

Insulin Production

The increased glucose supply to the fetus of the diabetic mother stimulates its endocrine pancreas to hypertrophy resulting in islets with hyperplasia of the beta cells, from at least day 20 of rat gestation[39]. Not only is the number of fetal beta cells increased, but also the biosynthetic activity of the individual beta cell is enhanced, as revealed by the ultrastructural appearance of its organelles and by the presence of an increased proportion of proinsulin-containing pale granules. These adaptations in islet and beta cell morphology are in accordance with a doubling of the insulin content in the fetal pancreas during the last two days of gestation. Also the insulin response to glucose stimulation is largely increased in these fetuses, both *in vivo* and *in vitro*[54,55]. No data are available yet on the relation between such an enhanced sensitivity and the presence of glucose transporters and metabolic enzymes in fetal beta cells that developed in a hyperglycaemic environment. In cultured neonatal islets, however, it has been demonstrated that increased glucose sensitivity is associated with an increased presence of $GLUT_2$ on the beta cell membranes[56]. All these adaptations of the fetal endocrine pancrease to the stimulation by maternal diabetes result in fetal hyperinsulinaemia[39,54,55,57].

In the human islet hypertrophy and beta cell hyperplasia have also been recognized for many years as typical features of fetuses and newborns of diabetic mothers. These features of beta cell stimulation are observed as early as 19 weeks of gestation[58–65]. From 32 weeks onwards, a positive correlation is present between the degree of islet and beta cell hyperplasia, with maternal glycaemia and body weight[66]. Increased birth weight is common in infants of diabetic mothers; insulin levels in the cord blood are high and related to the excess weight[67]; plasma amino acid levels are low[68]

Insulin Action

High levels of insulin are circulating in the fetus of the diabetic mother during the last trimester, the period in which the insulin receptors and post-receptor mechanisms generate in the liver and the peripheral tissues[48,49]. Little is known about the influence of this hyperinsulinaemia on the ontogenesis of the insulin receptor system.

Rabbit fetal tissues exposed to hyperinsulinaemia *in utero* have significantly greater numbers of insulin receptors than control fetal tissues[69,70]. In the human the increased glucose uptake by hyperinsulinaemic newborns of gestational diabetic and insulin-dependent diabetic women is also associated with an increased number of insulin receptors at the levels of the monocytes and the erythrocytes[71,72].

The combination of an excess of maternally derived metabolic fuels, fetal hyperinsulinaemia and an increased number of insulin receptors in the fetal tissues is in favour of accelerated fetal anabolism. Glucose utilization by fetal tissues is indeed stimulated[73]. Growth of adipose tissue and of the muscle tissue is enhanced through increased fetal glycogen synthesis, lipid deposition and protein synthesis[74,75]. Increased amino acid turnover results in hypoaminoacidaemia in the fetal rat[76]. In the fetal lamb, hyperinsulinaemia is also associated with stimulated glucose and oxygen consumption, and a significant increase in the net fetal protein synthesis, even at normal glucose levels[77–79]. Even a short (2 h) infusion of high insulin concentrations in the fetal lamb with clamped glucose levels promotes the entry of glucose into tissues, thereby increasing fetal glucose utilization and oxidation and substituting glucose oxidation for that of other substrates[80,81].

In the fetal monkey chronic insulin infusion also stimulates amino acid uptake and protein synthesis. In the presence of normal substrate concentrations this hyperinsulinaemia stimulates cellular hyperplasia in the soft tissues and causes macrosomia of the fetus, with an increased birth weight for normal length. When fetal substrate concentrations are also elevated, as in the fetus of the diabetic mother, both cellular hyperplasia and hypertrophy have been reported[82].

Nothing is known about the adaptation of glucose transporters in the fetal tissues to changes in glucose availability. In neonates, however, it has been shown that weaning onto a high-fat instead of a high-carbohydrate diet prevents the increase of $GLUT_4$ mRNA and protein, whereas $GLUT_1$ mRNA is not affected by the nutritional environment[50]. Although experimental data are not yet available, this allow the possibility that hyperglycaemia might also induce premature expression of the $GLUT_4$ glucose transporter in the fetus. Glucokinase gene expression in the liver has also been shown to be prematurely induced by glucose administration, at least in newborn rats[83].

Although many of the fine mechanisms at the cellular level have to be elucidated, the data grossly agree with the modified Pedersen hypothesis as described by Freinkel (1980): maternal fuels, with elevated glucose concentration, reach the fetus and stimulate beta cell development and secretion; as a consequence fetal fuels are consumed more intensively, resulting in near normal glycaemia and low amino acid levels, increased anabolism of fetal tissues and finally macrosomia[75].

MATERNAL DIABETES AND FETAL HYPOINSULINAEMIA

Insulin Production

When maternal hyperglycaemia is severe, the fetus is confronted with an enormous amount of circulating glucose. Fetal pancreatic islets are overstimulated, but the capacity of the islets to adapt to the increased insulin demands by islet hypertrophy and beta cell hyperplasia appears to be limited. In order to produce more insulin, the activity of individual beta cells is enhanced extremely, which may lead to beta cell overstimulation and exhaustion. Insulin secretion finally exceeds insulin production and the beta cells become degranulated, disorganized and incapable of reacting to any stimulus. The consequence is fetal hypoinsulinaemia[39,54]. This phenomenon has been described in the fetuses of badly controlled diabetic women[84].

Insulin Action

In this period of fetal hypoinsulinaemia, the development of the insulin receptor and the post-receptor system is retarded. A reduced number of insulin receptors on target cells has been described in fetuses of severely diabetic rats, leading to a reduction in fetal glucose uptake[85]. In the hypoinsulinaemic streptozotocin-injected fetal lamb, glucose uptake is also reduced[86,87]. The growth of the fetal protein mass is suppressed; fetal protein synthesis is consistently lower than in controls, whereas protein degradation increases sharply towards the end of gestation[88].

Thus in these fetuses of severely diabetic mothers the hypoinsulinaemia and hyposensitivity of the degranulated beta cells coincide with a deficient capacity of the fetal tissues to respond to insulin. The fetus of a severely diabetic mother therefore cannot profit from the abundant fuel supply for its growth and development and remains microsomic. In the human, small-for-dates infants are born to mothers with badly controlled diabetes, often complicated by vascular pathology.

MATERNAL MALNUTRITION

Insulin Production

Poor nutrition of the mother during pregnancy obviously leads to intrauterine growth retardation and microsomia in the human, as in experimental models. The decreased availability of nutrients for transplacental transport and a decreased placental blood flow[30] result in a decreased nutrient supply to the fetus. An inadequate stimulation of the fetal pancreas leads to hypoplasia of the pancreatic endocrine tissue, due to a smaller size of the islets of Langerhans; pancreatic insulin content is decreased and insulin response to stimuli is altered[89,90], resulting in fetal hypoinsulinaemia. The effect is similar whether the mothers were restricted in their total food intake, or whether only the protein component of the food was diminished, with or without complementing the diet up to isocaloric levels[89-91].

Insulin Action

Insulin deficiency affects umbilical uptake and utilization of glucose, resulting in proportionate growth retardation[35]. The combination of fetal hypoinsulinaemia and low substrate availability further decreases the fetal whole body glucose utilization rate in sheep[92] and rat[93], mainly due to a decrease in glucose uptake by the fetal skeletal muscles and heart, while glucose uptake by liver and brain is unaffected[93]. Also lipid deposition and protein breakdown are decreased, retarding the growth of muscle and adipose tissue[94]. No experimental data are available concerning the insulin receptor system in these conditions, but in the human growth retardation associated with the leprechaun syndrome shows evidence of insulin resistance in the fetal tissues at the post-receptor level[95]. A decreased glucose transporter activity, protein and mRNA has been reported in the lung of small-for-gestational-age fetuses in the rat[96].

The decreased insulin–glucagon ratio prematurely induces hepatic gluconeogenesis in the rat[97] and sheep fetuses[98] through induction of the gluconeogenic enzymes. The induction of fetal hepatic gluconeogenesis might be a mechanism to compensate for the decreased supply of glucose, although the increase in fetal hepatic glucose production remains modest[92,97].

FETAL INSULIN-LIKE GROWTH FACTORS

NORMAL AND INTRAUTERINE GROWTH RETARDATION PREGNANCY

Fetal insulin-like growth factors IGF-I and IGF-II are proinsulin-like polypeptides with molecular weights of 7 649 and 7 471 Da, respectively, and 62% homology in their DNA sequences. The IGFs are produced by almost all human fetal organs examined, in particular by connective tissue and cells of mesenchymal origin[99] from the first trimester of fetal life onwards. IGF-II expression has been identified as early as day 18 of human pregnancy; in rodents, IGFs are expressed in pre-implantation embryos. The discrepancy in distribution between the IGF mRNAs and the IGF peptides within the fetal tissues would indicate that the latter distribution also includes the sites of action of the IGFs[100]. Serum concentrations of the IGFs in the fetus or at birth are considered to be the 'overflow' of their tissue production, and it is generally assumed that the IGFs have a paracrine or autocrine rather than an endocrine mode of action in the fetus[99], in contrast to the endocrine action of IGF-I after birth. IGF-I and IGF-II are generally, but not always, co-expressed in the same cells[101]. The density of the IGF-II transcripts in the tissues[101], and the organ as well as the cord serum concentrations of IGF-II are many times higher than those of IGF-I in the fetus: the IGF-II/IGF-I ratio is between 1.6 and 7.8 for a number of human fetal organs at 14–16 weeks[102] and 6–10 for cord serum concentrations in third-trimester fetuses[103]. In many animal models (rats, guinea-pigs, sheep), IGF-II concentrations fall sharply after birth, so that IGF-II has been considered to be 'the fetal IGF'[104]. In human fetuses, however, both IGF-I and IGF-II concentrations rise with increasing gestational age, but remain lower than in children, adolescents or adults[102,105,106].

Experiments in mice have clearly shown that IGF-I and IGF-II play a crucial role in embryonic and fetal growth and development[107]. Fetal mice that are homozygous for the targeted disruption of the IGF-I gene and also have a paternally derived disruption of the IGF-II gene, so-called IGF-I $(-/-)$/IGF-II $(p-)$ double mutants, are severely growth retarded at birth (30% of normal weight) with marked developmental delay, and they do not survive after birth. Mice carrying one mutation, either IGF-I $(-/-)$ or IGF-II $(p-)$, have birth weights around 60% of normal and they can survive after birth, indicating some degree of 'redundancy' between the IGFs. In human fetuses, cord serum IGF-I concentrations are well correlated with their weight and length at birth[103,105,106]. IGF-I concentrations are clearly lower in cord serum of growth-retarded fetuses and higher in large-for-gestational age fetuses than in those with average weight[103,107,108]. Cord serum IGF-II concentrations have been found to be correlated with birth weight in some[103,105], but not in other[106,108] studies. We found normal concentrations of IGF-II in growth-retarded fetuses[103], confirming data by Lassare *et al.*[108], but increased IGF-II concentrations in large-for-gestational age fetuses. In experimental rat models of intrauterine growth retardation, by maternal starvation or by uterine artery ligation, IGF-I concentrations in fetal serum and tissue IGF-I gene expression are unequivocally decreased, whilst the results are discordant regarding IGF-II serum concentrations and tissue expression, showing either normal, increased or decreased concentrations[110–114].

Whereas the role of the IGFs in fetal growth and development is now undisputed, their potential role in anabolic/metabolic processes in the third trimester of fetal life is less certain. Thus far, experiments in fetal lambs suggest that the infusion of IGF-I results in augmented uptake of glucose and amino acids by the conceptus[115].

The regulation of IGF-I and IGF-II synthesis by the fetal tissues is not well understood. Fetal IGF-I and IGF-II do not appear to be growth hormone dependent, as IGF-I is after birth, because IGF-I and IGF-II are present in normal concentrations in sera of anencephalic fetuses[116]. However, since fetal IGF-I synthesis is invariably inhibited in both human pregnancies and animal model pregnancies with reduced uteroplacental blood flow, there is good evidence that the uteroplacental supply line to the fetus is an important determinant of fetal IGF-I synthesis. More specifically, the maternal–fetal transfer of oxygen and nutrients plays a pivotal role. Studies in sheep have demonstrated that hypoxaemia in mother and fetus lowers fetal IGF-I concentrations[117], and that the infusion of glucose—but not amino acids—to the fetus after a period of starvation restores fetal IGF-I concentrations to normal[118]. The regulation of the IGF-II synthesis is unknown, but local factors (adrenocorticotrophic hormone synthesis in the adrenal glands) may be involved.

The IGFs circulate bound to a number of IGF binding proteins (IGFBPs). It has become clear that the IGFBPs not only serve as carrier proteins for the IGFs in the circulation, but that they also modulate (stimulate or inhibit) the bioactivity of the IGFs. Six IGFBPs (IGFBP1 to IGFBP6) have been cloned or sequenced. All IGFBPs are expressed in human fetal tissues, but IGFBP1 and IGFBP2 appear to be the most abundantly expressed in the human fetus. IGFBP1 (molecular weight 25–26 kDa) is produced mainly or exclusively by the fetal liver in rodents[119,120]. On immunohistochemistry of human fetal tissues, however, IGFBP1 is distributed in the same cells as the IGF peptides[121], which lends support to the contention that IGFBP1 modulates bioactivity of the IGFs at the target tissue level. Serum concentrations of IGFBP1 decline with increasing gestational age in the third-trimester fetuses[103], and even further in the first month after birth[122]. IGFBP1 concentrations in cord serum are negatively correlated with birth weight[103,123]. In addition, cord serum IGFBP1 concentrations are markedly increased in small or growth-retarded fetuses[103,109,123], and there is a sharp rise of IGFBP1 serum concentrations as well as IGFPB1 gene expression in the liver of fetal animal models (rats and sheep) with experimental intrauterine growth retardation or hypoxaemia[112,117,124,127]. High mid-trimester amniotic fluid IGFBP1 concentrations predict the later development of intrauterine growth retardation in human fetuses[128]. It would, therefore, seem that IGFBP1 inhibits the growth-stimulatory action of the IGFs in the fetus[129] and IGFBP1 may well be the 'somatomedin (IGF) inhibitory substance' that was characterized by Tató *et al.*[130] with a bioassay in the plasma of preterm and small-for-gestational age fetuses. The same factors that regulate fetal IGF-I synthesis, the maternal–fetal supply of oxygen and nutrients, also regulate IGFBP1 production in the fetal liver, but in an inverse manner. Even transient fetal hypoxaemia stimulates IGFBP1 synthesis: fetuses with signs of distress in labour (abnormal cardiotocogram, meconium-stained liquor) have higher IGFBP1 concentrations, and there is an inverse correlation between cord serum IGFBP1 and cord pH[131,132].

IGFBP2 (molecular weight 31 kDa) is produced by a variety of fetal organs in rodents[119,120]. The regulation and biological significance of IGFBP2 are more uncertain than those of IGFBP1. IGFBP2 concentrations in cord serum have been found to be equally increased in growth-retarded pregnancies[133], but fetal IGFBP2 serum concentrations and tissue mRNA concentrations are variably altered in animal models of intrauterine growth retardation or hypoxia: either increased[114,125,134], normal[112,127] or decreased[126]. The serum concentrations of IGFBP3 (molecular weight of the IGFBP3 complex: 150 kDa)—the most abundant and growth hormone-dependent IGFBP after birth—are low during fetal life but slowly increase during the second half of fetal life[135], and IGFBP3 concentrations are decreased in small-for-gestational age fetuses compared with normal-weight fetuses[109].

The biological effects of the IGFs are receptor mediated, through two different IGF receptors. Both type 1 and type 2 IGF receptors are expressed during embryonic and fetal life. The type 1 IGF receptor resembles the insulin receptor, contains intracellular tyrosine kinase domains, and binds IGF-I as well as IGF-II and insulin; the type 2 IGF receptor is also known as the mannose 6-phosphate receptor, is devoid of tyrosine kinase activity, and binds only IGF-II. Fetal mice carrying a null mutation of the type I IGF receptor gene show severe growth retardation (45% of normal weight), and cannot survive after birth[136]; thus, the type 1 IGF receptor is essential for normal fetal growth and development. At least in mice, the effects of both IGF-I and IGF-II are mediated through the type 1 IGF receptor, but IGF-II also appears to interact with an unknown receptor which is not the type 2 IGF receptor.

DIABETIC PREGNANCY

Because cord serum IGF-I concentrations correlate well with birth weight and cord serum IGF-I is higher in large-for-gestational age fetuses of non-diabetic mothers than in average-weight fetuses[103,109], it is to be expected that the macrosomic fetuses of diabetic mothers also have increased cord serum IGF-I concentrations. This has indeed been shown to be the case in a number of studies in which IGF-I concentrations were measured either in cord serum or in amniotic fluid of fetuses of diabetic mothers with proven macrosomia, or whose mothers had poor diabetes control during pregnancy[103,137–139]; this was not, however, confirmed in all studies[140]. Whether the hyperinsulinaemia present in macrosomic infants of diabetic mothers or even in large-for-gestational age infants of non-diabetic mothers[103,109] is involved in this increase of fetal IGF-I synthesis is less certain at present. Arguments in favour of such a cause–effect relationship are: (1) data that cord serum C peptide and IGF-I concentrations are correlated in normal as well as diabetic pregnancies[103,139]; (2) data showing that pancreatectomized fetal lambs have a 25% drop in serum IGF-I concentrations[141]; (3) the well-known stimulation of hepatic IGF-I gene expression by insulin after birth[142].

However, pancreatectomized fetal lambs weigh less than normal (71% of controls), and fetal IGF-I synthesis is not predominantly in the liver as in children but widespread in all fetal organs. Therefore, the correlation that exists between cord serum C peptide and IGF-I may be an association rather than a cause–effect relationship, and simply a reflection of differences in weight.

The effects of maternal diabetes on fetal IGF-II and IGFBP concentrations are poorly understood. Normal or increased concentrations of IGF-II have been reported[103,140,143], as well as normal cord serum concentrations of IGFBP1[103]. In children and adults, there is an inverse correlation between serum concentrations of insulin and IGFBP1, and insulin suppresses IGFBP1 gene expression in rat liver[142]; diabetic subjects have increased serum IGFBP1 levels and exogenous insulin suppresses IGFBP1 levels[129,144]. However, we found no differences in cord serum IGFBP1 levels of fetuses with either high or low C peptide concentrations, nor did we find an inverse correlation between cord serum C peptide and IGFBP1[103]. It seems, therefore, that the relationship between insulin and IGFBP1 does not hold in fetal life.

LONG-TERM EFFECTS

From the previous discussion it is clear that the maternal metabolic condition substantially determines fetal growth and development. Alterations in the maternal circulating substrates will induce alterations in placental and fetal metabolism, involving structural and functional adaptations. The question then arises as to whether this offspring, modulated during its fetal development by an abnormal intrauterine milieu, will experience lasting consequences for its glucose metabolism throughout its life.

Offspring of rats which were hyperglycaemic throughout the last week of gestation, at adulthood appear as normal healthy animals with a normal body weight, normal basal glucose and insulin levels and morphologically normal endocrine pancreas[145,146]. When stressed, however, glucose tolerance appears to be impaired, and the effect is divergent whether the youngster had passed its intrauterine life in a mildly or in a severely diabetic mother. When the maternal hyperglycaemia was mild and resulted in fetal hyperinsulinaemia, the induced increase in amino acid turnover is maintained in adulthood, and the beta cell response to glucose stimulation is deficient, while the insulin receptor system appears to be unaffected[146-148]. When the maternal hyperglycaemia was severe and resulted in fetal hypoinsulinaemia, the adult offspring not only displays a deregulation of the stimulated insulin output, but also insulin resistance in the liver and the peripheral tissues[147,149]. When the mothers were malnourished during pregnancy, whether in a qualitative (protein deficiency) or a quantitative (50% restriction) way, glucose tolerance is also impaired in the offspring[90,91].

Pregnancy causes a considerable stress on the glucose and insulin metabolism of the mother and implies important adaptations of the endocrine pancreas at the structural and functional level. The mass of islet tissue doubles and the activity of the beta cells is enhanced[150]. Normal pregnancy is associated with hyperinsulinaemia and insulin resistance. When these youngsters of diabetic or malnourished mothers, with impaired glucose tolerance, become pregnant, they develop gestational diabetes[74,146,151]. This implies that their fetuses also will develop in an abnormal intrauterine milieu and have to adapt to it. Indeed they display the typical features of fetuses from mildly diabetic mothers, and when they become adult they develop impaired glucose tolerance and gestational diabetes[74,146]. A diabetogenic tendency is thereby transmitted from one generation to another, without any genetic involvement, but as a result of the fact that the fetus developed in an abnormal intrauterine milieu.

In the human a number of epidemiological studies also point to the importance of the intrauterine milieu for the development of the fetus. A higher incidence of non-insulin-dependent diabetes and of gestational diabetes is reported in children from diabetic mothers than from diabetic fathers[152], and a higher incidence of diabetes is present in offspring from diabetic great-grandmothers via the maternal than via the paternal line[153]. Systematic treatment of diabetic mothers during pregnancy may result in a decreased incidence of diabetes in their children[154]. The most convincing data on the intrauterine transmission of the diabetogenic tendency in the human derive from studies of Pettitt and co-workers on the Pima Indians, a population with a high incidence of diabetes. Glucose tolerance is much more frequent in children from mothers who had diabetes during pregnancy than in children from mothers who developed diabetes only after that pregnancy. The difference is convincing: 33% versus 1%[155]. Recent epidemiological studies, relating birth files from 50 years ago with the health condition of these people now, also demonstrate a significant relationship between body weight at birth, whether or not related to a known metabolic pathology of the mother, and the incidence of impaired glucose tolerance and diabetes in adulthood[156].

We can conclude that even a minor disturbance in maternal metabolism induces alterations in the fetal metabolism with lasting consequence for the offspring, even over several generations. The effect is situated at the level of insulin secretion (number, sensitivity, synthesis and secretion of beta cells) but also at the level of the insulin receptor system (number and sensitivity of receptors and post-receptor mechanisms).

REFERENCES

1 Bridgman J. A morphological study of the development of the placenta of the rat: II. An histological and cytological study of the development of the chorioallantoic placenta of the white rat. *J Morphol* 1949; **83:** 195–224.
2 Robertson WB, Brosens I, Dixon G. Uteroplacental vascular pathology. *Eur J Obstet Gynaecol Reprod Biol* 1975; **5:** 47–65.
3 Devaskar SU, Mueckler MM. The mammalian glucose transporters. *Pediatr Res* 1992; **31:** 1–13.
4 Takata K, Kasahara T, Kasahara M *et al.* Immunolocalization of glucose transporters GLUT$_1$ in the rat placental barrier: possible role of GLUT$_1$ and the gap junction in the transport of glucose across the placental barrier. *Cell Tissue Res* 1994; **276:** 411–18.
5 Hauguel-De Mouzon S, Boileau P, Girard J. Structural localization and regulation of glucose transporter expression in placentae of diabetic rats. *Diabetes* 1994; **43:** 135A.
6 Zhou J, Bondy CA. Placental glucose transporter gene expression and metabolism in the rat. *J Clin Invest* 1993; **91:** 845–52.
7 Arnott G, Coghill G, McArdle HJ, Hundal HS. Immunolocalization of GLUT$_1$ and GLUT$_3$ glucose transporters in human placenta. *Biochem Soc Trans* 1994; **22:** 272S.
8 Challier JC, Hauguel S, Desmaizieres V. Effect of insulin on glucose uptake and metabolism in the human placenta. *J Clin Endocrinol Metab* 1986; **62:** 803–7.
9 Hauguel S, Desmaizieres V, Challier JC. Glucose uptake, utilization, and transfer by the human placenta as functions of maternal glucose concentration. *Pediatr Res* 1986; **20:** 269–73.
10 Vasilenko P. Diabetic alterations of uterine and placental function. In: Shafrir E (ed.), *Frontiers in Diabetes Research. Lessons from Animal Diabetes III* 1990; **XI.4:** 538–44.
11 Emmrich P, Birke R, Gödel E. Beitrag zur Morphologie der myometrialen und dezidualen Arterien bie normalen Schwangerschaften, EPH-Gestosen und mütterlichem Diabetes mellitus. *Pathol Microbiol* 1975; **43:** 38–61.
12 Björk O, Persson B, Stangenberg M, Vaclavinkova V. Spiral artery lesions in relation to metabolic control in diabetes mellitus. *Acta Obstet Gynecol Scand* 1984; **63:** 123–7.
13 Pinkerton JMH. The placental bed arterioles in diabetes. *Proc R Soc Med* 1963; **56:** 1021–2.
14 Khong TY. Acute atherosis in pregnancies complicated by hypertension, small-for-gestational-age infants, and diabetes mellitus. *Arch Pathol Lab Med* 1991; **115:** 722–5.
15 Salvesen DR, Higueras MT, Mansur CA *et al.* Placental and fetal Doppler velocimetry in pregnancies complicated by maternal diabetes mellitus. *Am J Obstet Gynecol* 1993; **168:** 645–52.

92   *Diabetes and Pregnancy*

16 Zimmermann P, Kujansuu E, Tuimala R. Doppler flow velocimetry of the uterine and uteroplacental circulation in pregnancies complicated by insulin-dependent diabetes mellitus. *J Perin Med* 1994; **22:** 137–47.
17 Abramovici A, Sporn J, Prager K *et al.* Glycogen metabolism in the placenta of streptozotocin diabetic rats. *Horm Metab Res* 1978; **10:** 195–9.
18 Diamant YZ, Shafrir E. Placental enzymes of glycolysis, glucogenesis and lipogenesis in the diabetic rat and in starvation: comparison with maternal and fetal liver. *Diabetologia* 1979; **15:** 481–5.
19 Gewolb IH, Barret G, Warshaw IB. Placental growth and glycogen metabolism in streptozotocin diabetic rats. *Pediatr Res* 1983; **17:** 587–91.
20 Aerts L, Holemans K, Van Assche FA. Impaired insulin response and action in offspring of severely diabetic rats. In: Shafrir E (eds.), *Frontiers in Diabetes Research. Lessons from Animal Diabetes III.* 1990; **XI.8:** 561–6.
21 Davies J, Glasser SR. Histological and fine structural observations on the placenta of the rat. *Acta Anat* 1968; **69:** 542–608.
22 Prager R, Abramavici A, Liban E, Laron Z. Histopathological changes in the placenta of stretozotocin induced diabetes rats. *Diabetologia* 1974; **10:** 89–91.
23 Shafrir E, Barash V. Placental glycogen metabolism in diabetic pregnancy. *Isr J Med Sci* 1991; **73:** 888–893.
24 Desoye G, Hofmann HH, Weiss PA. Insulin binding to trophoblast plasma membranes and placental glycogen content in well-controlled gestational diabetic women treated with diet or insulin, in well-controlled overt diabetic patients and in healthy control subjects. *Diabetologia* 1992; **35:** 45–55.
25 Schmon B, Hartmann M, Jones CJ, Desoye G. Insulin and glucose do not affect the glycogen content in isolated and cultured trophoblast cells of human term placenta. *J Clin Endocrinol Metab* 1991; **73:** 888–93.
26 Fox H. *Pathology of the Placenta.* Saunders, London, 1978; 223–30.
27 Teasdale F, Jean-Jacques G. Morphometry of the microvillous membrane of the human placenta in maternal diabetes mellitus. *Placenta* 1986; **7:** 81–8.
28 Boyd PA, Scott A, Keeling JW. Quantitative structural studies on placentas from pregnancies complicated by diabetes mellitus. *Br J Obstet Gynaecol* 1986; **63:** 123–7.
29 Mayhew TM, Sorensen FB, Klebe JG, Jackson MR. Growth and maturation in villi in placentae from well-controlled diabetic women. *Placenta* 1994; **15:** 57–65.
30 Rosso P, Kava R. Effect of food restriction on cardiac output and blood flow to the uterus and placenta in the pregnant rat. *J Nutr* 1980; **110:** 2350–4.
31 Koshy TS, Sara VR, King TL, Lazarus L. The influence of protein restriction imposed at various stages of pregnancy on fetal and placental development. *Growth* 1975; **39:** 497–506.
32 Rosso P. Placental growth, development, and function in relation to maternal nutrition. *Fed Proc* 1980; **39:** 250–4.
33 Lechtig A, Yarbrough C, Delgado H *et al.* Effect of moderate maternal malnutrition on placenta. *Am J Obstet Gynecol* 1975; **123:** 191–201.
34 Mukherjee NK, Mitra NK. The effect of malnutrition on placenta. *Indian J Pathol Microbiol* 1990; **33:** 314–22.
35 Fowden AL. The role of insulin in fetal growth. *Early Hum Dev* 1992; **29:** 177–81.
36 Pictet R, Rutter W. Development of the endocrine pancreas. In: Steiner DF, Freinkel N (eds), *Handbook of Physiology*, Sect 7, Vol. I. *Endocrine Pancreas.* Williams & Wilkins, Baltimore, 1972; 25–66.
37 Pang K, Mukonoweshuro C, Wang GG. Beta cells arise from glucose transporter type 2 (GLUT$_2$)-expressing epithelial cells of the developing rat pancreas. *Proc Natl Acad Sci USA* 1994; **91:** 9559–63.
38 Finegood DT, Seaphia L, Bonner-Weis S. Dynamics of β-cell mass in the growing rat pancreas: estimation with a simple mathematical model. *Diabetes* 1995; **44:** 249–56.
39 Aerts L, Van Assche FA. Rat fetal endocrine pancreas in experimental diabetes. *J Endocrinol* 1977; **73:** 339–46.
40 Perrier-Barta H. A morphometric study of the secretory process in the endocrine pancreas of the fetal rat. *Cell Tissue Res* 1983; **229:** 651–71.

41 Sodoyez-Goffaux F, Sodoyez JC, De Vos CJ, Foá PP. Insulin and glucagon secretion by islets isolated from fetal and neonatal rats. *Diabetologia* 1979; **16:** 121–3.

42 Kervran A, Randon J, Girard J. Dynamics of glucose-induced plasma insulin increase in the rat fetus at different stages of gestation. *Biol Neonate* 1979; **35:** 242–8.

43 Hole RL, Pian-Smith MCM, Sharp GWG. Development of the biphase response to glucose in fetal and neonatal rat pancreas. *Am J Physiol* 1988; 254 (*Endorcrinol Metab* 17): E167–74.

44 Otonski T. Insulin and glucagon secretory responses to arginine, glucogen, and theophylline during perifusion of human islet-like cell clusters. *J Clin Endocrinol Metab* 1988; **67:** 734–40.

45 Grasso S, Messina A, Saporito N, Reitano Y. Serum insulin response to glucose and amino-acids in the premature infant. *Lancet* 1968; **ii:** 755–6.

46 Hughes SJ. The role of reduced glucose transporter content and glucose metabolism in the immature secretory response of fetal rat pancreatic islets. *Diabetologia* 1994; **37:** 134–40.

47 Mally MI, Otonski T, Lopez AD, Hayek A. Developmental gene expression in the human fetal pancreas. *Pediatr Res* 1994; **36:** 537–44.

48 Sodoyez-Goffaux F, Sodoyez JC, De Vos CJ. Maturation of liver handling of insulin in the rat fetus. *Diabetes* 1982; **31:** 60–9.

49 Sodoyez-Goffaux F, Sodoyez JC, De Vos CJ. Insulin receptors in the gastro-intestinal tract of the rat fetus: quantitative autoradiographic studies. *Diabetologia* 1985; **28:** 45–50.

50 Leturque A, Postic C, Ferré P, Girard J. Nutritional regulation of glucose transporter in muscle and adipose tissue of weaned rats. *Am J Physiol* 1991; **260:** E588–93.

51 Walker DC, Saton SW. Regulation of development of hepatic glucokinase in the neonatal rat by the diet. *Biochem J* 1967; **105:** 771–7.

52 Wang C, Hu SM. Developmental regulation in the expression of rat heart glucose transporters. *Biochem Biophys Res Commun* 1991; **177:** 1095–1100.

53 Santalucia T, Camps M, Castello A. *et al.* Developmental regulation of $GLUT_1$ and $GLUT_4$ glucose transporter expression in rat heart, skeletal muscle and brown adipose tissue. *Endocrinology* 1992; **130:** 837–46.

54 Kervran A, Guillaume A, Jost A. The endocrine pancreas of the fetus from diabetic pregnant rat. *Diabetologia* 1978; **15:** 387–99.

55 Bihoreau MT, Ktorza A, Kervran A, Picon L. Effect of gestational hyperglycemia on insulin secretion in vivo and in vitro by fetal rat pancreas. *Am J Physiol* 1986; **251:** (*Endocrinol Metab* 14): E86–91.

56 de Mazancourt P, Carneiro EM, Atroater I, Bosehero AC. Prolactin treatment increases $GLUT_2$ but not the G protein subunit content in cell membranes from cultured neonatal rat islets. *FEBS Lett* 1994; **343:** 137–40.

57 Stevens D, Alexander G, Bell AW. Effect of prolonged glucose infusion into fetal sheep on body growth, fat deposition and gestational length. *J Dev Physiol* 1990; **13:** 277–81.

58 Dubreuil G, Anderodias J. Ilöts de Langerhans géants chez un nouveauné issue de mère glucosurique. *CR Sesanc Soc Biol Paris* 1920; **24:** 1940–1; also in Steiner DF, Freinkel N. (eds), Williams and Wilkins, Baltimore, 1972; 25–66.

59 Miller HC. Effect of diabetic and prediabetic pregnancy on fetuses and newborn infants. *Pediatrics* 1946; **19:** 445–52.

60 Cardell BS. Hypertrophy and hyperplasia of the pancreatic islets in newborn infants. *J Pathol Bacteriol* 1953; **66:** 335–46.

61 Jackson WPU, Woolf N. Maternal prediabetes as a cause of unexplained stillbirth. *Diabetes* 1958; **7:** 446–54.

62 D'Agostino AN, Bahn RC. A histopathology study of the pancreas of infants of diabetic mothers. *Diabetes* 1963; **121:** 327–31.

63 Naeye RL. Infants of diabetic mothers: quantitative morphologic study. *Paediatrics* 1965; **35:** 980–9.

64 Van Assche FA. A morphological study of Langerhans islets of the fetal pancreas in late pregnancy. *Biol Neonate* 1968; **12:** 331–42.

65 Van Assche FA, Gepts W, Aerts L. The fetal endocrine pancreas in diabetes (human). *Diabetologia* 1976; **12:** 423.

66 Hultquist GT, Olding L. Pancreatic islet fibrosis in young infants of diabetic mothers. *Lancet* 1975; **ii:** 1015–16.

67 de Gasparo M, Hoet JJ. Normal and abnormal fetal weight gain. In: Rodriguez RR, Valence J (eds), *Diabetes Mellitus: Proceedings of the Seventh Congress of the IDF 1971*. Excerpta Medica, Amsterdam, 1971; 667–676.

68 Vejtorp M, Pedersen J, Klebbe JC, Lund E. Low concentrations of plasma amino-acids in newborn babies of diabetic mothers. *Acta Paedriatr Scand* 1977; **66:** 53–8.

69 Neufeld ND, Corbo LM, Kaplan SA. Plasma membrane insulin receptors in fetal rabbit lung. *Pediatr Res* 1981; **15:** 1058–62.

70 Neufeld ND, Corbo L. Increased fetal insulin receptors and changes in membrane fluidity and lipid composition. *Am J Physiol* 1982; **243:** E246–50.

71 Neufeld ND, Kaplan SA, Lippe BM, Scott M. Increased monocyte receptor binding of ^{125}I-insulin in infants of gestational diabetic mothers. *J Clin Endocrinol Metab* 1978; **47:** 590–5.

72 Pederson O, Beck-Nielsen H, Klebe JG. Insulin receptors in the pregnant diabetic and her newborn. *J Clin Endocrinol Metab* 1981; **53:** 1160–6.

73 Leturque A, Revelli JP, Hauguel S. *et al*. Hyperglycemia and hyperinsulinemia increase glucose utilization in fetal rat tissues. *Am J Physiol* 1987; **253:** E616–20.

74 Aerts L, Holemans K, Van Assche FA. Maternal diabetes during pregnancy: consequences for the offspring. *Diabetes Metab Rev* 1990; **6:** 147–67.

75 Freinkel N. Of pregnancy and progeny. *Diabetes* 1980; **29:** 1023–35.

76 Aerts L, Van Bree R, Feytons V *et al*. Plasma amino-acids in diabetic pregnant rats and in their fetal and adult offspring. *Biol Neonate* 1989; **56:** 31–9.

77 Philipps AF, Dubin JW, Raye JR. Effect of endogenous insulin release on fetal alanine concentration and uptake. *Am J Obstet Gynecol* 1981; **139:** 22–32.

78 Philipps AF, Rosenkrantz TS, Raye JR. Consequences of perturbations of fetal fuels in ovine pregnancy. *Diabetes* 1985; **34:** 32–5.

79 Philipps AF, Rosenkrantz TS, Lemons JA *et al*. Insulin-induced alterations in amino-acid metabolism in the fetal lamb. *J Physiol* 1990; **13:** 251–9.

80 Hay Jr WW, Meznarich HK, Sparks JW *et al*. Effect of insulin on glucose uptake in near-term fetal lambs. *Proc Soc Exp Biol Med* 1985; **178:** 557–64.

81 Hay Jr WW, Meznarick HK. The effect of hyperinsulinemia on glucose utilization and oxidation and on oxygen consumption in the fetal lamb. *Q J Exp Physiol* 1986; **71:** 689–98.

82 Susa JB, Schwartz R. Effects of hyperinsulinemia in the primate fetus. *Diabetes* 1985; **34:** 36–41.

83 Bossard P, Parsa D, Decaux JF *et al*. Glucose administration induces the premature expression of liver glucokinase gene in newborn rats. *Eur J Biochem* 1993; **215:** 883–92.

84 Van Assche FA, Aerts L, De Prins F. Degranulation of the insulin-producing beta cells in an infant of a diabetic mother: case report. *Br J Obstet Gynaecol* 1983; **90:** 182–5.

85 Mulay S, Philip A, Salomon S. Influence of maternal diabetes on fetal rat development: alteration of insulin receptors in fetal liver and lung. *J Endocrinol* 1983; **98:** 401–10.

86 Philipps AF, Rozenkrantz TS, Grunnet ML *et al*. Effect of fetal insulin secretory deficiency on metabolism in fetal lamb. *Diabetes* 1986; **35:** 964–72.

87 Philipps AF, Rosenkrantz TS, Clark RM *et al*. Effects of fetal insulin deficiency on growth and development in fetal lambs. *Diabetes* 1991; **40:** 20–7.

88 Canavan JP, Goldspink DF. Maternal diabetes in rats II. Effects on fetal growth and protein turnover. *Diabetes* 1988; **37:** 1671–7.

89 Snoeck A, Remache C, Reusens B, Heet JJ. Effect on low-protein diet during pregnancy on the fetal rat endocrine pancreas. *Biol Neonate* 1990; **57:** 107–18.

90 Dahri S, Snoeck A, Reusens-Billen B *et al*. Islet function in offspring of mothers on low-protein diet during gestation. *Diabetes* 1991; **40:** 115–20.

91 Holemans K, Verhaeghe J, Dequeker J, Van Assche FA. Insulin sensitivity in adult female rats subjected to malnutrition during perinatal period. *J Soc Gynecol Invest* 1995; **3:** 71–7.

92 Dalinghaus M, Rudolph CD, Rudolph AM. Effects of maternal fasting on hepatic gluconeogenesis and glucose metabolism in fetal lambs. *J Dev Physiol* 1991; **16:** 267–75.

93 Leturque A, Hauguel S, Revelli J-P *et al*. Fetal glucose utilization in response to maternal starvation and acute hyperketonemia. *Am J Physiol* 1989; **256:** E699–703.

94 Liechty EA, Lemons JA. Changes in ovine fetal hindlimb amino acid metabolism during maternal fasting. *Am J Physiol* 1984; **246:** E430–5.

95 Fowden AL. The role of insulin in prenatal growth. *J Dev Physiol* 1989; **12:** 173–82.

96 Simmons RA, Gounis AS, Bangalore SA, Ogata ES. Intrauterine growth retardation: fetal glucose transport is dimished in lung but spared in brain. *Pediatr Res* 1992; **31:** 59–63.

97 Girard J, Ferré P, Gilbert M *et al.* Fetal metabolic response to maternal fasting in the rat. *Am J Physiol* 1977; **232:** E456–63.

98 Lemons JA, Moorehead HC, Hage GP. Effects of fasting on gluconeogenic enzymes in the ovine fetus. *Pediatr Res* 1986; **20:** 676–9.

99 Han VKM, D'Ercole AJ, Lund PK. Cellular localization of somatomedin (insulin-like growth factor) messenger RNA in the human fetus. *Science* 1987; **236:** 193–7.

100 Han VKM, Hill DJ, Strain AJ *et al.* Identification of somatomedin/insulin-like growth factor immunoreactive cells in the human fetus. *Pediatr Res* 1987; **22:** 245–9.

101 Han VKM, Lund PK, Lee DC, D'Ercole AJ. Expression of somatomedin/insulin-like growth factor messenger ribonucleic acids in the human fetus: identification, characterization, and tissue distribution. *J Clin Endocrinol Metab* 1988; **66:** 422–9.

102 Hill DJ. Relative abundance and molecular size of immunoreactive insulin-like growth factors I and II in human fetal tissues. *Early Hum Dev* 1990; **21:** 49–58.

103 Verhaeghe J, Van Bree R, Van Herck E *et al.* C-peptide, insulin-like growth factors I and II, and insulin-like growth factor binding protein-1 in umbilical cord serum: correlations with birth weight. *Am J Obstet Gynecol* 1993; **169:** 89–97.

104 Moses AC, Nissley SP, Short PA *et al.* Increased levels of multiplication-stimulating activity, an insulin-like growth factor, in fetal rat serum. *Proc Natl Acad Sci USA* 1980; **77:** 3649–53.

105 Bennett A, Wilson DM, Liu F *et al.* Levels of insulin-like growth factors I and II in human cord blood. *J Clin Endocrinol Metab* 1983; **57:** 609–12.

106 Gluckman PD, Johnson-Barrett JJ, Butler JH *et al.* Studies of insulin-like growth factor-I and -II by specific radioligand assays in umbilical cord blood. *Clin Endocrinol* 1983; **19:** 415–13.

107 Liu JP, Baker J, Perkins AS *et al.* Mice carrying null mutations of the genes encoding insulin-like growth factor I and type 1 IGF receptor. *Cell* 1993; **75:** 59–72.

108 Lassarre C, Hardouin S, Daffos F *et al.* Serum insulin-like growth factors and insulin-like growth factor binding proteins in the human fetus: relationships with growth in normal subjects and in subjects with intrauterine growth retardation. *Pediatr Res* 1991; **29:** 219–25.

109 Giudice LC, de Zegher F, Gargosky SE *et al.* Insulin-like growth factors and their binding protein in the term and preterm human fetus and neonate with normal and extremes of intrauterine growth. *J Clin Endocrinol Metab* 1995; **80:** 1548–55.

110 Vileisis RA, D'Ercole AJ. Tissue and serum concentrations of somatomedin-C/insulin-like growth factor I in fetal rats made growth retarded by uterine artery ligation. *Pediatr Res* 1986; **20:** 126–30.

111 Davenport ML, D'Ercole AJ, Underwood LE. Effect of maternal fasting on fetal growth, serum insulin-like growth factors, and tissue IGF messenger ribonucleic acids. *Endocrinology* 1990; **126:** 2062–7.

112 Straus DS, Ooi GT, Orlowski CC, Rechler MM. Expression of the genes for insulin-like growth factor-I, IGF-II, and IGF-binding proteins-1 and -2 in fetal rat under conditions of intrauterine growth retardation caused by maternal fasting. *Endocrinology* 1991; **128:** 518–25.

113 Bernstein IM, DeSouza MM, Copeland KC. Insulin-like growth factor I in substrate-deprived, growth-retarded fetal rats. *Pediatr Res* 1991; **30:** 154–7.

114 Price WA, Rong L, Stiles AD, D'Ercole AJ. Changes in IGF-I and -II IGF binding protein, and IGF receptor transcript abundance after uterine artery ligation. *Pediatr Res* 1992; **32:** 291–5.

115 Harding JE, Liu L, Evans PC, Gluckman PD. Insulin-like growth factor I alters feto-placental protein and carbohydrate metabolism in fetal sheep. *Endocrinology* 1994; **134:** 1509–14.

116 Ashton IK, Zapf J, Einschenk I, MacKenzie IZ. Insulin-like growth factors 1 and 2 in human foetal plasma and relationship to gestational age and foetal size during midpregnancy. *Acta Endocrinol* 1985; **110:** 558–63.

117 Iwamoto HS, Murray MA, Chernausek SD. Effects of acute hypoxemia on insulin-like growth factors and their binding proteins in fetal sheep. *Am J Physiol* 1992; **263:** E1151–6.

118 Oliver MH, Harding JE, Breier BH *et al.* Glucose but not a mixed amino acid infusion regulates plasma insulin-like growth factor-I concentrations in fetal sheep. *Pediatr Res* 1993; **34:** 62–5.

119 Ooi GT, Orlowski CC, Brown AL *et al.* Different tissue distribution and hormonal regulation of messenger RNAs encoding rat insulin-like growth factor-binding proteins-1 and -2. *Mol Endocrinol* 1990; **4:** 321–8.

120 Schuller AGP, Zwarthoff EC, Drop SLS. Gene expression of the six insulin-like growth factor binding proteins in the mouse conceptus during mid- and late gestation. *Endocrinology* 1993; **132:** 2544–50.

121 Hill DJ, Clemmons DR, Wilson S *et al.* Immunological distribution of one form of insulin-like growth factor-binding protein and IGF peptides in human fetal tissues. *J Mol Endocrinol* 1989; **2:** 31–8.

122 Bernardini S, Spadoni GL, Póvoa G *et al.* Plasma levels of insulin-like growth factor binding protein-1 and growth hormome binding protein activity from birth to the third month of life. *Acta Endocrinol* 1992; **127:** 313–18.

123 Wang HS, Lim J, English J *et al.* The concentration of insulin-like growth factor-I and insulin-like growth factor-binding protein-1 in human umbilical cord serum at delivery: relation to fetal weight. *J Endocrinol* 1991; **129:** 459–64.

124 Unterman T, Lascon R, Gotway MB *et al.* Circulating levels of insulin-like growth factor binding protein-1 and hepatic mRNA are increased in the small for gestational age fetal rat. *Endocrinology* 1990; **127:** 2035–7.

125 Gallaher BW, Breier BH, Oliver MH *et al.* Ontogenic differences in the nutritional regulation of circulating IGF binding proteins in sheep plasma. *Acta Endocrinol* 1992; **126:** 49–54.

126 McLellan KC, Hooper SB, Bocking AD *et al.* Prolonged hypoxia induced by the reduction of maternal uterine blood flow alters insulin-like growth factor-binding protein-1 and IGFBP-2 gene expression in the ovine fetus. *Endocrinology* 1992; **131:** 1619–28.

127 Osborn BH, Fowlkes J, Han VKM, Freemark M. Nutritional regulation of insulin-like growth factor-binding protein gene expression in the ovine fetus and pregnant ewe. *Endocrinology* 1992; **131:** 1743–50.

128 Hakala-Ala-Pietilä TH, Koistinen RA, Salonen RK, Seppälä MT. Elevated second-trimester amniotic fluid concentration of insulin-like growth factor-binding protein-1 in fetal growth retardation. *Am J Obstet Gynecol* 1993; **169:** 35–9.

129 Taylor AM, Dunger DB, Preece MA. The growth hormone independent insulin-like growth factor-I binding protein BP-28 is associated with serum insulin-like growth factor-I inhibitory bioactivity in adolescent insulin-dependent diabetics. *Clin Endocrinol* 1990; **32:** 229–39.

130 Tató L, Dal Moro A, Piemonte G *et al.* A longitudinal study on plasma somatomedin activity in full-term, preterm and small-for-gestational age newborns. *Biol Neonate* 1981; **39:** 160–4.

131 Hills FA, Crawford R, Harding S *et al.* The effects of labor on maternal and fetal levels of insulin-like growth factor binding protein-1. *Am J Obstet Gynecol* 1994; **171:** 1292–5.

132 Crawford RAF, Hills FA, Farkas A, Chard T. Elevated levels of insulin-like growth factor binding protein-1 in fetal distress. *Br J Obstet Gynaecol* 1995; **102:** 538–40.

133 Crystal RA, Giudice LC. Insulin-like growth factor binding protein profiles in human fetal cord sera: ontogeny during gestation and differences in newborns with intrauterine growth retardation and large for gestational age newborns. In: Spencer EM (ed.), *Modern Concepts for Insulin-like Growth Factors.* Elsevier, New York, 1991; 395–408.

134 Tapanainen PJ, Bang P, Wilson K *et al.* Maternal hypoxia as a model for intrauterine growth retardation: effects on insulin-like growth factors and their binding proteins. *Pediatr Res* 1994; **36:** 152–8.

135 Bang P, Westgren M, Schwander J *et al.* Ontogeny of insulin-like growth factor-binding protein-1, -2 and -3: quantitative measurements by radioimmunoassay in human fetal serum. *Pediatr Res* 1994; **36:** 528–36.

136 Baker J, Liu JP, Robertson EJ, Efstratiadis A. Role of insulin-like growth factors in embryonic and postnatal growth. *Cell* 1993; **75:** 73–82.

137 Bhaumick B, Danilkewich AD, Bala RM. Insulin-like growth factors I and II in diabetic

pregnancy: suppression of normal pregnancy-induced rise of IGF-I. *Diabetologia* 1986; **29:** 792–7.

138 Delmis J, Drazanzic A, Ivanisevic M, Suchanek E. Glucose, insulin HGH and IGF-I levels in maternal serum, amniotic fluid and umbilical venous serum: a comparison with late normal pregnancy and pregnancies complicated with diabetes and fetal growth retardation. *J Perinat Med* 1992; **20:** 47–56.

139 Simmons D. Interrelation between umbilical cord serum sex hormones, sex hormone-binding globulin, insulin-like growth factor I, and insulin in neonates from normal pregnancies and pregnancies complicated by diabetes. *J Clin Endocrinol Metab* 1995; **80:** 2217–21.

140 Susa JB, Widness JA, Hintz R *et al.* Somatomedins and insulin in diabetic pregnancies: effects on fetal macrosomia in the human and Rhesus monkey. *J Clin Endocronol Metab* 1984; **58:** 1099–105.

141 Gluckman PD, Butler JH, Comline R, Fowden A. The effects of pancreatectomy on the plasma concentrations of insulin-like growth factors 1 and 2 in the sheep fetus. *J Dev Physiol* 1987; **9:** 79–88.

142 Pao C-I, Farmer PK, Begovic S *et al.* Expression of hepatic insulin-like growth factor-I and insulin-like growth factor-binding protein-1 genes is transcriptionally regulated in steptozotocin-diabetic rats. *Mol Endocrinol* 1992; **6:** 969–77.

143 Hall K, Hansson U, Lundin G *et al.* Serum levels of somatomedin and somatomedin-binding protein in pregnant women with type I or gestational diabetes and their infants. *J Clin Endocrinol Metab* 1986; **63:** 1300–6.

144 Suikkari AM, Koivisto VA, Rutanen EM *et al.* Insulin regulates the serum levels of low molecular weight insulin-like growth factor-binding protein. *J Clin Endocrinol Metab* 1988; **66:** 266–72.

145 Aerts L, Van Assche FA. Endocrine pancreas in the offspring of rats with experimentally induced diabetes. *J Endocrinol* 1981; **88:** 81–8.

146 Ktorza A, Gauguier D, Bihoreau MT *et al.* Adult offspring from mildly hyperglycemic rats show impairment of glucose regulation and insulin secretion which is transmissible to the next generation. In: Shafrir E (ed.) *Frontiers of Diabetes Research. Lessons from Animal Diabetes III.* Smith-Gordon, London, 1990; 555–60.

147 Aerts L, Sodoyez-Goffaux F, Sodoyez JC *et al.* The diabetic intrauterine milieu has a long-lasting effect on insulin secretion by β-cells and on insulin uptake by target tissues. *Am J Obstet Gynecol* 1988; **5:** 1287–92.

148 Susa JB, Boylan JM, Seghal P, Schwartz R. Persistence of impaired insulin secretion in infant rhesus markers that had been hyperinsulinemic in utero. *J Clin Endocrinol Metab* 1992; **75:** 265–9.

149 Holemans K, Aerts L, Van Assche FA. Evidence for an insulin resistance in the adult offspring of pregnant steptozotocin-diabetic rats. *Diabetologia* 1991; **34:** 81–5.

150 Van Assche FA, Aerts L. Morphologic and ultrastructural modifications in the endocrine pancreas of pregnant rats. In: Davlos C (ed.), *Early Diabetes in Early Life.* Academic Press, New York, 1975; 333–41.

151 Holemans K, Van Bree R, Verhaeghe J *et al.* In vivo glucose utilization by individual tissues in virgin and pregnant offspring of severely diabetic rats. *Diabetes* 1993; **42:** 530–6.

152 Martin AO, Simpson JL, Ober C, Freinkel N. Frequency of diabetes mellitus in probands with gestational diabetes: possible maternal influence on the predisposition to diabetes. *Am J Obstet Gynecol* 1985; **151:** 471–3.

153 Dörner G, Plagemann A, Reinagel H. Familial diabetes aggregation in type 2 diabetics: gestational diabetes as apparent risk factor for increased diabetes susceptibility in the offspring. *Exp Clin Endocrinol* 1987; **89:** 84–90.

154 Dörner G, Steindel E, Thoelke H, Sehliak V. Evidence for decreasing prevalence of diabetes mellitus in childhood apparently produced by prevention of hyperinsulinism in the foetus and newborn. *Exp Clin Endocrinol* 1984; **84:** 134–42.

155 Pettitt DJ, Aleck KA, Baird HR *et al.* Congenital susceptibility to NIDMM. Role of intrauterine environment. *Diabetes* 1988; **37:** 622–8.

156 Phipps K, Barker DJP, Hales CN *et al.* Fetal growth and impaired glucose tolerance in men and women. *Diabetologia* 1993; **36:** 225–8.

Part II
PREGNANCY

6

Pre-pregnancy Care

JUDITH M. STEEL

Victoria Hospital, Kirkcaldy, UK

Before the discovery of insulin, when pregnancy occurred in a woman with diabetes the maternal morbidity and mortality were high and only a few babies survived. In the early days of insulin treatment there was a dramatic improvement in maternal mortality but perinatal mortality remained as high as 50%. Retrospectively, it is interesting that the poor outcome of pregnancy in those early years was one of the first indications that injections of insulin were not going to solve all the problems for people with diabetes.

A major step forward was the description by Jørgen Pedersen in Copenhagen of his simple hyperglycaemia–hyperinsulinism hypothesis. In his now famous book *The Pregnant Diabetic and her Newborn* first published in 1967 he stated: 'Maternal hyperglycaemia results in fetal hyperglycaemia and hence, in hypertrophy of fetal islet tissue with insulin hypersecretion. This again means a greater fetal utilisation of glucose. This phenomenon will explain several abnormal structures and changes found in the newborn'[1].

From this it was logical that good control would reduce many of the abnormal changes in the infants of diabetic mothers. Karlson and Kjellmer showed a direct relationship between the degree of control and the perinatal mortality[2]. Early delivery reduced the number of stillbirths, and the opening of special care baby units improved the outcome for premature babies and those with neonatal problems. Obstetric monitoring and better anaesthetics also contributed to improvements but, despite all these advances, in the 1970s the perinatal mortality in many centres remained high, often well over 10% even in specialized centres[3].

Diabetes and Pregnancy: An International Approach to Diagnosis and Management.
Edited by A. Dornhorst and D. R. Hadden.
© 1996 John Wiley & Sons Ltd

RATIONALE OF PRE-PREGNANCY CARE

In the 1970s there appeared to be three major problems all of which, it seemed, might be improved by pre-pregnancy counselling and care[4].

Problems related to patients presenting late for antenatal care

These women were often unsure of their dates, which made assessment of gestation difficult. They frequently had unplanned pregnancies, poorly controlled diabetes and tended to be poor clinic attenders.

Problems in women with long-term complications of diabetes

In 1950 Beetham had reported on the occurrence of retinopathy in a group of 200 pregnant diabetic subjects, many of whom had deteriorated during pregnancy, including 12 patients with proliferative retinopathy who experienced visual deterioration progressing to blindness[5]. As a result of this and a few other studies it was felt by some doctors that proliferative retinopathy was a contraindication to pregnancy[6]. Since then, the advent of laser therapy has meant that retinopathy is no longer a contraindication to pregnancy but it may be appropriate to treat some patients before conception[7].

Women with severe nephropathy, particularly those who were also hypertensive, were known to have very high-risk pregnancies[8]. Again, the outlook for pregnancy in these women has improved a great deal over the years but it is desirable to carry out careful assessment and optimize treatment before conception[9].

The danger of maternal death in women with severe ischaemic heart disease was recognized in the 1970s[10] and the severe autonomic neuropathy causing repeated vomiting in pregnancy was described in the 1980s[11].

The high incidence of major congenital malformations

In 1964 Mølsted-Pedersen had described a high incidence of congenital malformations in infants of diabetic mothers[12]. Kucera reviewed the world literature between 1930 and 1964; the incidence of congenital malformations in diabetic pregnancies was 4.8% compared with 1.6% in the general population[13]. Although Pedersen initially thought that macrovascular complications were important in the aetiology, he also observed that: 'The occurrence of hypoglycaemic reactions and insulin coma during the first trimester was low in mothers with malformed infants, indicating a poor compensation of the diabetes at that time'.[14]

Our pre-pregnancy clinic in Edinburgh was started in 1976 when it seemed likely that good control in early pregnancy might reduce the incidence of major malformations. Over the next few years there were many more reports of the increased incidence of abnormalities, from 4% to 11%, and showing that they tended often to be severe, multiple and fatal[15-17]. Mills *et al.* showed that the abnormalities tended to be cardiac, neural tube and skeletal and that varieties of the caudal regression syndrome were particularly related to maternal diabetes (Table 6.1). They also pointed out that these abnormalities occur by the eighth week of pregnancy (six weeks post conception; Table 6.2)[18].

Table 6.1. Congenital malformations in infants of diabetic mothers

Anomaly	Ratios of incidence
Causal regression	252
Situs inversus	84
Renal anomalies	
Ureter duplex	23
Agenesis	6
Cystic kidney	4
Cardiac anomalies	4
Anencephaly	3
Spina bifida hydrocephalus	2

Adapted from Mills *et al.*[18].

Table 6.2. Timing of congenital malformations

Weeks		
0	←	Ovulation
1		
2		
3	←	Caudal regression
4	←	Spina bifida, anencephalys
5	←	Transposition, renal abnormalities
6	←	Ventricular septal defect, anal atresia

In 1978 Deuchar's work on rats suggested that hyperglycaemia in early pregnancy was associated with a high rate of abnormal development in the fetus[19]. Baker *et al.*[20] demonstrated subsequently that congenital abnormalities in rats could be prevented by meticulous control during the early stages of pregnancy, while others working on rat embryos showed that incubation with increasing concentrations of glucose raised the frequency of developmental abnormalities[21]. Glucose is not the only factor; somatostatin and β-hydroxybutyrate act additively with glucose. The precise mechanisms by which hyperglycaemia leads to abnormal development are incompletely understood. However, one possible mechanism suggested for rats is that glucose competitively inhibits the cellular uptake of *myo*-inositol. This is supported by the observation that some yolk sac abnormalities in rats can be prevented by adding arachidonic acid to the culture media. A great deal of laboratory animal work has been done and is continuing to be done.

Measurement of haemoglobin A_1 (glycated haemoglobin, HbA_1) provides an integrated retrospective index of blood glucose control over the preceding six to eight weeks and makes it possible to look at control in early human diabetic pregnancy. Leslie *et al.*[22] at King's College London in 1978 observed that three of five women with markedly elevated HbA_1 levels in the first trimester delivered infants with malformations; none occurred in 20 infants of mothers with lower HbA_1 values. Miller *et al.*[23], working at the Joslin Clinic in Boston, published a much larger series in 1981 of 116 insulin-dependent diabetic women who had had HbA_1 levels measured in the first trimester. The frequency of major malformations was 22% in infants of 58 mothers with markedly elevated HbA_1 levels (>1.7 times the median for the non-diabetic population) compared with 3% in infants of 58 mothers with lower HbA_1 values. Ylinen *et al.*[24] reached a similar conclusion in 1984 when they found that the malformation rate ranged from 4.8% to 35.2%, respectively, in groups with the best and worst control. These observations have been confirmed by several other groups[25-27]. The title of the paper by the US National Institute of Child Health and Human Development appears to throw some doubt on the subject, but the study itself supports the view that hyperglycaemia in early pregnancy is associated with a high incidence of malformations[28,29]. There may be a graded risk but a large study by Greene *et al.*[30] suggests a threshold effect. They showed an extremely high risk of both spontaneous abortions and major congenital malformations in women whose HbA_1 was greater than 12 standard deviations above the mean and stated that there may be a broad range of 'acceptable' diabetic control.

PURPOSES OF A PRE-PREGNANCY CLINIC

If pregnancies are to be planned contraceptive advice is essential. This must be addressed well before the stage of planning a pregnancy. Pregnancy and diabetes, family planning and the importance of pre-conception care should be discussed with all women with diabetes of childbearing age. This is sometimes called pre-pre-pregnancy care.

When a patient declares that she is planning a pregnancy the following objectives should be addressed:

1. Assess the patient's suitability for pregnancy, relative to the complications of diabetes.
2. Obtain maximum co-operation from the patient and her partner, stressing the reasons for and the importance of good control, teaching

them to achieve it and explaining the pregnancy programme.
3. Obtain optimal diabetic control at the time of conception.
4. Identify any gynaecological abnormality.
5. Avoid infection with rubella.
6. Advise against and treat obesity.
7. Check thyroid function.
8. Provide folic acid supplementation in early pregnancy.
9. Discuss the inheritance of diabetes.
10. Identify the time of conception, by asking the women to note the dates of her menstrual periods. Possibly also identify the time of ovulation using a suitable kit. Do an early pregnancy test and ensure the patient comes early for an ultrasound scan.
11. Identify and treat infertility as early as possible.

These objectives have changed very little since their original description[4].

PRACTICE OF PRE-PREGNANCY CLINICS

THE EDINBURGH CLINIC

The author ran a pre-pregnancy clinic in a teaching hospital in Edinburgh between 1976 and 1993 and is now running a similar clinic in a district general hospital in Kirkcaldy.

In Edinburgh all women with insulin-dependent diabetes attend a hospital clinic as there is no private practice in diabetes. There is therefore a complete cohort of women to target. Initially, all were invited to come to the clinic; posters were put up in the Department of Diabetes, articles about it were included in the clinic newsletter and colleagues were asked to refer patients. After the first few years, diabetes nurse specialists mentioned pregnancy, contraception and the pre-pregnancy clinic to all women of childbearing age attending the clinic or seen at home. As a physician working for 24 years in the same department, in a children's clinic, an adolescent clinic and in several general diabetic clinics, the author already knew a large proportion of the patients, so it was fairly easy to get to know them all. The couples were seen by special appointment at a time suitable both to the author and the couple, and were usually also seen by one obstetrician with a special interest in pregnancy and diabetes. The clinic was run on an outpatient basis; only very rarely was a women admitted to hospital to improve control.

At the first visit a full medical, obstetric and gynaecological history, including a full history of current medications, was taken. Complications of diabetes were assessed by examining fundi, blood pressure and renal function and, in women with long-standing diabetes, autonomic function tests and electrocardiography were carried out. Retinopathy was treated before conception, if this was indicated, and hypertension was treated if necessary. Many young diabetic patients are being treated with angiotensin converting enzyme (ACE) inhibitors in order to protect their kidneys from serious vascular disease. These agents are not safe during pregnancy and women should change to a more appropriate drug before conception[31].

Diabetic control was assessed by home blood glucose monitoring four times daily (before breakfast, before lunch, before the evening meal and before the late night snack)[1] and by measuring HbA_1. Over the years an increasing proportion of patients were on multiple injection regimes, given short-acting insulin using a pen device, before each meal with a long- or intermediate-acting insulin before bed. On the grounds that the degree of control is more important than the way in which it is achieved, patients well controlled on short and intermediate insulin twice daily continued on that regime, sometimes given the intermediate insulin before bed. The aim was to obtain HbA_1 in the normal non-diabetic range (6–8% in the author's laboratory), but women were considered individually. Some women, particularly those with very long-standing diabetes, find it difficult to achieve a 'normal' HbA_1. The author felt that it was very important not to put too much pressure on women or to make them feel guilty, so the aim was to achieve the best possible HbA_1 without too much risk of hypoglycaemia.

Dietary advice was provided by an experienced dietitian, emphasizing accuracy in carbohydrate intake and adequacy in the essential nutrients needed during pregnancy. Overweight women were encouraged to lose weight before conception. Recently folic acid supplements have been advised, following the British government guidelines, which recommend 400 μg folic acid over the period of conception until the 12th week of pregnancy[32].

Partners, and sometimes other relatives and friends, were taught how to recognize and treat hypoglycaemia, including the use of subcutaneous glucagon. The importance of testing for urinary ketones and the dangers of ketoacidosis to a fetus were stressed. All women were instructed to test their urine for ketones if their blood glucose was high, if they were ill for any reason and particularly if vomiting. They were instructed to report high ketones immediately, as ketoacidosis is a preventable condition. They were all given the appropriate hospital or home telephone contact number, so they could obtain advice at any time of day or night.

Rubella antibodies and thyroid function were checked and women were strongly advised against smoking if this was relevant. The inheritance of diabetes was also discussed and couples were invited to ask questions and were given written information.

All couples came for a second visit, and the programme was then individualized; some were well controlled with no complications, while others required many sessions to optimize diabetic control and treat their complications. At the appropriate time contraception was stopped. Some patients identified the time of ovulation and all were asked to send off a pregnancy test five weeks after their last menstrual period and to contact the department directly as soon as the result was positive.

OTHER PRE-PREGNANCY CLINICS

Many of those running pre-pregnancy clinics do not publish their methods or experience; but the author knows that other enthusiasts in Britain at centres in Belfast, Aberdeen, Leeds and King's College London run their clinics on similar lines[33-35]. Inevitably there are minor variations; some like to measure postprandial blood glucose levels and some occasionally use fixed-mix insulins. In some centres couples are seen in designated pre-pregnancy clinic sessions, sometimes in antenatal or gynaecology clinics and sometimes during routine diabetic clinics. In each case this choice depends on the local needs and facilities available. In all, the patients are identified by the diabetes team, who have the great advantage of already knowing them.

The first pre-pregnancy clinic to publish results demonstrating a reduction in congenital malformations was run by Fuhrmann in Karlsburg, Germany[36]. At that centre women were admitted to hospital every three months before conception and again from 16 days after their menstrual period until at least eight weeks of gestation. This length of hospitalization would not be acceptable to women in many other countries.

The objectives for pre-pregnancy care recommended by the American Diabetes Association are identical to those described earlier in this chapter[37]. As a result of differences between methods of delivering health care to women with diabetes in the USA and Britain, those organizing pre-pregnancy care use rather different methods of enrolling patients but the objectives and methods are very similar. The programmes in most American centres appear to follow the American Diabetes Association Guidelines. Kitzmiller *et al.*[38] have published details of their practice, which differs in only a few very minor ways from our own. They have about a quarter of their patients on subcutaneous insulin infusion pumps, have a counsellor–social worker as a member of their team and use basal body temperature for detecting ovulation. The organizers of the Maine Diabetes in Pregnancy Program have published their 'Guide for Preconception Care of Women with established Diabetes Mellitus' giving details of a similar nature[39]. The objectives of Goldman's clinic in Israel are identical to those originally described[40].

EXPERIENCE OF PRE-PREGNANCY CLINICS

ATTENDANCE AT PRE-PREGNANCY CLINICS

At the Edinburgh clinic, between 1976 and 1993 the author's team saw 294 couples. Twenty-six were advised against pregnancy, nine decided not to become pregnant, 39 had been investigated for infertility, 11 moved away, and five left their partners. At the end of 1993 some were pregnant and others were still trying to conceive: 196 pregnancies had progressed beyond 26 weeks.

It was 1977 before the first patients who attended the pre-pregnancy clinic actually delivered. By 1979 it was running well. From 1979 to 1993 there were a total of 277 pregnancies, 188 (68%) in women who had come through the pre-pregnancy clinic. Of the 89 patients not coming through the clinic, 36 had come already pregnant from other centres; if these patients are excluded, 78% of our patients have come through the pre-pregnancy clinic. This is a considerably higher proportion than in other centres; only 28% of Fuhrmann's patients in Karlsburg kept to his programme[36]. Goldman *et al.* compared 44 (59%) women coming through a pre-pregnancy clinic with 31 who did not[40]. Kitzmiller recruited his patients by advertising and it is, therefore, perhaps invalid to calculate the proportion of women attending, but only 84 out of their total group of 194 had attended for pre-conception care[39]. In Cousins' California Diabetes and Pregnancy Program, only 8% enrolled prior to conception[41]. In the Maine programme, of the total of 185 pregnancies, 62 (34%) occurred in women who received pre-conception counselling[39]. In Rosenn's study, 28 had attended a pre-conception clinic and 71 had enrolled after conception. Thirty-three women had dropped out of their pre-pregnancy programme[42].

All those running this type of service are very aware that, as with any form of preventive medicine, those who most need to come may be least likely to do so. In the author's experience, non-attenders were significantly younger, less likely to be married, and much more likely to smoke. They were also more likely to be primigravid and were of slightly lower social class but these differences were not significant[43]. Janz *et al.* have looked in detail at factors associated with seeking pre-conception care[44]. In a multicentre study, they compared 57 women attending for pre-conception care with 97 who had not. Pre-conception care subjects were significantly more likely to be married and employed, and to have higher education and income. They were more knowledgeable about diabetes, perceived greater benefits on pre-conception care, and received more instrumental support.

PATIENTS ADVISED AGAINST PREGNANCY

In the author's series 26 patients were advised against pregnancy; one had severe retinopathy, three had ischaemic heart disease, 11 nephropathy and hypertension and the others miscellaneous problems. The single patient advised against pregnancy on the grounds of retinopathy was seen in 1976. Since then retinopathy has not been considered a contraindication to pregnancy, but may require treatment before pregnancy. If adequate laser treatment has been given it is very rare for retinopathy to deteriorate during pregnancy and it does not appear to deteriorate after successful vitrectomy[45]. In the pre-pregnancy group 20 patients were treated before pregnancy, 15 were treated with a laser for proliferative retinopathy and four of these also had a vitrectomy. Five were treated with a laser for pre-proliferative retinopathy. Only one of these 20 patients required further laser treatment during pregnancy. There were seven other patients who required treatment during pregnancy; two of these had not attended the pre-pregnancy clinic, three were referred from other centres because of retinopathy, and one, who had only background retinopathy before pregnancy, developed pre-proliferative retinopathy during pregnancy. No patient in the whole series suffered significant loss of visual acuity during pregnancy.

Renal disease, especially in association with hypertension, used to be the commonest reason for advising against pregnancy, but the management of mothers and premature babies has improved so much that no one with renal disease has been advised against pregnancy for several years and one women had a successful pregnancy after renal transplantation.

Ischaemic heart disease has replaced renal disease as the commonest cause of death in young people with diabetes, and women with diabetes do not have the protection generally afforded by being female. Severe ischaemic heart disease is a contraindication to pregnancy because of the risk of maternal death.

CONTROL IN WOMEN RECEIVING PRE-PREGNANCY CARE

As would be expected, published series show that patients receiving pre-pregnancy care are better controlled than those not attending[38,40–42]. Each year the author compared HbA_1 levels in those coming through the pre-pregnancy clinic with those who did not. Although patients coming through the clinic were self-selected, before starting the pre-pregnancy regime they were only slightly better controlled than those not attending. Motivation towards pregnancy was not necessarily associated with good control; some pre-pregnancy clinic patients had been very poorly controlled but they tended to improve before conception and attended early for antenatal care[46–48]. Over the years the two groups (pre-pregnancy clinic patients and non-attenders) became increasingly similar, due to the marked improvement in those not coming through the clinic. It became rare to see any patient later than seven weeks gestation at the antenatal clinic and the first scan usually had to be delayed to the second or third visit. The reason for this change was the increased awareness of the importance of good control in pregnancy in those who did not actually come to the clinic because they had been told, often repeatedly, about the importance of good control in pregnancy and of attending early for antenatal care. Detailed interviewing of 50 women who were already attending the diabetic clinic but did not request an appointment at the pre-pregnancy clinic revealed that seven had not heard about the clinic, six had attended before in a previous pregnancy and did not see the need to come again and four thought that the only reason to come was to achieve good control and correctly judged themselves to be well controlled. There were six chronic defaulters who were poorly controlled and four of these had abnormal babies. It is interesting that there were only three genuinely unplanned pregnancies. There was a fairly large group of 20 women who improved their control, then stopped contraception, and came early for antenatal care. These women did not wish to declare their intention to conceive to the clinic – and in several cases not to their partner either!

This raises the question as to whether it is necessary to have formalized pre-pregnancy care at all. Gregory and Tattersall in Nottingham, UK feel that the results from their own centre are so good that no further improvement is possible[49]. They do have excellent nurses who advise all women about pregnancy and good control and so to some extent they already provide pre-pregnancy counselling. The editorial in the same issue of *The Lancet* suggested that pre-pregnancy care is a waste of time. The beneficial effect of increasing awareness of good control, improving the outlook in diabetic pregnancy, is supported by the Copenhagen group, who have shown a reduction in congenital malformations in the period 1982–1986 compared with the period 1967–1981[50]. In Sweden improved diabetic control has been associated with a fall in congenital malformations over the last two decades[51]. It is true that in an ideal world all women with diabetes would be perfectly controlled and all fully informed about pregnancy. However, we have not reached that stage yet and, as already discussed, there are reasons other than achieving good control for attending for pre-pregnancy care.

There is considerable confusion over the use of the word 'clinic'. Special visits may be arranged in different ways in different places but I prefer to continue to use the word 'clinic' rather than 'counselling' to define the specific provision for those who declare a wish to become pregnant and come through a formal system as described, which is different from that offered to all the other women attending the diabetes department who are told in passing about the importance of pregnancy. Many would agree that both these stages are important and complementary. For some, only the first stage may be necessary but those coming through the formal clinic are easier to manage and, in the case of women with complications of diabetes, those who are difficult to control, those taking medications and those with previous obstetric or gynaecological problems, special provision is essential. The fact that the programmes attract highly motivated women is a reason for targeting those less motivated, not a reason for withdrawing the service for everyone. These issues are discussed in the correspondence columns of *The Lancet*[35,52–54].

SPONTANEOUS ABORTION RATES

Several studies have shown that spontaneous abortion in women with diabetes is related to poor glycaemic control in early pregnancy. Combs *et al.*[55] showed that the risk of spontaneous abortion was 12.4% with first trimester HbA_1 >9.3% (>6 standard deviations above the mean) and 37.5% with first trimester HbA_1 >14.4% (>15 standard deviations above the mean). Mills *et al.*[30] found that, among diabetic women, those who had spontaneous abortions had higher first trimester fasting and postprandial glucose levels than women whose pregnancies continued to delivery[56].

Dicker reported a beneficial effect of pre-conception glycaemic control on the spontaneous abortion rate (8.4% in a group of 59 women with mean HbA_1 of 7.5% at the time of conception, and 28% in 10 of 35 women presenting in the first trimester with mean HbA_1 of 10.5%)[57]. Rosenn reported a spontaneous abortion rate of 7% in women attending for pre-pregnancy counselling compared with 24% in the group that did not[42].

CONGENITAL MALFORMATIONS

Fuhrmann and colleagues[36] were the first to report that improving control in early pregnancy can reduce the congenital abnormality rate. They only had two malformations in 185 insulin-dependent women attending their clinic (1.1%) compared with 31 in 473 not attending (6.6%). They made numerous blood glucose measurements, but HbA_1 was, unfortunately, not measured.

In the author's whole series, there have been 14 abnormalities in 117 pregnancies where the mother has not come through the pre-pregnancy clinic (12%), compared with three (1.5%) in 196 women who have come through the pre-pregnancy clinic. The overall incidence was 5.4% and the difference between the two groups is highly significant ($p \leq 0.0001$). Details are shown in Table 6.3. All those who did not come through the clinic but had HbA_1 measured in the first trimester were poorly controlled to the extent of frequently omitting insulin in the first trimester. However, two women who came through the clinic but had abnormal babies were fairly well controlled. This may reflect the background incidence of malformations, or it may be that blood glucose variations or other metabolites are important. One of the patients attending the clinic did become well controlled, but then, owing to family and social problems, decided to delay a pregnancy. Unfortunately she conceived as a result of failed contraception. Some investigators would have considered that she had left the pre-pregnancy group. However, the author has included all patients who attended at any time before the index pregnancy, because of a great interest in the practicalities of running a service rather than organizing a research project. Only two other patients became poorly controlled as they became discouraged by the time it took to become pregnant, but fortunately they had normal babies.

Only three of the abnormal babies died in the perinatal period, indicating that the outcome of pregnancy for women with diabetes is much worse than crude perinatal mortality figures would suggest. It is also important to

Table 6.3. Edinburgh Royal Infirmary: diabetes pregnancy clinic. Major congenital abnormalities, 1976–1993

No.	HbA$_1$ First trimester	Defect	Outcome
Non-attenders, pre-pregnancy clinic			
1	Before assay	Encephalocele	Major surgery
		Survived, retarded	
2	Too late	Anencephaly	Aborted
	Omitted insulin		
3	Too late	Sacral hypoplasia	Urinary incontinence
	Omitted insulin		
4	Too late	Microcephaly	Survived, retarded
5	13.4%	Sirenomelia	Died
		Renal agenesis	
6	11.6%	Kyphoscoliosis	Major surgery
		Deafness	Survived
7	11.4%	Monomelia	Died
		Renal agenesis	
8	13.8%	Kyphoscoliosis	Major surgery
		Deafness	Survived
9	13.7%	Single ventricle	Died
		Mitral atresia	
10	14.9%	Fallot's tetralogy	Shunt, for surgery
11	12.2%	Encephalocele	Aborted
12	Too late	Anencephaly	Aborted
	Omitted insulin		
13	12.9%	Sacral agenesis	Severely handicapped
14	11.7%	Situs inversus	For surgery
		atrial septal defect,	
		ventricular septal defect	
Attenders at pre-pregnancy clinic			
15	8.8%	Anencephaly	Aborted
16	9.5%	Transposition great	Diagnosed 6 weeks
		vessels	Died surgery 8 weeks
17	12.0%	Pulmonary atresia	IUD 14 weeks
		Left atrial isomerism	

note that if congenital abnormalities had been defined as those detected at birth, or if the patients had not been followed up, four of the abnormalities would have been missed: no. 3 was diagnosed at three years, no. 6 at six months, no. 8 at 18 months and no. 10 at six weeks.

Other investigators have found a reduced number of congenital malformations in women attending before conception (Table 6.4). The title

Table 6.4. The influence of pre-pregnancy counselling on the occurrence of major congenital malformations

Author	Pre-conception care group		No pre-conception care group	
	No.	%	No.	%
Fuhrmann et al.[36,70]	1/128	0.8	22/292	7.5
Goldman et al.[40]	0/44	0.0	3/31	9.7
Mills et al.[28]	17/347	4.9	25/279	9.0
Steel et al.[43]	2/143[a]	1.4	10/96[a]	10.4
Kitzmiller et al.[38]	1/84	1.2	12/100	10.9
Rosenn et al.[42]	0/28	0.0	1/71	1.4
Cousins et al.[41]	0/27	0.0	23/347	6.6
Drury and Doddridge[35]	1/100	1.0	10/244	4.1
Willhotte et al.[39]	1/62	1.6	8/123	6.5
Steel[71]	3/196	1.5	14/117	12.0
Total	24/1016	2.4	118/1604	7.4

[a]Figures for Steel et al.[43] were not included in the total as Steel[71] is an extension of the same experience.

of the paper by Mills *et al.* 'Lack of relation of increased malformation rates in infants of diabetic mothers to glycaemic control during organogenesis', suggests that it does not agree with all the other studies, but the study itself supports the view that hyperglycaemia in early pregnancy is associated with a high incidence of malformations[28]. Kitzmiller's group reported an abnormality rate of 1.2% in 84 women recruited before conception, compared with 12 out of 110 (10.9%) seen after conception[38]. These figures are similar to those of the Edinburgh series and probably reflect the fact that they followed a high proportion of their babies for a year.

Willhotte *et al.* had one abnormality out of 62 pregnancies in the pre-pregnancy group (1.6%) and eight out of 122 in the other group (6.5%). They also found a great difference in pregnancy outcome in the two groups; there were four neonatal deaths (6.4%) in the pre-pregnancy group and 26 (21.6%) in the other group[39].

Over the last few years work on rats has shown that rat embryos develop abnormalities if exposed to hypoglycaemia at a stage equivalent to days 32–38 in human pregnancy[58]. Looking prospectively at days 28–42 in 101 consecutive pregnancies, the author found that 48 women had symptomatic hypoglycaemia during this period, 46 had mild episodes, 16 had severe episodes (defined as requiring help from someone) and 12 required glucagon. Nevertheless, all these women had normal babies. Over the same study period six women had abnormal babies and none of them had experienced any hypoglycaemia. This lack of association between first trimester hypoglycaemia and fetal abnormality is supported by Mills *et al.*[28]

and Kitzmiller *et al.*[38], who reported similar findings. Thus, there is no evidence that hypoglycaemia in early pregnancy causes malformations in human embryos.

INFERTILITY

Women with diabetes tend to have irregular cycles; defects of the pituitary axis have been described and women with diabetes are more prone to infection including pelvic inflammatory disease. Despite this, there is very little evidence that women who have diabetes are any less fertile than women who do not[59]. In the author's series, 39 women were investigated for infertility (Table 6.5). The large number and high proportion with no identifiable cause may reflect the fact that some couples were investigated after just over a year of infertility. Long delays in conception are a problem when running a pre-pregnancy clinic[47]. The risks of pregnancy in a woman with diabetes are related to the presence of complications (and hence to the duration of diabetes). In many areas adoption is difficult and new and better methods of treating infertility are available so, time being of the essence, it is important to investigate infertility at an early stage.

Table 6.5. Infertile couples who had attended at the Edinburgh pre-conception clinic

Diagnosis	No.	Treatment	No.	Pregnancies
Anovulation	7	Ovulation induction	5	3
Blocked fallopian tubes	4	Salpingolysis	2	2
Oligospermia	6	AIH	2	1
		AID	2	2
		None	2	1
Azoospermia	2	AID	1	1
No cause found	20	GIFT	1	1
		None	19	5
Total	39			16

AIH, artificial insemination by husband; AID, artificial insemination by donor; GIFT, gamete intrafallopian transfer.

COST EFFECTIVENESS OF PRE-PREGNANCY CARE

Elixhauser *et al.* analysed the costs and savings of a hypothetical pre-conception care programme. They calculated that the 1993 costs of pre-conception plus prenatal care were $17 519 per delivery, whereas the costs of prenatal care alone were $13 843 per delivery. Taking into account maternal and neonatal adverse outcomes, the net savings of pre-conception care were $1720 per enrollee, over prenatal care only, giving a significant benefit : cost ratio of 1.86[60].

Sceffler *et al.* worked out the cost effectiveness of the California Diabetes and Pregnancy Program in 1992. They matched 90 enrollees and 90 control cases. It was found that hospital charges were about 30% less for programme participants and days in hospital were 25% less. The programme effects were larger for women who enrolled before eight weeks gestation. More severely affected diabetic subjects were also found to have larger reduction in charges and days. After adjusting for inflation and differences in charges across hospitals it was calculated that $5.10 was saved for every dollar spent on the programme[61].

PRE-PREGNANCY CARE IN WOMEN WITH NON-INSULIN-DEPENDENT DIABETES

In Scotland there are few women of childbearing age with non-insulin-dependent diabetes. The majority are overweight and are strongly advised to lose weight before conception. Most authorities feel that oral hypoglycaemic agents are contraindicated at the time of conception and during pregnancy. If it is not possible to obtain good glycaemic control with diet and exercise, insulin should be given before conception.

In some parts of the world non-insulin-dependent diabetes is very common and pre-pregnancy counselling for this group is therefore important. Some studies have grouped those with non-insulin-dependent diabetes with insulin-dependent diabetic subjects but have not analysed the results separately. Rowe and co-workers[62,63] have stressed the importance of pre-pregnancy counselling in non-insulin-dependent diabetes and previous gestational diabetes, and have shown improvement in pregnancy outcome in a small group of Asian women receiving pre-pregnancy counselling. Mølsted-Pedersen and Damm have drawn attention to the high percentage of women with gestational diabetes who go on to develop diabetes, and the importance of contraceptive advice and pre-conception counselling in this group (see page 341).

HOW CAN WE INCREASE THE NUMBER OF WOMEN WITH DIABETES WHO RECEIVE PRE-PREGNANCY CARE?

Although the purposes of pre-pregnancy care were published in 1980 and since then many enthusiasts have recommended this approach[4,64,65], it is disappointing that many centres still do not offer the service and, where it is offered, the proportion of women attending tends to be small.

A survey of the care of women with diabetes in Britain carried out by the British Diabetic Association in 1989 showed that only 22 (12%) of the 182 districts who replied offered pre-conception counselling. It seemed rather unlikely that it was offered by many of the 57 districts which did not reply.

In 1988 an American survey, sent to obstetricians with an interest in diabetes, showed that only 17.8% (48/269) of the respondents consulted with an internist or diabetologist in the care of pregnancies complicated by diabetes and noted that 20% or less of their patients seek pre-conceptual care[66]. In 1989 the American Diabetes Association included pre-pregnancy counselling in its standards of medical care for patients with diabetes mellitus[67]. In 1992 the European Division of the International Diabetes Federation recommended pre-pregnancy care in its St Vincent Declaration Action Programme[68]. A recent survey by the St Vincent Joint Task Force of the UK Department of Health and the British Diabetic Association Pregnancy Subgroup revealed that 87% of hospitals provide pre-pregnancy counselling and 12% provide a special pre-pregnancy clinic. Sometimes the counselling is simply a nurse telling a women that pregnancies should be planned and that good control is important. Nevertheless, there does seem to be increasing awareness, which is encouraging.

The high attendance rate in Edinburgh came about because all insulin-dependent women attend a hospital clinic and one enthusiastic physician working in the same department for over 20 years was able to get to know all the women and had the support of diabetes nurse specialists who shared her enthusiasm and were able to visit defaulters at home. Many centres do not have these advantages. Some of the American programmes have gone to enormous lengths to recruit women. In Maine they registered all women in the childbearing age group who attended a physician and sent them detailed information. They developed public service television announcements, an education seminary, education brochures and a free telephone service[39]. Janz's group took a similar approach, using numerous education programmes, journal advertisements, newsletters, posters, etc.[44]. Greenspoon has suggested that a label should be placed on all diabetic equipment warning that poor control of diabetes can cause birth defects and advising women to see their physician before becoming pregnant[69].

It is clearly essential to get the message over, loud and clear, to both carers and women with diabetes. Janz's group recommend that providers should regard every visit with a diabetic woman as a pre-conception visit. Contraception must be explicitly discussed, and pregnancies should be planned. The benefits of pre-conception care should be stressed and the support of families should be elicited. Added to that should be special resources and effort directed to those who do not attend for diabetes care as these comprise the highest-risk group.

REFERENCES

1 Pedersen J. *The Pregnant Diabetic and her Newborn*. Munksgaard, Copenhagen, 1967; 128.
2 Karlsson K, Kjellmer LO. The outcome of diabetic pregnancies in relation to mothers blood sugar level. *Am J Obstet Gynecol* 1972; **112**: 213–20.

3 Gabbe SG. Medical complications of pregnancy management of diabetes in pregnancy: six decades of experience. In: Pitkin RM, Zlatnik RJ (eds), *Year Book of Obstetrics and Gynecology*. Year Book Medical Publishers, Chicago, 1980; 37–49.
4 Steel JM, Parboosingh J, Cole RA, Duncan LJP. Pre-pregnancy counselling: a logical prelude to the management of the pregnant diabetic. *Diabetes Care* 1980; 3: 371–3.
5 Beetham WP. Diabetic retinopathy in pregnancy. *Trans Am Ophthalmol Soc* 1950; 48: 205–11.
6 White P. Pregnancy and diabetes: medical aspects. *Med Clin North Am* 1965; 49: 1115–24.
7 Price JH, Hadden DR, Harley DG. Diabetic retinopathy in pregnancy. *Br J Obstet Gynaecol* 1984; 91: 11–17.
8 Pedersen J. *The Pregnant Diabetic and her Newborn*, 2nd edn. Munksgaard, Copenhagen, 1977; 97.
9 Kitzmiller JL, Brown LR, Phillippe M *et al*. Diabetic nephropathy and perinatal outcome. *Am J Obstet Gynecol* 1981; 141: 741–51.
10 Hare JW, White P. Pregnancy in diabetes complicated by vascular disease. *Diabetes* 1977; 26: 953–5.
11 Steel JM. Autonomic neuropathy in pregnancy. *Diabetes Care* 1989; 12: 170–1.
12 Mølsted-Pedersen L, Tygstrup I, Pedersen J. Congenital malformations in new born infants of diabetic women. *Lancet* 1964; i: 1124–6.
13 Kucera J. Rate and type of congenital anomalies among offspring of diabetic women. *J Reprod Med* 1971; 7: 61–70.
14 Pedersen J. Congenital malformations. In: *The Pregnant Diabetic and her Newborn*, 2nd edn. Munksgaard, Copenhagen, 1977; 196.
15 Soler NG, Walsh CH, Malins JM. Congenital malformations in infants of diabetic mothers. *Q J Med* 1976; 45: 303–13.
16 Gabbe SG. Congenital malformations in infants of diabetic mothers. *Obstet Gynecol Survey* 1977; 32: 125–32.
17 Glasgow ACA, Harley JMG, Montgomery DAD. Congenital malformations in infants of diabetic mothers. *Ulster Med J* 1979; 48: 109–17.
18 Mills JL, Baker L, Goldman AS. Malformations in infants of diabetic mother occur before the seventh gestational week: implications for treatment. *Diabetes* 1979; 28: 292–3.
19 Deuchar E. Experimental evidence relating foetal anomalies to diabetes. In: Sutherland HW, Stowers JM (eds), *Carbohydrate Metabolism in Pregnancy and the Newborn*. Springer-Verlag, Berlin, 1978; 247–63.
20 Baker L, Engler J, Kein S, Goldman AS. Meticulous control of diabetes during organogenesis prevents congenital lumbo-sacral defects in rats. *Diabetes* 1981; 30: 955–9.
21 Sadler TW, Horton WE, Hunter ES. Mechanisms of diabetes-induced congenital malformations as studies in mammalian embryo culture. In: Jovanovic L, Peterson CM, Fuhrmann K (eds), *Diabetes and Pregnancy, Teratology, Toxicity and Treatment*. Praeger, New York, 1986; 51–71.
22 Leslie RDG, John PN, Pyke DA, White JM. Haemoglobin A$_1$ in diabetic pregnancy. *Lancet* 1978; ii: 958–9.
23 Miller E, Hare JW, Cloherty JP *et al*. Elevated maternal haemoglobin A$_1$ in early pregnancy and major congenital anomalies in infants of diabetic mothers. *N Engl J Med* 1981; 303: 1331–4.
24 Ylinen K, Rawo K, Teramo K. Haemoglobin A$_1$ predicts the perinatal outcome in insulin-dependent diabetic pregnancies. *Br J Obstet Gynaecol* 1981; 88: 961–7.
25 Key TC, Giuffrida R, Moore TR. Predictive value of early pregnancy glycohemoglobin in the insulin-treated diabetic patient. *Am J Obstet Gynecol* 1987; 156: 1096–100.
26 Stubbs SM, Doddridge MC, John JN *et al*. Haemoglobin A$_1$ and congenital malformation. *Diabetic Med* 1987; 4: 156–9.
27 Miodovnik M, Mimouni F, Dignan PSJ *et al*. Major malformations in infants of IDDM women; vasculopathy and early first-trimester poor glycaemic control. *Diabetes Care* 1988; 11: 713–18.
28 Mills JL, KnoppRH, Simpson JL *et al*. Lack of relation of increased malformation rates in infants of diabetic mothers to glycaemic control during organogenesis. *N Engl J Med* 1988; 318: 671–6.
29 Editorial. Congenital abnormalities in infants of diabetic mothers. *Lancet* 1988; i: 1313–14.

30 Greene MI, Hare JW, Cloherty JP *et al*. First-trimester haemoglobin A₁ and risk for major malformation and spontaneous abortion in diabetic pregnancy. *Teratology* 1989; **39**: 225–31.

31 Hanssens M, Keirse MJ, Bankelecom F, Van-Assche FA. Fetal and neonatal effects of treatment with angiotensin-converting enzyme inhibitors in pregnancy. *Obstet Gynecol* 1991; **1**: 128–35.

32 MRC Vitamin Study Research Group. Prevention of neural tube defects: results of the medical research council vitamin study. *Lancet* 1991; **338**: 131–7.

33 Hadden DR. Pre-pregnancy counselling in endocrine and metabolic disorders. In: Harley JMG (ed.), *Pre-pregnancy Counselling in Obstetrics. Clin Obstet Gynaecol.* 1982; **9**(1): 29–57.

34 Tindall H, Vinall PS, Stickland M, Wales JK. Improved results for diabetic pregnancies after pre-pregnancy counselling. *Practical Diabetes* 1986; **3**: 250–2.

35 Drury PL, Doddridge M. Pre-pregnancy clinics for diabetic women. *Lancet* 1992; **340**: 919.

36 Fuhrmann K, Reiher H, Semmler K *et al*. Prevention of congenital malformations in infants of insulin dependent diabetic mothers. *Diabetes Care* 1983; **6**: 219–23.

37 Miller E. Pre-pregnancy counselling and management of women with pre-existing diabetes or previous gestational diabetes in medical management of pregnancy complicated by diabetes. American Diabetes Association, 1993.

38 Kitzmiller JL, Gavin LA, Gin GD *et al*. Pre-conception care of diabetes: glycaemic control prevents congenital anomalies. *JAMA* 1991; **265**: 731–6.

39 Willhotte MB, Bennert HW, Palomaki GE *et al*. The impact of pre-conception counselling on pregnancy outcomes. *Diabetes Care* 1993; **16**: 450–5.

40 Goldman JA, Dicker D, Feldberg D *et al*. Pregnancy outcome in patients with insulin-dependent diabetes mellitus with pre-conceptional diabetic control: A comparative study. *Am J Obstet Gynecol* 1986; **155**: 293–7.

41 Cousins L. The California Diabetes and Pregnancy Program: a statewide collaborative program for the pre-conception and prenatal care of diabetic women. *Baillieres Clin Obstet Gynaecol* 1991; **5**: 443–59.

42 Rosenn B, Miodovnik M, Combs CA *et al*. Pre-conception management of insulin dependent diabetes: improvement in pregnancy outcome. *Obstet Gynecol* 1991; **77**: 846–9.

43 Steel JM, Johnstone FD, Hepburn DA, Smith FA. Can pre-pregnancy care of diabetic women reduce the risk of abnormal babies? *Br Med J* 1990; **301**: 1070–4.

44 Janz NK, Herman WH, Becker MP *et al*. Diabetes and pregnancy: factors associated with seeking pre-conception care. *Diabetes Care* 1995; **18**: 157–65.

45 Young LB, Steel JM, West CP, Chawla H. Pregnancy after vitrectomy for proliferative diabetic retinopathy. *Diabetic Med* 1987; **4**: 77–8.

46 Steel JM, Johnstone FD, Smith AF, Duncan LJP. Five years experience of a pre-pregnancy clinic for insulin-dependent diabetes. *Br Med J* 1982; **285**: 355–6.

47 Steel, JM. Pre-pregnancy counselling and contraception in the insulin dependent diabetic patient. *Clin Obstet Gynaecol* 1985; **28**: 553–6.

48 Steel JM, Johnstone FD, Smith AF. Pre-pregnancy preparation. In: Sutherland HW, Stowers JM, Pearson DWM (eds), *Carbohydrate Metabolism in Pregnancy and the Newborn*, Vol IV. Springer-Verlag, Berlin, 1989; 129–39.

49 Gregory R, Tattersall RB. Are diabetic pre-pregnancy clinics worthwhile? *Lancet* 1992; **340**: 656–8.

50 Damm P, Mølsted-Pedersen L. Significant decrease in congenital malformations in newborn infants of an unselected population of diabetic women. *Am J Obstet Gynecol* 1989; **161**: 1163–7.

51 Persson B, Bjork O, Hanson U, Stangenberg M. Neonatal management 1982. In: Sutherland HW, Stowers JM (eds), *Carbohydrate Metabolism in Pregnancy and the Newborn*. Churchill Livingstone, Edinburgh, 1994; 133–43.

52 Steel JM, Johnstone FD. Pre-pregnancy clinics for diabetic women. *Lancet* 1992; **340**: 918–19.

53 Kitzmiller JL, Buchanan T, Coustan D. Pre-pregnancy care in diabetes. *Lancet* 1992; **340**: 919–20.

54 Baird JD, Bellman O, Eriksson U *et al*. Pre-pregnancy care in diabetes. *Lancet* 1992; **340**: 1106–7.

55 Combs CA, Kitzmiller JL. Spontaneous abortion and congenital malformations in diabetes. *Baillieres Clin Obstet Gynaecol* 1991; **5**: 315–11.

56 Mills JL, Van Allen M, Piarons JH *et al*. Incidence of spontaneous abortion among normal women and insulin-dependent diabetic women whose pregnancies were identified within 21 days of conception. *N Engl J Med* 1988; **319**: 1617–23.
57 Dicker D, Feldberg D, Samuel N. Spontaneous abortion in patients with insulin-dependent diabetes mellitus: the effects of pre-conceptual diabetic control. *Am J Obstet Gynecol* 1988; **158**: 1161–4.
58 Buchanan TA, Schemmer JK, Freinkel N. Embryotoxic effects of brief maternal insulin-hypoglycaemia during organogenesis in the rat. *J Clin Invest* 1986; **78**: 645–9.
59 Randall JM, Hesham A, Templeton AA. Diabetes mellitus and infertility. In: Sutherland HW, Stowers JM, Pearson DWM (eds), *Carbohydrate Metabolism in Pregnancy and the Newborn*, Vol. IV. Springer-Verlag, Berlin, 1989; 65–73.
60 Elixhauser A, Weschler JM, Kitzmiller JL *et al*. Cost–benefit analysis of pre-conception care for women with established diabetes mellitus. *Diabetes Care* 1993; **16**: 1146–56.
61 Scheffler RM, Feuchtbaum LB, Phibbs CS. Prevention: the cost effectiveness of the California Diabetes and Pregnancy Program. *Am J Public Health* 1992; **82**: 168–75.
62 Rowe BR, Rowbotham CJ, Barnett AH. Pre-conception counselling, birthweight, and congenital abnormalities in established and gestational diabetic pregnancy. *Diabetic Res* 1987; **6**(1): 33–5.
63 Rowe BR, Barnett AM. Pre-conception counselling in Asian women with non-insulin-dependent diabetes and impaired glucose tolerance. *Diabetes Res* 1988; **8**(1): 35–8.
64 Hadden DR. Pre-pregnancy counselling in diabetes mellitus. *Midwives Chron* 1987; **100**: 30–2.
65 Hare JW. *Diabetes Complicating Pregnancy: The Joslin Clinic Method*. New York, 1989; 33–51.
66 Bryce FC, Bodansky HJ, Redmond S, Buchan PC. A survey of UK diabetic pregnancy management. *Diabetic Med* 1991; **8**: 382–4.
67 American Diabetic Association. Standards of medical care for patients with diabetes mellitus. *Diabetes Care* 1989; **12**: 368.
68 Krans HMJ, Porta M, Keen H (eds). *Diabetes Care and Research in Europe: The St Vincent Declaration Action Programme*. WHO, Geneva, 1992; 39.
69 Greenspoon JS, Morgan BR. A product warning label to encourage pre-pregnancy control of diabetes. *JAMA* 1991; **266**: 2225.
70 Fuhrmann R, Reiher H, Semmler RK, Glockner E. The effect of intensified conventional insulin therapy before and during pregnancy on the malformation rate in offspring of diabetic mothers. *Exp Clin Endocrinol* 1984; **83**: 173–7.
71 Steel JM. Personal experience of pre-pregnancy care in women with insulin dependent diabetes. *Aust NZ J Obstet Gynaecol* 1994; **34**(2): 135–9.

7

Insulin Therapy in Diabetic Pregnancy

RICHARD G. FIRTH

Mater Misericordiae Hospital, Dublin, Eire

Prior to the discovery of insulin in 1921, pregnancy in what later became known as insulin-dependent diabetes was uncommon, since such women lost weight, were infertile, and most had died within two years of the diagnosis. The majority that did become pregnant lost their babies and often their own lives in diabetic ketoacidosis[1]. Since then, with progressively earlier and stricter diabetic control, both perinatal mortality and morbidity in insulin-dependent diabetic pregnancy have approached and in some cases surpassed the outcomes in non-diabetic pregnancy, thereby fulfilling one of the specific goals of the St Vincent Declaration of the European Association for the Study of Diabetes and the World Health Organization.

A few major challenges remain. These include reduction in the still unacceptably high risks of congenital malformation, and the risk of progression of maternal diabetic microvascular complications by eliminating unplanned pregnancy, by pre-conception counselling, and by allowing progression towards spontaneous onset of labour and normal delivery in such patients. The issues in gestational diabetes are much less clear, and identification of such at-risk pregnancies and their optimal management remain major problems worldwide.

How then have such excellent results been achieved? Undoubtedly, centralization of care, better education of both patients and carers, improved diet and social conditions, improved communications and better maternal and fetal monitoring have all played a part in achieving better metabolic control in diabetic pregnancy, which has been the chief determinant of pregnancy outcome.

Diabetes and Pregnancy: An International Approach to Diagnosis and Management.
Edited by A. Dornhorst and D. R. Hadden.
© 1996 John Wiley & Sons Ltd.

The maternal hyperglycaemia–fetal hyperinsulinaemia–macrosomia hypothesis[2,3] remains unchallenged although it has been extended to include increased transplacental flux of amino acids and fats[4]. Post-absorptive and fasting plasma glucose levels are reduced in normal pregnancy, as are circulating amino acid levels. Serum cholesterol and triglyceride levels rise particularly in the second trimester[5]. In the insulin-deficient state of poorly controlled insulin-dependent diabetes or the insulin-resistant/relative insulin-deficient state of gestational diabetes, elevated maternal plasma glucose, amino acids, free fatty acids and ketone levels can be demonstrated and correlated with fetal macrosomia[6]. The rise in serum cholesterol and triglyceride levels is blunted in diabetic pregnancy[7].

The relative contribution of these perturbations to fetal macrosomia is unknown and measurement of most of these various metabolites is impractical in the antenatal clinic. It is thus reassuring that intensive glycaemic control has been shown to result in return of maternal glycogenic and branched-chain amino acids, free fatty acids, cholesterol, triglycerides and ketone levels to normal, albeit at the expense of hyperinsulinaemia[8].

MANAGEMENT OF INSULIN-REQUIRING DIABETIC PREGNANCY

In view of the foregoing it is important to tell the patient that 'satisfactory' glycaemic goals for the non-pregnant state are much too high in pregnancy and will adversely affect the outcome. Glycaemic targets must be lowered to mimic those found in normal pregnancy.

The strategies adopted in the author's unit in order to achieve such control with safety will be described below. Exclusive delivery of care of diabetic pregnancy by a single unit to the three Dublin maternity hospitals (combined delivery rate 24 000 deliveries per year) has allowed policies to become uniform and routine. Intensity of follow-up and care may be considered excessive or beyond local resources, but has produced a perinatal mortality rate below that of non-diabetic pregnancy, despite 68% of insulin-dependent diabetic pregnancies entering labour spontaneously and 58% being delivered at 40 weeks or later, with mean birth weight and ponderal index identical to the general population[9]. Maternal and neonatal morbidity have also fallen (Table 7.1)[10].

Centralization of care, and experience in the management of diabetic pregnancy, are of proven benefit[11]. The combined antenatal clinic should have a minimum staffing requirement of diabetologist, obstetrician, nurse/educator and dietitian with access to ophthalmologist, nephrologist, counsellor and social worker. Most importantly, personnel should be as constant as possible to provide continuity of care and to establish a close medical/social relationship with the patient. Ideally, all diabetic pregnancies should be planned pregnancies, and all patients 'graduates' of pre-pregnancy clinics, with early referral on to the combined antenatal clinic. Here, full obstetrical,

Table 7.1. Diabetes in pregnancy 1981–1990

(a) Antenatal complications

	81–82 $n = 71$	83–84 $n = 50$	85–86 $n = 61$	87–88 $n = 47$	89–90 $n = 47$	Total $n = 276$
Pre-eclampsia	21%	16%	15%	13%	9%	15%
Suspected hydramnios	15%	12%	15%	4%	0%	10%
Suspected macrosomia	4%	12%	18%	15%	0%	10%
Maternal hypoglycaemia	17%	4%	7%	11%	8%	10%
Amniocentesis	15%	12%	3%	8%	4%	9%
L/S ratio						

(b) Neonatal complications

	81–82 $n = 71$	83–84 $n = 50$	85–86 $n = 61$	87–88 $n = 47$	89–90 $n = 48$	Total $n = 277$
Macrosomia (>90%)	39%	34%	39%	23%	2%	29%
Admission to special care nursery	38%	26%	39%	26%	32%	33%
Respiratory distress syndrome	$n = 3$	$n = 2$	$n = 1$	–	–	2%
Neonatal hypoglycaemia	17%	14%	13%	6%	6%	12%
Neonatal jaundice	11%	16%	10%	2%	4%	9%

Antenatal complications and neonatal complications in 276 pre-gestational insulin-dependent diabetic pregnancies at the National Maternity Hospital, Dublin, 1981–1990. Table shows figures for each successive two-year period over the decade and the mean for the decade as a whole. Obstetrical policies remained unchanged over this period. The reduction in complications seen is chiefly due to more modern individualized insulin regimen and diabetes care, allowing euglycaemia with less risk of hypoglycaemia. No pregnancy terminations took place during this period. L/S = lecithin/sphingomyelin. Adapted from Rasmussen et al.[10]. Fetal morbidity in IDDM. *Diabetes News*. Excerpta Medica 1995; **16**: 6–8.

metabolic and social/domestic assessment can be undertaken.

Combined antenatal clinics are held weekly. After initial booking, subsequent visits take place at least every second week and then weekly from 36 weeks in uncomplicated cases. Home blood glucose monitoring results during non-visit weeks are telephoned or telefaxed to the clinic for insulin dose adjustment. A twice-weekly or even daily facility for dose changes by the consultant physician exists in cases of poor or unstable control or other intercurrent problems.

MONITORING AND INDICES OF CONTROL

Patients are lent reflectance meters, memory equipped for date, time and result. This practice has benefits in terms of verification and data collection and has allowed us to discontinue laboratory venous blood glucose checks in those patients on insulin. We have found verification laboratory glucose values to be misleading and to correlate poorly with haemoglobin A_{1c} (HbA$_{1c}$) and fructosamine values due to logistic problems such as timing of samples, and patients' 'training' for blood tests[12].

Home blood glucose monitoring is performed seven times daily throughout the pregnancy, 30 min prior to and 1 h after each of the three main meals and before the bedtime snack. The attempted blood glucose goals are <5 mmol/l (90 mg/dl) before meals and bedtime snack and <7 mmol/l (126 mg/dl) 1 h postprandially. Corresponding guidelines of fasting blood glucose <5.6 mmol/l (<100 mg/dl) and postprandial values <8.0 mmol/l (145 mg/dl) are given by the European IDDM Policy Group[13].

Fructosamine estimation corrected for serum albumin concentration is performed at each two-weekly clinic visit and provides a retrospective index of control for the previous two-week period. HbA$_{1c}$ is assayed every four weeks as a further check on the previous four to six weeks' performance. The goals for fructosamine and HbA$_{1c}$ are to achieve values as low as possible without subjective or objective hypoglycaemia and certainly well within the non-diabetic normal range.

In order to achieve such goals safely, individualized complex multiple daily injection regimes are required, which in turn require the intensive monitoring and management offered. In general, compliance is extremely good and patients prefer the security for their own and their baby's health offered by such a regimen.

TYPES OF INSULIN

Human insulins have several theoretical and practical advantages. In gestational diabetic mothers requiring insulin for the duration of the index pregnancy only, the lower insulin antigenicity of human insulin decreases the likelihood of insulin binding antibody formation, which may reduce endogenous insulin secretion as well as posing potential problems with control should insulin therapy be required in the future[14-17]. Transplacental antibody-bound insulin might theoretically lead to fetal hyperinsulinaemia and macrosomia, but this suggestion has not been confirmed; studies suggest instead that improved glycaemic control, lower insulin requirements, and better postprandial profiles in subjects using human insulin influence birth weight, rather than absent insulin binding antibodies[18,19]. Only human insulin is presently available in convenient pen injection devices. Finally, there is no convincing evidence that human insulin promotes hypoglycaemic unawareness[20].

ROUTE AND MODES OF INSULIN DELIVERY

Open-loop continuous subcutaneous insulin infusion pumps appear to confer no advantage over individualized multiple-dose regimens in pregnancy[21], in terms of HbA$_{1c}$ levels, hypoglycaemia or pregnancy outcome.

They may indeed have certain inherent disadvantages, including the potential for rapid development of hyperglycaemia and ketosis during needle or catheter blockage[22] quite apart from their inherent inconvenience. The value of jet injection devices remains unclear. The American Diabetes Association position statement on such devices focuses on the potential for insulin denaturation and consequent enhanced antigenicity after passing rapidly through a tiny port[23]. However, one report suggests a decreased antibody response, less postprandial glycaemic variability and better acceptance during jet injection therapy[24].

The subcutaneous injection sites usually recommended do not differ during pregnancy. Insulin absorption from the abdomen is the most consistent irrespective of exercise[25], and rotation of sites across a wide area between the upper and lower abdomen should be used for daytime injection, while the thigh or buttock may be used at night. To ensure maximal consistency of insulin absorption rates we discourage mixing of insulins in the syringe and encourage the use of soluble and isophane insulins given separately by pen injection devices.

INSULIN DOSES AND REGIMENS

Insulin resistance in pregnancy falls during the first trimester and then increases progressively about three-fold from gestational week 20 onwards[26]. As a result all groups – insulin-dependent, non-insulin-dependent and insulin-requiring gestational diabetic mothers – are likely to require large and increasing doses of insulin as pregnancy progresses[27], until the last month of gestation when the requirement may fall slightly in insulin-dependent mothers (but perhaps not in gestational diabetes)[28]. A significant number of women lose hypoglycaemic awareness in pregnancy, perhaps as a result of intensification of control. This together with very large doses of insulin is a potentially dangerous combination.

Absorption rates of intermediate-acting insulin can vary by as much as 20–100% on a day-to-day basis in the same individual under basal conditions[29]. Clinically this becomes even more readily apparent with long-acting insulin–zinc suspensions (Ultratard, Ultralente). Although intermediate-acting insulins will obviously be required, very long-acting insulin should be avoided except in a very small group of non-hypoglycaemia-prone patients who have proven stability on this type of insulin.

The size of individually administered doses is also important, and the rate of absorption of subcutaneously administered insulin varies inversely with the volume of the dose[30]. In practical terms this means that there is a limit (probably around 20 units) above which the peak effect (6–10 h) of the injected insulin becomes attenuated and delayed and ceases to 'target' a particular blood glucose – the effect is simply prolonged, leading to possible inappropriate late hyperinsulinaemia and hypoglycaemia, and weight gain. Large single doses can be avoided partly by using unmixed injections, giving virtually simultaneous separate injections of soluble and isophane insulin. Where progressively larger doses fail to control glucose levels at a particular time point, dietary manipulation either by calorie restriction or by simply moving carbohydrate exchanges back and forth can have limited success in achieving the stringent goals required. We feel that factory pre-mixed insulins should not be used in pregnancy. As in all situations where insulin requirements are in a state of flux (such as the 'honeymoon period' following diagnosis) pre-mixed insulins do not confer the flexibility required in pregnancy.

Finally, the rate at which euglycaemia is achieved may be important in the person with microvascular disease, particularly retinopathy. There is little to be gained and much to be lost in the rapid restoration of euglycaemia in the poorly controlled individual with unstable maculopathy, pre-proliferative or proliferative retinopathy, since such action may accelerate deterioration in the unstable fundus[31]. Provided the patient is seen early in the first trimester, gradual institution of control over a period of four to six weeks with close retinal surveillance may be the sensible option.

TWICE DAILY INSULIN REGIMENS

Traditional 'mixed-split' insulin regimens consisting of soluble and intermediate-acting insulins given twice daily (Figure 7.1a)[32] are of value in only a handful of patients requiring moderate dose levels. These include those with 'mild' gestational diabetes and a few 'non-brittle' insulin-dependent diabetic patients, some of whom may have residual insulin secretion. In most pregnant diabetic women the large insulin requirements make such regimens insufficiently sensitive, for the reasons discussed

---

Figure 7.1. (*opposite*) Insulin regimens used in pregnancy. (a) The conventional 'mixed-split' regimen of a twice-daily mixture of soluble (regular) insulin and intermediate-acting (isophane (NPH)/Lente) insulin. (b) A modification of the above in which the evening intermediate-acting insulin is given separately at 10 p.m. instead of with the soluble insulin at the evening meal. This counteracts the waning basal insulin in the early morning. (c) The 'conventional' multiple daily injection regimen. In general basal insulin levels during the day are insufficient to control preprandial glycaemia during pregnancy. (d) A complex multiple daily injection regimen. The conventional multiple dose regimen above is modified by the addition of intermediate-acting (isophane) insulin at any or all of the mealtimes to control preprandial glycaemia. Isophane given with B controls glycaemia at S. Isophane given with L controls glycaemia at HS. Isophane given at S controls glycaemia overnight and at B if isophane at HS is unable to do so. (B, breakfast; L, lunch; S, evening meal; HS, 10 p.m.) Adapted from Schade DS, Santiago JV, Skyler JS, Rizza RA. *Intensive insulin therapy*. Excerpta Medica 1983; 209–11

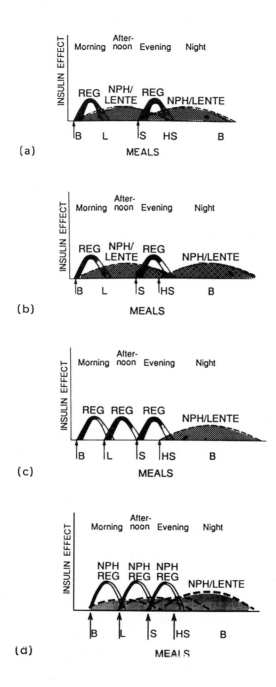

above. Furthermore, the pre-evening meal glucose level may not fall and will require additional lunchtime soluble insulin. The inability to control early morning (fasting) glycaemia may require splitting the evening injection by moving the isophane component to 10 p.m. (Figure 7.1b). In general, however, we find that twice-daily regimens or modifications of these are unable to achieve blood glucose levels comparable to non-diabetic pregnancy in most insulin-dependent diabetic mothers, or in insulin-requiring gestational diabetes.

MULTIPLE DAILY INJECTION REGIMENS

Regimens such as the breakfast soluble/lunchtime soluble/dinnertime soluble/10 p.m. intermediate insulin (Figure 7.1c) have gained widespread use in the non-pregnant diabetic by conferring lifestyle flexibility and reducing unpredictable glycaemic swings, especially those toward hypoglycaemia. Because of their tendency to cause unpredictable hypoglycaemia, we find that UltraLente and Ultratard-based regimens have little place in diabetic pregnancy.

However, such 'simple' conventional regimens do not provide enough basal insulin in the context of the 'accelerated catabolism' of diabetic pregnancy to maintain post-absorptive or preprandial glycaemia below 5 mmol/l (Figure 7.1c). Progressive increments in preprandial soluble insulin will simply cause postprandial hypoglycaemia without solving the problem. We therefore devise individualized complex regimens by the addition of isophane insulin to any or all of the mealtimes as required (Figure 7.1d). No soluble insulin is given at night. Initiation of such a regimen in a person on a conventional twice-daily insulin regimen generally takes the following route: (1) addition of lunchtime soluble insulin (if pre-evening meal glucoses remain high); (2) 'splitting' the evening dose by moving the evening isophane insulin to 10 p.m. (to control morning fasting glycaemia); (3) addition of breakfast and/or lunchtime isophane (if increasing bolus mealtime soluble insulin cannot control preprandial values without postprandial hypoglycaemia); (4) addition of pre-evening meal isophane insulin if the fasting pre-breakfast glucose remains above 5 mmol/l despite 20–26 units of isophane insulin at 10 p.m.; (5) simultaneous compensatory adjustment in soluble insulin doses is described below.

As shown in Figure 7.1(d), the chief effect of the soluble insulin is on the immediate next postprandial glycaemic excursion, and that of the isophane insulin is on the next two preprandial values, especially the second (isophane given at breakfast will affect preprandial values at the evening mealtime more than at lunch). Ideally, the soluble insulins are adjusted to maintain the next postprandial value below 7 mmol/l and the next preprandial value below 5 mmol/l. If this preprandial value cannot be controlled by soluble insulin, isophane is added to or increased in the *previous* injection and the soluble insulin adjusted to a maximum dose allowing a postprandial glycaemic excursion of 2–3 mmol/l. The morning isophane is adjusted to provide an evening mealtime glucose of less than 5 mmol/l, and the lunchtime soluble adjusted to allow glycaemic excursion of 2–3 mmol/l.

Frequently, fasting pre-breakfast hyperglycaemia cannot be controlled by up to 26 units of isophane insulin given at 10 p.m. We find that the addition of isophane at the evening meal will invariably achieve the target. Occasional 3 a.m. readings should be taken to disclose nocturnal hypoglycaemia. Postprandial hyperglycaemia can occasionally prove problematical and may require an increase in the injection/mealtime interval and/or dietary manipulation to correct.

Numerous centres commence and change insulin regimens on an ambulatory care basis. However, our belief in centralized care leads to difficulties with distance, and we therefore admit a significant number of patients to hospital for rapid institution of an individualized regimen, intensive education and nocturnal monitoring, especially in those who are hypoglycaemia prone. Once satisfactory profiles are obtained, 'fine-tuning' can be performed by telephone or day centre contact.

INITIATING INSULIN THERAPY IN NON-INSULIN-DEPENDENT AND GESTATIONAL DIABETES

In known non-insulin-dependent diabetic pregnancy, planning allows intensification of management aimed particularly towards dietary and exercise optimization and achievement of ideal body weight. In such circumstances where diet alone is insufficient to achieve and maintain HbA_{1c} levels as near the non-diabetic range as possible, patients should be commenced on insulin, and oral hypoglycaemic agents discontinued prior to pregnancy. Most such patients will achieve adequate peri-conception control on twice-daily insulin unless large insulin doses are required or the patient is hypoglycaemia prone (unlikely in this subset of patients). Following the onset of pregnancy, if a more complex multiple daily injection regime is required to achieve the more stringent goals desired, this can be initiated as described above. Those non-insulin-dependent diabetic patients initially achieving adequate glycaemic control on diet alone are likely to require insulin during the second half of pregnancy. Initiation of twice daily insulin and subsequent intensification is described below.

In gestational diabetes, the majority of those requiring insulin to achieve the glycaemic goals will commence therapy sometime after 20 weeks of pregnancy. The decision when to start insulin is beyond the scope of this chapter but varies greatly from centre to centre, even within the same country[33], and is based on many factors including effectiveness of screening, local incidence, mode and intensity of surveillance, individual obstetrical, medical and psychosocial factors, goal ascertainment and local resources. We would consider sustained preprandial plasma glucose values above 6.0 mmol/l and/or 1–2 h postprandial values over 8.0 mmol/l to be absolute indications for commencing insulin therapy.

The trend in recent studies appears to be towards intensification of surveillance with progressively stricter criteria for initiating insulin therapy, and more intensive insulin regimens to achieve glycaemic goals once on insulin therapy. Such intensification leads to significantly improved outcome approaching that of non-diabetic pregnancy[34]. Perhaps the most important component of the care of these patients is their identification[35] since untreated or undertreated gestational diabetes is associated with adverse outcome[36].

Unless blood glucose levels constitute an emergency, diurnal profiles by capillary blood glucose monitoring obtained either by the patients themselves or in hospital are likely to be available as a guide to the individual insulin requirements in terms of total dose and insulin type. In general, a conventional twice-daily regimen is initiated and subsequently intensified if necessary as in insulin-dependent diabetic pregnancy, to achieve similar goals (preprandial under 5 mmol/l, and postprandial under 7 mmol/l). Initial doses may be based empirically on capillary blood glucose monitoring profiles or on body weight and subsequently adjusted. Since most gestational diabetic patients require an insulin dose upwards of 0.6 U/kg body weight, they may safely be given an initial total daily dose of 0.4 U/kg divided two-thirds in the morning and one-third in the evening. Each of these doses is divided into one-third soluble and two-thirds isophane insulin. Subsequent adjustment and, if necessary, intensification to a complex multiple-dose regimen is achieved as described above.

MANAGEMENT DURING LABOUR

In general, only insulin-requiring pregnancies will require insulin during labour. The aims during this period are euglycaemia (blood glucose < 6.0 mmol/l) in the mother to prevent neonatal hypoglycaemia in the infant, and to prevent ketosis which inhibits uterine contractility with the potential consequence of prolonged labour. Once the mother is in established labour and fasting, 5% dextrose or a mixture of 0.18% saline and 4% dextrose given at a rate of 1 litre over 8 h will provide sufficient carbohydrate; 10–20 mEq of potassium chloride may be added. Insulin may be delivered by either of two methods:

1. *Insulin/dextrose infusion:* Soluble insulin equivalent to 2/9 of the most recent total daily insulin requirement is added to each litre of the above fluid and given over 8 h. This is repeated until delivery. Provided the

daily requirement is reasonably stable and appropriate this simple regimen usually results in euglycaemia during labour. Two-hourly capillary blood glucose monitoring is performed and supplemental subcutaneous insulin given as necessary (4 U soluble insulin every 2 h if the blood glucose exceeds 6 mmol/l).

2. *Continuous variable insulin infusion:* 50 U of soluble insulin is diluted in 50 ml of normal saline in a 50 ml syringe and delivered by syringe pump (calibrated in millilitres per hour in intervals of 0.1 ml/h; thus 1 ml/h equates to 1 U of insulin per hour). Capillary blood glucose monitoring is performed hourly and the pump rate adjusted according to an algorithm such as that given in Table 7.2.

It must be stressed that no algorithm will be the same for different patients, and it will need to be adjusted according to response to maintain maternal glucose levels between 4.0 and 6.0 mmol/l. Simultaneous glucose and potassium administration is mandatory (see also pages 262 and 300).

Table 7.2. Algorithm for insulin infusion rate in labour. Capillary blood glucose is monitored hourly and the pump rate adjusted as shown (suggested figures for a typical patient)

Blood glucose (mmol/l)	Pump rate (ml/h = units/h)
Under 4	0
4–6	0.5
6–8	1.0
8–10	2.0
10–12	3.0
12–14	5.0
14–16	6.0
16–18	7.0
18–20	8.0
20–22	10.0
Over 22	12.0

If subcutaneous depot insulin has been given prior to labour, the same intravenous fluids may be given without added insulin to prevent hypoglycaemia. When capillary blood glucose values approach 6 mmol/l (indicating waning depot insulin) insulin may be restarted.

POSTNATAL INSULIN REQUIREMENTS

Following delivery, a dramatic fall in insulin requirement is seen almost immediately, particularly if breastfeeding is chosen. Most mothers with gestational diabetes are unlikely to require insulin postnatally, but blood glucose monitoring may be performed for 24–48 h to confirm this. Some of these patients, however, particularly those requiring insulin prior to 20 weeks gestation (suggesting pre-gestational glucose intolerance), and some pre-gestational non-insulin-dependent diabetic patients may remain hyperglycaemic postnatally and require insulin or oral hypoglycaemic therapy, as the case may be, if diet alone fails.

For insulin-dependent diabetic mothers where delivery has been uncomplicated, a subcutaneous insulin regimen at a dose approximating their pre-pregnancy dose or slightly less is reinstituted, perhaps with a supplemental scale in case of hyperglycaemia. In the case of operative delivery ongoing intravenous insulin and dextrose will be required until oral intake is re-established. Regimens similar to either of the two outlined above for labour may be used, and where a combined insulin/dextrose regimen is chosen ⅔th of the total daily *pre-pregnancy* dose should be added to each litre of fluid.

DIABETIC KETOACIDOSIS

Diabetic ketoacidosis may result in fetal losses of up to 25–35%. The cause of fetal death is not known, but appears to be associated with later gestational age, more extreme hyperglycaemia, increased osmolality and biochemical evidence of dehydration, higher insulin requirements and slowness of resolution[37]. Other series suggest that fetal loss occurs predominantly in the first trimester, suggesting hyperglycaemia-induced lethal congenital malformations[38].

This complication is unusual in an intensively managed, well-educated and closely monitored pregnant diabetic subject. The commonest precipitating factors in pregnancy appear to be emesis (often with a background of diabetic gastroenteropathy), the use of tocolytic β-sympathomimetic drugs in premature labour, infection, poor maternal compliance and management error[39,40]. A third of all episodes of ketoacidosis in one series occurred in previously undiagnosed diabetic subjects, and accounted for 57% of all fetal deaths. No fetal losses occurred once treatment had commenced[37].

The management of ketoacidosis in pregnancy differs little from the intensive modern management in insulin-dependent diabetes and is beyond the scope of this chapter. However, certain points should be stressed. Diabetic ketoacidosis should be anticipated in those with a history of diabetic gastroparesis, poor compliance or where tocolytic β-adrenergic agents are used. Careful patient education regarding the symptoms and setting in which ketoacidosis occurs should be given. Monitoring for urinary ketones even in the absence of profound hyperglycaemia should be ensured where symptoms occur. The mother should maintain close contact with the diabetes care team, with early hospitalization; routine 'sick day' regimens are inappropriate in pregnancy. If necessary, rapid, in-hospital institution of therapy with combined medical and obstetrical care should take place. Intravenous and not intramuscular insulin should always be used, wherever possible using a syringe pump.

HYPOGLYCAEMIA

Significant maternal hypoglycaemia has been reported as occurring in 19–41% of pregnant insulin-dependent diabetic women[41], particularly in those with a history of severe hypoglycaemia prior to pregnancy. It occurs principally during the first half of pregnancy[42]. A reduction in insulin dose requirement during the first trimester frequently occurs and should be anticipated. The reason for this increased insulin sensitivity has never been adequately explained and is seen even in the absence both of emesis and of overtreatment prior to the pregnancy. The high incidence of severe hypoglycaemia and of asymptomatic hypoglycaemia may in part be explained by blunted glucagon[43,44], adrenergic[43] and cortisol[44] responses in diabetic pregnancy.

Full and careful education on prevention, recognition and treatment of hypoglycaemia is a prerequisite, especially in those with a history of severe hypoglycaemia. Optimized and individualized insulin regimens are perhaps the most important factor. Maintenance of normal blood glucose levels in the non-diabetic individual obviously requires an exquisitely functioning glucose/insulin counter-regulatory system, and to fully reproduce this in diabetic pregnancy requires a complex insulin regimen to ensure an optimal bolus/basal insulin balance.

Careful monitoring and frequent contact are essential. The dangers of driving whilst hypoglycaemic must be carefully explained and the woman should *always* check her blood glucose prior to driving. Occasionally this problem is severe enough for the physician to advise her not to drive.

Treatment of hypoglycaemia does not differ substantially from insulin-induced hypoglycaemia outside pregnancy. In the conscious state, one exchange (10 g) of rapidly absorbed simple soluble carbohydrate is taken for adrenergic symptoms. Neuroglycopenic symptoms require two exchanges. If symptoms persist for more than 10–15 min, the dose is repeated. In the absence of impending helplessness, hypoglycaemia may be confirmed by blood glucose monitoring, although symptoms may depend on the rate of decline of blood glucose as well as on the absolute value. Symptoms should always be treated. If the reaction occurs within 30 min of a meal, it should be treated and the next insulin injection delayed until after the meal. Asymptomatic hypoglycaemia discovered preprandially should be treated and the insulin dose also delayed.

If unconscious, 1 mg glucagon given subcutaneously or intramuscularly almost anywhere on the body should be administered by appropriately trained family members or friends. This should result in recovery of consciousness within 5–10 min and a second dose can be given if necessary. Following recovery of consciousness two carbohydrate exchanges may be given orally. If a trained professional is present, 25 ml of 50% dextrose may be given intravenously, repeated 5 min later if necessary, which is a more direct and reliable course.

An explanation for the hypoglycaemic attacks should always be sought and corrected. Overadministration of insulin must be assumed if a diet or exercise-related cause cannot be found. Here a reduction in or redistribution of insulin is required. HbA_{1c} and fructosamine levels are a guide to total insulin requirement.

The early post-implantation embryo is dependent on glycolysis for energy and thus theoretically vulnerable to hypoglycaemia. Despite the demonstration of teratogenicity of hypoglycaemia and the interruption of glycolysis in rodent embryos[45,46], no untoward effects have ever been demonstrated in the human, in terms of congenital malformation or fetal mortality, despite a vast clinical experience. Furthermore, controlled studies have failed to demonstrate alteration in fetal heart rate or reactivity in placental blood flow during maternal hypoglycaemia[43,44].

ORAL HYPOGLYCAEMIC AGENTS

Oral hypoglycaemic agents fall broadly into two categories: those that are enterally active such as guar gum and α-glucosidase inhibitors, and those that act systemically, such as sulphonylureas and biguanides.

The enterally active agents function by delaying digestion and/or absorption of nutrients, particularly carbohydrate. Guar gum is a viscous gel-forming polysaccharide which predominantly inhibits convective mixing of intestinal contents, thus inhibiting digestive enzyme and brush border contact with ingested nutrient[47]. Acarbose is a synthetic α-glucosidase inhibitor of poly- and disaccharidases, thus inducing a state of chemical carbohydrate malabsorption. Both agents have been successfully used in both insulin-dependent and non-insulin-dependent patients, where they may blunt postprandial glycaemic excursions or even improve fasting glycaemia[48–51]. No data exist on their use in diabetic pregnancy and they will not be discussed further.

The mode of action of sulphonylureas is to increase beta cell insulin secretion directly as well as enhancing the sensitivity of the beta cell to glucose[52]. The biguanides may reduce glucose absorption by the gut and appear to inhibit hepatic glucose production through a reduction in gluconeogenesis, as well as enhancing tissue insulin sensitivity[52]. Phenformin is no longer generally available and data available in pregnancy are confined to metformin.

Pregnancy is currently regarded as a contraindication to the use of oral hypoglycaemic agents in Western society. However, difficulties in obtaining and managing patients on insulin have enforced their use in many Third World countries. Experience has been gained using both sulphonylureas and metformin particularly in gestational diabetes, but data exist on their inadvertent use in early pregnancy in non-insulin-dependent diabetes.

Apart from efficacy, the chief issue is that of placental transfer to the fetus, which may then have certain consequences, including teratogenicity and congenital anomalies, sulphonylurea-induced fetal hyperinsulinism with macrosomia, or sulphonylurea-induced neonatal hypoglycaemia[53]. The first-generation sulphonylureas (tolbutamide and chlorpropamide) appear to cross the placenta in appreciable amounts, whereas in similar studies using full term human placentae glyburide did not[54,55]. However, during *in vivo* studies, significant amounts of isotopically labelled glyburide, a second-generation sulphonylurea, can be demonstrated in rat fetuses when administered to the mother[56]. Whether or not this is a species-specific feature is unclear. Studies using embryo culture have found tolbutamide, chlorpropamide and phenformin to be teratogenic[57-59] independent of their hypoglycaemic activity, whereas metformin did not cause fetal anomalies.

Earlier studies using first-generation sulphonylureas gave conflicting results, with some suggesting embryotoxicity and others reporting a favourable outcome. However, these data are bedevilled by the confounding influence of the teratogenic potential of poor metabolic control during organogenesis.

An alarming report in 1991 showed a 50% incidence of congenital anomalies in a group of children born to Mexican-American women taking oral hypoglycaemic agents whilst pregnant[60]. However, 25% of the children had anomalies involving the ear, a pattern not normally associated with offspring of diabetic mothers. The authors also found more hyperbilirubinaemia, polycythaemia and hyperviscosity syndrome amongst the exposed infants. The influence of poor metabolic control, however, and the inability to demonstrate a dose-related effect have cast doubt on the causal role of the oral agents in this study[53]. A more recent report of inadvertent consumption of oral agents in early pregnancy showed a more favourable outcome. Here the infants of 25 women who had taken sulphonylureas and/or metformin during organogenesis had no major congenital malformations and only one had a minor anomaly[61].

The issue of teratogenicity does not arise if the use of these drugs is confined to true gestational diabetes. Coetzee in South Africa[62] routinely administers metformin (250 mg twice daily) in dietary failure with subsequent addition of glibenclamide (5 mg twice daily) if necessary. No teratogenesis or severe neonatal hypoglycaemia was found in their series. The rate of macrosomia and other neonatal complications was acceptable. A similar favourable outcome of combined insulin/sulphonylurea use has been reported recently in Israel[63]. Earlier reports of severe neonatal hypoglycaemia involved the use of first-generation sulphonylureas, particularly chlorpropamide[64,65].

Ideally, insulin should be used to control glycaemia in gestational diabetic or non-insulin-dependent diabetic pregnancies where diet and exercise alone are inadequate. Where insulin availability or use is a problem then oral therapy is justified but should be avoided in the organogenetic phase. The value of these drugs either alone or in combination with insulin would appear to be greatest in gestational diabetes. From the point of view of teratogenicity and neonatal hypoglycaemia, only second-generation sulphonylureas (glyburide, glibenclamide) and/or metformin should be used in moderate dosage. Where inadvertent consumption of all oral agents in early pregnancy has taken place, the mother should be switched to insulin where possible and reassured, particularly if glycaemic control has been adequate. Metabolic control both in early and later pregnancy would still appear to be the chief determinant of fetal outcome.

REFERENCES

1 Gabbe SG. Pregnancy in women with diabetes mellitus: the beginning. *Clin Perinatol* 1933; **20**: 507–15.
2 Mintz D, Chez R, Hutchinson D. Sub-human primate pregnancy complicated by streptozotocin-induced diabetes mellitus. *J Clin Invest* 1972; **51**: 837–47.
3 Pedersen J. *The Pregnant Diabetic and her Newborn*, 2nd edn, Williams & Wilkins, Copenhagen, 1977; 211–20.
4 Freinkel N, Metzger B. Pregnancy as a tissue culture experience: the critical implications of maternal metabolism for fetal development. In: *Pregnancy Metabolism, Diabetes and the Fetus*. Ciba Foundation Symposium No. 63 (New Series). Excerpta Medica, Amsterdam, 1979; 3–28.
5 Reece EA, Homko C, Wiznitzer A. Metabolic changes in diabetic and non diabetic subjects during pregnancy. *Obstet Gynecol Surv* 1994; **49**: 64–71.
6 Kalkhoff RK. Impact of maternal fuels and nutritional state on fetal growth. *Diabetes* 1991; **40** (Suppl. 1): 61–5.
7 Peterson CM, Jovanovic-Peterson L, Mills JL *et al*. The diabetes in early pregnancy study: changes in cholesterol, triglycerides, body weight and blood pressure. *Am J Obstet Gynecol* 1992; **166**: 513–18.
8 Reece EA, Coustan R, Sherwin RS *et al*. Does intensive glycaemic control in diabetic pregnancies result in normalisation of other metabolic fuels? *Am J Obstet Gynecol* 1991; **165**: 126–30.
9 National Maternity Hospital, Dublin. Annual Reports 1987–1994.
10 Rasmussen MHJ, Firth R, Foley M, Stronge JM. The timing of delivery in diabetic pregnancy: a 10 year review. *Aust NZ J Obstet Gynaecol* 1992; **32**: 313–17.
11 Lowy C, Beard RW, Goldschmidt J. The UK Diabetic Pregnancy Survey. *Acta Endocrinol* 1986; **277** (Suppl.): 86–9.
12 Scanlan P, Stronge J, Greene AT *et al*. Pregnancy in the clinical diabetic: glycaemic control and outcome. *Diabetologia* 1991; **34** (Suppl. 2): 793.
13 European IDDM Policy Group. Consensus guidelines for management of insulin-dependent (type 1) diabetes. *Diabetic Med* 1993; **10**: 990–1005.
14 Ludvigsson J, Heding L. C-peptide in patients with juvenile diabetes: a preliminary report. *Diabetologia* 1976; **12**: 627–30.
15 Andersen O, Egeberg J. The clinical significance of insulin antibodies. *Acta Paediatr Scand*

1977; Suppl. 270: 63–8.
16 Dickson K, Exon P. Hughes H. Insulin antibodies in etiology of labile diabetes. *Lancet* 1972; i: 343–7.
17 Roy B, Chou M, Field J. Time–action characteristics of regular and NPH insulin in insulin-treated diabetics. *J Clin Endocrinol Metab* 1980; **50**: 475–9.
18 Rosen B, Miodovnik M, Combs CA *et al*. Human vs. animal insulin in the management of insulin dependent diabetes: lack of effect on fetal growth. *Obstet Gynecol* 1991; **78**: 590–3.
19 Jovanovic-Peterson L, Kitzmiller JL, Peterson CM. Randomised trial of human vs. animal species insulin in diabetic pregnant women: improved glycaemic control, not fewer antibodies to insulin, influences birth weight. *Am J Obstet Gynecol* 1992; **167**: 1325–30.
20 Cryer PE. Hypoglycaemia unawareness in IDDM. *Diabetes Care* 1993; **16** (Suppl. 3): 40–7.
21 Litwak LE, Mileo-Vaglio R, Fried T *et al*. Intensified insulin therapy in the management of gestational diabetes. *Medicina* 1992; **52**: 523–33.
22 Mecklenburg R, Benson J Jr, Becker N *et al*. Clinical use of the insulin infusion pump in 100 patients with type 1 diabetes. *N Engl J Med* 1982; **307**: 513–18.
23 American Diabetes Association. Positional statement on jet injector devices. *Diabetes Care* 1988; **11**: 600.
24 Jovanovic-Peterson L, Sparks S, Palmer JP, Peterson CM. Jet-injected insulin is associated with decreased antibody production and postprandial glucose variability when compared with needle-injected insulin in gestational diabetic women. *Diabetes Care* 1993; **16**: 1479–84.
25 Koivisto VA, Gelig P. Effects of exercise on insulin absorption. *N Engl J Med* 1978; **298**: 79–83.
26 Kuhl C. Etiology of gestational diabetes. *Baillieres Clin Obstet Gynaecol* 1991; **5**: 279–92.
27 Jovanovic L, Druzin N, Peterson C. Effect of euglycaemia on the outcome of pregnancy in insulin dependent diabetic women as compared with normal control subjects. *Am J Med* 1981; **71**: 921–7.
28 McManus RM, Ryan EA. Insulin requirements in insulin dependent and insulin requiring GDM women during final month of pregnancy. *Diabetes Care* 1992; **15**: 1323–7.
29 Lauritzen T, Farber O, Binder C. Variation in 125 I-insulin absorption and blood glucose concentrations. *Diabetologia* 1979; **17**: 291–5.
30 Binder C. Absorption of injected insulin. *Acta Pharmacol Toxicol* 1969; **27** (Suppl. 2): 1–86.
31 Diabetes Control and Complications Trial Research Group. The effect of intensive treatment of diabetes on the development and progression of long-term complications in insulin-dependent diabetes mellitus. *N Engl J Med* 1993; **329**: 977–86.
32 Schade DS, Santiago JV, Skyler JS, Rizza RA. *Intensive insulin therapy*. Excerpta Medica, Amsterdam, 1983; 209–11.
33 Bryce FC, Bodansky HJ, Redmond S, Buchan PC. A survey of UK diabetic pregnancy management. *Diabetic Med* 1991; **8**: 382–4.
34 Langer O, Rodriguez DA, Xenakisem EM *et al*. Intensified versus conventional management of gestational diabetes. *Am J Obstet Gynecol* 1994; **170**: 1036–46.
35 Coustan DR. Management of gestational diabetes. *Clin Obstet Gynecol* 1991; **34**: 558–64.
36 Sunehag A, Berne C, Lindmark G, Ewald U. Gestational diabetes: perinatal outcome with a policy of liberal and intensive insulin therapy. *Ups J Med Sci* 1991; **96**: 185–98.
37 Montoro MN, Meyers VP, Mestman JH *et al*. Outcome of pregnancy in diabetic ketoacidosis. *Am J Perinatol* 1993; **10**: 17–20.
38 Kilvert JA, Nicholson HO, Wright AD. Ketoacidosis in diabetic pregnancy. *Diabetic Med* 1993; **10**: 278–81.
39 Rodgers BD, Rodgers DE. Clinical variables associated with diabetic ketoacidosis during pregnancy. *J Reprod Med* 1991; **36**: 797–800.
40 Harvey MG. Diabetic ketoacidosis during pregnancy. *J Perinat Neonatal Nurse* 1992; **6**: 1–13.
41 Persson B, Hansson U. Hypoglycaemia in pregnancy. *Baillieres Clin Endocrinol Metab* 1993; **7**: 731–9.
42 Kimmerle R, Heinemann L, Delecki A, Berger M. Severe hypoglycaemia incidence and predisposing factors in 85 pregnancies of type 1 diabetic women. *Diabetes Care* 1992; **15**: 1034–7.
43 Diamond MP, Reece EA, Caprio S *et al*. Impairment of counterregulatory hormone responses to hypoglycaemia in pregnant women with insulin dependent diabetes mellitus.

Am J Obstet Gynecol 1992; **166**: 70–7.

44 Nisell H, Persson B, Hanson U *et al*. Hormonal, metabolic and circulatory responses to insulin-induced hypoglycaemia in pregnant and non pregnant women with insulin-dependent diabetes. *Am J Perinatol* 1994; **11**: 231–6.

45 Freinkel N, Lewis NJ, Akazawa S *et al*. The honeybee syndrome: implications of the teratogenicity of mannose in rat-embryo culture. *N Engl J Med* 1984; **310**: 223–30.

46 Sadler TW, Hunter ES. Hypoglycaemia: how little is too much for the embryo? *Am J Obstet Gynecol* 1987; **157**: 190–3.

47 Blackburn NA, Redfern JS, Jarjis H *et al*. The mechanism of action of guar gum in improving glucose tolerance in man. *Clin Sci* 1984; **86**: 645–53.

48 Jenkins DJA, Wolever TM, Leeds AR *et al*. Dietary fibres, fibre analogues and glucose tolerance: importance of viscosity. *Br Med J* 1978; **i**: 1992–4.

49 Fuessl HS, Wilkanis G, Adrian TE, Bloom SR. Guar sprinkled on food: effect on glycaemic control, plasma lipids and gut hormones in non insulin dependent diabetes mellitus. *Diabetic Med* 1986; **4**: 463–8.

50 Walton RJ, Sheriff IT, Noy GA, Alberti KGMM. Improved metabolic profiles in insulin-treated diabetic patients given an alpha-glucosidase inhibitor. *Br Med J* 1979; **i**: 220–1.

51 Sachse G, Willms B. Effect of the alpha-glucosidase inhibitor Bay g 5421 on blood glucose control of sulphonylurea-treated diabetics and insulin-treated diabetics. *Diabetologia* 1979; **17**: 287–90.

52 Williams G. Management of NIDDM. *Lancet* 1994; **343**: 95–100.

53 Hod M, Sahfrir E. Oral hypoglycaemic agents as an alternative therapy for gestational diabetes. *Isr J Med Sci* 1995; **31**: 640–3.

54 Elliott B, Langer O, Schenker S *et al*. Insignificant transfer of glyburide occurs across the human placenta. *Am J Obstet Gynecol* 1991; **165**: 807–12.

55 Elliott B, Schenker S, Langer O *et al*. Oral hypoglycaemic agents: profound variation exists in their rate of human placental transfer. *Proceedings of the 13th Annual Meeting of the Society of Perinatal Obstetricians*, San Francisco, February 1993.

56 Sivan E, Feldman B, Dolitzri M *et al*. Glyburide crosses the placenta in vivo in pregnant rats. *Diabetologia* 1993; **38**: 753–6.

57 Smithburg M, Runner MN. Teratogenic effects of hypoglycaemic treatments in inbred strains of mice. *Am J Anat* 1963; **113**: 479–89.

58 Smoak TW. Teratogenic effects of chlorpropamide in mouse embryos in vitro. *Teratology* 1992; **45**: 474.

59 Denno KM, Saddler TW. Effects of the biguanide class of oral hypoglycaemic agents on mouse embryogenesis. *Teratology* 1994; **49**: 260–6.

60 Piacquadio K, Hillingsworth DR, Murphy H. Effects of in-utero exposure to oral hypoglycaemic drugs. *Lancet* 1991; **338**: 866–9.

61 Hellmuth E, Damm P, Mølsted-Pedersen L. Congenital malformations in offspring of diabetic women treated with oral hypoglycaemic agents during embryogenesis. *Diabetic Med* 1994; **11**: 471–4.

62 Coetzee EJ. Oral hypoglycaemic agents in the treatment of gestational diabetes. In: Jovanovic L (ed), *Endocrinology and Metabolism Controversies in Diabetes and Pregnancy*. Springer-Verlag, Berlin, 1988; 57–76.

63 Ravina A. Non-insulin-dependent diabetes of pregnancy treated with the combination of sulfonylurea and insulin. *Isr J Med Sci* 1995; **31**: 623–5.

64 Zucker P, Simon G. Prolonged symptomatic neonatal hypoglycaemia associated with maternal chlorpropamide therapy. *Paediatrics* 1968; **42**: 824–5.

65 Kemball MI, Melver C, Milmer RDG *et al*. Neonatal hypoglycaemia in infants of diabetic mothers given sulphonylurea drugs in pregnancy. *Arch Dis Child* 1970; **45**: 696–701.

8

The Dietary Management of Diabetes and Pregnancy

CAROLINE PIMBLETT

Dulwich Hospital, London, UK

The goals of the dietary management of diabetes in pregnancy are to ensure adequate nutrition to meet the needs of mother and fetus, to maintain blood glucose levels within the normal range, and to ensure an appropriate maternal weight gain. Dieticians base the dietary management of pregnant women with diabetes on the principles of the nutrient requirements of pregnancy combined with the principles of the dietary management of diabetes.

For women with diabetes before pregnancy, pre-pregnancy nutritional assessment and advice from a dietician will help to achieve the best possible diabetes control before conception. To achieve excellent blood glucose control throughout pregnancy it is important that every woman is offered individualized dietary advice and that this is reviewed at frequent intervals as pregnancy progresses.

This chapter is divided into three sections. The first section gives an account of nutrition in normal pregnancy, including energy and protein requirements, and gestational weight gain. The second section describes the dietary recommendations for diabetes and how these apply in pregnancy. The third section looks at some current approaches to the dietary management of the different types of diabetes in pregnancy.

NUTRITION AND NORMAL PREGNANCY

THE ENERGY COST OF PREGNANCY

A theoretical energy cost of pregnancy has been calculated as the sum of the energy involved in all of the changes caused by pregnancy: the

Diabetes and Pregnancy: An International Approach to Diagnosis and Management.
Edited by A. Dornhorst and D. R. Hadden.
© 1996 John Wiley & Sons Ltd.

production of the fetus and the placenta, increased mass of maternal organs, increased blood volume, deposition of maternal adipose tissue, increased maternal basal metabolic rate, and the higher energy cost of movement of the heavier mother. Hytten and Leitch calculated the theoretical energy cost for the whole of pregnancy as 334 MJ (80 000 kcal)[1]. Until recently, international recommendations for energy intake in pregnancy have been derived from these theoretical calculations. For example, in 1985 a joint FAO/WHO/UNU Expert Consultation on Energy and Protein Requirements stated that the extra energy costs of pregnancy (i.e. 334 MJ) should be met by an average addition to the daily food intake of 1190 kJ per day (285 kcal per day). This was reduced to 840 kJ per day (200 kcal per day) if women were to reduce energy expended in physical activity[2]. Investigations into actual energy intake during pregnancy have rarely demonstrated an increase to parallel these theoretical increased requirements. There are two possible ways that women could modify the energy cost of pregnancy to explain this apparent discrepancy; they could reduce their physical activity or they could make energy-sparing metabolic adaptations.

A longitudinal study of the energy requirements of pregnant women from five countries (Scotland, the Netherlands, the Gambia, Thailand and the Philippines), living under very different environmental and socioeconomic circumstances, has made important contributions to our understanding of the energy requirements of pregnancy[3-5]. Measurement of the average total energy cost of pregnancy in well-nourished Dutch and Scottish women by indirect calorimetry found it to be 288 MJ (69 000 kcal), a figure only slightly less than the theoretical calculation of Hytten and Leitch. Whilst the women showed a steady increase in basal metabolic rate from around the 16th week of gestation, reaching approximately 1670 kJ per day (400 kcal per day) in the final stages of pregnancy, actual extra dietary energy intake was in the order of only 420 kJ per day (100 kcal per day) during the second and third trimesters. Small, but hard to detect, reductions in physical activity might account for the difference between the actual extra energy intake and the measured energy costs of pregnancy[3].

A study of the energy balance of Dutch women before and during pregnancy found an increase in 24 h energy expenditure at weeks 12, 23 and 34 of gestation to an extent that was predictable from changes in resting metabolic rate and concluded that in these women there was little scope for adaptive metabolic mechanisms[6]. However, there is some evidence to suggest energy-sparing metabolic adaptations even in well-nourished pregnant women. Twenty-four-hour whole body calorimetry found that some pregnant women showed a highly significant depression of metabolism up to 24 weeks of gestation, a finding in support of an energy-sparing adaptation, whereas other women showed no such response[7]. An important fact demonstrated by this study is that the metabolic response to pregnancy varies widely between individuals.

Energy-sparing adaptations to pregnancy are likely to have a greater bearing on the outcome of pregnancy in women living under the constraints of limited food supply and physical hard work. Using direct calorimetry in pregnant Gambian women with strictly controlled levels of physical activity it has been shown that basal metabolic rate can adapt to meet the energy cost of pregnancy[8]. It would seem that, unable to increase her food supply or decrease her physical work, and with little in the way of fat reserves to mobilize, the only 'option' for the Gambian woman to meet the energy cost of pregnancy is to depress her basal metabolic rate.

In summary, energy metabolism differs enormously among pregnant women, and this variation is largely, but not exclusively, dependent on their pre-pregnancy nutritional status, and food availability and physical activity during pregnancy. It would seem that no extra dietary energy may be required by the malnourished woman, whereas the well-nourished woman may have an extra energy requirement of several thousand kilojoules per day above her pre-pregnancy requirement. However, two women of similar nutritional status from the same socioeconomic background can show very different metabolic responses to pregnancy. This variability makes it difficult to advise the individual woman on her diet during pregnancy and has implications for governments and nutritional agencies setting nutritional recommendations for a population. For example, in 1991 the UK Committee on Medical Aspects of Food Policy (COMA) published *Dietary Reference Values for Food Energy and Nutrients for the United Kingdom*[9]. COMA considered the evidence and concluded that the true additional dietary energy requirement of pregnancy under the conditions prevailing in Western societies is probably modest. However, they warned that caution should be exercised in coming to such a conclusion because of the apparent disparity between the calculations and the experimental findings. They agreed that pregnant women should be recommended to take an additional 0.8 MJ per day (200 kcal per day) only during the last trimester, but that women who are underweight at the beginning of pregnancy, and those who do not reduce activity, may need more.

WEIGHT GAIN IN PREGNANCY

A review of the determinants and consequences of gestational weight gain was undertaken by the US Institute of Medicine in 1990[10]. In general, the strongest determinant of gestational weight gain is pre-pregnancy body mass index (BMI) (weight/height^2)—women who are overweight at conception tend to gain less weight than do thinner women. A range of other maternal characteristics (e.g. age, race, socioeconomic status) may act together to influence weight gain.

On the consequences of gestational weight gain, the US Institute of Medicine found a large body of evidence to indicate that weight gain, particularly in the second and third trimesters, is an important determinant of fetal growth. Low gestational weight gain is associated with an increased risk of giving birth to an infant with a low birth weight. Very high weight gain is associated with a high birth weight (macrosomia), which may have adverse consequences for mother and infant[11,12]. The effect of gestational weight gain on fetal growth is modified by the nutritional status of the mother; the effect of a given weight gain is greatest in thin women. Among obese women, the measured effect of weight gain on birth weight is very weak. Above and beyond any effect of gestational weight gain, pre-pregnancy weight is a determinant of fetal growth; women who are thinner before pregnancy tend to have babies that are smaller than heavier women with the same gestational weight gain.

As a result of this review the US Institute of Medicine made recommendations for weight gain in pregnancy on the basis of pre-pregnancy weight for height. It recommended that underweight women with a pre-pregnancy BMI < 19.8 should gain 12.5–18 kg, normal weight women with a BMI 19.8–26.0 should gain 11.5–16 kg, and overweight women with a BMI > 26.0–29.0 should gain 7–11.5 kg. A lower limit on gestational weight gain of 6.8 kg was set for obese women with a pre-pregnancy BMI of > 29.0, although it was acknowledged that many obese women with good pregnancy outcomes gain less than 6.8 kg (Table 8.1). On the rate of weight gain, women with a normal pre-pregnancy weight were recommended to gain weight at a rate of approximately 0.4 kg per week in the second and third trimesters of pregnancy. Underweight women were recommended to gain at a slightly higher rate and overweight women at a slightly lower rate.

Much of the variation in gestational weight gain is due to variation in the amount of fat that women deposit during the course of pregnancy. Fat deposition occurs primarily in the second trimester of pregnancy and is thought to provide an energy reserve for later pregnancy when the energy demands of the fetus are greatest, and for lactation. Based on an average gestational weight gain of 12.5 kg, the theoretical amount of fat that a

Table 8.1. Recommended weight gains for pregnant women[a]

Weight for height category	Recommended weight gain (kg)
Low (BMI < 19.8)	12.5–18.0
Normal (BMI 19.8–26.0)	11.5–16.0
High (BMI > 26.0–29.0)	7.0–11.5

[a]Young adolescents and black women should strive for gains at the upper end of the recommended range. Short women (< 157 cm) should strive for gains at the lower end of the range. The target gain for obese women (BMI > 29.0) is at least 6.8 kg.
Reprinted with permission from *Nutrition During Pregnancy*. Copyright 1990 by the National Academy of Sciences. Courtesy of the National Academy Press, Washington, DC.

women will gain is 3–4 kg[13]. Gestational weight gain and fat deposition are correlated in studies of well-nourished women in developed countries, which suggests that large weight gains during pregnancy increase the risk of women laying down excess deposits of fat that may increase the risk of obesity in the future[14].

With the observation of the US Institute of Medicine that amongst obese women the measured effect of weight gain is weak, and the acknowledgement that many obese women with good pregnancy outcomes gain less than 6.8 kg, one is led to ask whether an obese women who becomes pregnant should be advised to restrict her energy intake during the second and third trimesters of her pregnancy to lessen the amount of fat that she lays down. This question has been the subject of considerable controversy. Epidemiological studies in the UK that have suggested that poor maternal nutrition results in small infants with increased risk of disease later in life[14] have added to concerns about possible effects of restricting maternal nutrition on fetal growth. However, the lower birth weights in these studies reflected poor maternal nutrition both before and during pregnancy, which cannot be likened to a mild energy restriction for obese mothers in the latter months of pregnancy. There are also concerns that energy restriction may promote maternal ketosis, with potential teratogenic effects of maternal ketonaemia. A study correlating measures of metabolism in pregnant diabetic and non-diabetic women with intellectual development in their offspring found an association between maternal gestational ketonaemia and lower IQ in the child[16]. The degree of energy restriction has been shown to be important in preventing maternal ketosis[17]. Research must continue to show the effects of energy restriction on the obese pregnant woman and her child.

Health professionals have a strong influence over the amount of weight that women gain during pregnancy[18] and so pregnant women must be given unambiguous messages about weight gain. There is obviously a wide range of weight gains that result in good pregnancy outcome. Dietary energy restriction in the normal-weight mother should be avoided, and normal weight women who try to restrict their weight gain should be warned of the possible harm to their child. Women who are overweight at conception should be warned against severe 'dieting' but should be encouraged to gain less weight than thinner women.

THE PROTEIN REQUIREMENTS OF PREGNANCY

The protein requirements of pregnancy are calculated to allow for protein retained in the products of conception and in the growth of maternal tissues. The 1985 FAO/WHO/UNU expert consultation gave a recommendation for the protein requirements of pregnant women of an additional 6 g per day of high-quality protein throughout pregnancy[2]. The quality of a protein food is determined by its content of amino acids; proteins that contain all the essential amino acids in sufficient amounts to support growth or maintain nutritional status are termed high-quality proteins. To apply the recommendation to populations obtaining protein from mixed diets the amount is adjusted to allow for the digestibility of the diet and for the quality of the protein consumed. For the typical Western diet, based on refined cereals, a correction of 95% is applied for digestibility, but the amino acid profile is such that no correction for protein quality is required[9]. For diets that contain considerable amounts of unrefined cereals and vegetables, and diets that contain only a limited selection of low-quality protein foods, then greater correction factors are applied.

For women of childbearing age the WHO recommended daily protein intake is 45 g. Adding the recommended increment of 6 g during pregnancy this figure rises to 51 g. Studies of the actual diets of pregnant women in the UK have consistently shown that UK women consume in excess of this amount[19–21]. The recommendation that pregnant women need an extra 6 g of protein per day above their pre-pregnancy requirements assumes that protein metabolism remains unaltered. This assumption has been questioned following work that discovered that the pregnant rat has protein-sparing metabolic adaptations[22]. If women were to be shown to demonstrate such adaptations then the protein requirement of pregnancy may be less than that currently recommended[23].

DIETARY RECOMMENDATIONS FOR PEOPLE WITH DIABETES AND HOW THEY APPLY IN PREGNANCY

INTRODUCTION

The dietary management of diabetes has a history that can be traced back over many centuries. The major changes in management strategy have centred around the percentage of the total dietary energy that should be derived from carbohydrate. Traditionally diabetes was managed using diets low in carbohydrate, which inevitably resulted in much of the dietary energy being provided by fat. Such diets were eventually seen to conflict with the evolving nutritional recommendations for the general population. It is no longer believed that a carbohydrate-restricted diet is necessary to achieve good diabetes control. In the late 1970s and early 1980s both the British and American Diabetic Associations published policy statements on nutrition which marked the abandoning of carbohydrate-restricted diets for people with diabetes, recommending instead a diet restricted in fat and higher in complex carbohydrate and fibre[24,25]. Later updated versions of these policy statements have upheld most of the earlier recommendations[26,27]. Essentially similar policies have been introduced by many other countries, for example by the Nutrition Study Group of the European Association for the Study of Diabetes[28].

ENERGY AND OVERWEIGHT

The most fundamental aspect of the dietary treatment of diabetes is to ensure an appropriate energy intake. Achieving an appropriate long-term energy intake probably has the greatest dietary influence on diabetes control.

About 75% of people newly diagnosed with non-insulin-dependent diabetes are overweight[29,30]. In the short term, energy restriction in the overweight non-insulin-dependent diabetic subject rapidly leads to improved blood sugar control even before any substantial loss in weight has occurred[31]. Although the amount of weight loss necessary to normalize blood glucose is often very large, weight loss has been shown to be the only treatment that improves the life expectancy of the overweight non-insulin-dependent patient[29].

The energy requirements for normal pregnancy have been described in full above and equally apply to the pregnant woman with diabetes. The use of dietary energy restriction as a management strategy for gestational diabetes is discussed later.

COMPLEX CARBOHYDRATE AND FAT

The diabetic diet is now relatively high in carbohydrate foods, with carbohydrate contributing about half of the total dietary energy. Most of this carbohydrate should come from complex sources, and preferably from foods high in dietary fibre. The inclusion of foods rich in cereal fibre (found in whole-grain cereal foods) and soluble fibre (found largely in fruit, vegetables and pulses) in the diets of people with diabetes has small but detectable blood glucose-lowering effects. Soluble fibre has the additional benefit of improving the blood lipid profile[32].

The relative glycaemic responses following the ingestion of different carbohydrate foods are classified as glycaemic indices[33]. Factors that influence the glycaemic index of a food include its fibre content, but there are many other possible influences, such as the physical form of the food (e.g. boiled versus mashed potatoes). There has been debate about whether the glycaemic index of an individual food changes when taken as part of a mixed meal, but it has now been demonstrated that the glycaemic index of a mixed meal reflects the individual glycaemic indices of the carbohydrates that make up that meal[33]. There may, therefore, be beneficial effects on blood glucose control of recommending low glycaemic index staple carbohydrate foods.

Respected reports have recommended a stringent dietary fat restriction to below 30% of total energy for individuals at high risk of ischaemic vascular disease, which would include people with diabetes. Indeed, the general dietary recommendation for the US population is to decrease total dietary fat to 30% or less of energy, although pregnant and lactating women and children under two years of age are excluded from this recommendation[34,35]. The main aim of these recommendations to restrict total fat intake is to reduce the intake of saturated fat, regarded as an important goal to reduce the risk of cardiovascular disease. A reduction in saturated fat intake to below 10% of total energy is recommended for people with diabetes[26-28]. Indeed, a reduction in saturated fat has been described as the most important dietary change for people with diabetes, particularly those with non-insulin-dependent diabetes[26].

A diet deriving less than 30% of energy from fat is by nature a diet that derives most of its energy from carbohydrate. There is some evidence that in people with diabetes some very high-carbohydrate diets can worsen glycaemic control and have deleterious effects on blood lipid levels[36,37]. Controversy has therefore arisen over whether a reduction in saturated fat energy should be replaced by carbohydrate, unsaturated (mono-unsaturated and poly-unsaturated) fat or both. In recent years the potential benefits of diets rich in mono-unsaturated fat have been investigated and people with diabetes are being increasingly encouraged to eat fats rich in mono-unsaturates (e.g. olive oil) in place of some saturated fat. Very high intakes of poly-unsaturated fats are discouraged because of the potentially damaging effects of an increased production of lipid peroxidases[38].

There are some variations in the recommendations made by international diabetes organizations regarding the actual percentage of dietary fat, but all are based on a compromise between the above considerations. For example, the British Diabetic Association[26] recommends that dietary fat should be restricted to below 35% of total energy, with no more than 10% from saturates, 10% from poly-unsaturates and the remainder from mono-unsaturates. The American Diabetes Association recommends that normal-weight individuals with normal lipid levels should consume less than 30% of energy from fat, but adjusts this recommendation for the overweight and those with hyperlipidaemia[27]. In practice, the advice to an individual regarding fat intake should always take into account blood lipid levels, blood glucose control, desirable energy intake, and cultural and individual food preferences.

As regards the pregnant woman with diabetes, diets that are relatively high in carbohydrate and low in fat have a nutrient density at least as good as a traditional British diet. Very low-fat diets (less than 30% fat) are not recommended because of a possible risk of nutrient deficiency, particularly essential fatty acids and fat-soluble vitamins. Today's dietary advice for people with diabetes shares much in common with the healthy eating guidelines advocated for the whole population. During pregnancy women have frequent contact with health professionals and may be motivated towards making health-related changes to their lifestyle. Pregnancy may therefore be an appropriate time to offer women dietary advice that may have beneficial effects on their own and their families' long-term health.

SUGAR AND SWEETENERS

In recent years recommendations regarding refined sugars have relaxed. Scientific evidence shows that the use of moderate amounts of sucrose does not impair blood glucose control in people with diabetes. Very high sucrose intakes may contribute to the development of obesity and hyperlipidaemia. A moderate daily consumption of sucrose, as recommended in healthy eating guidelines for the general population, is acceptable for people with diabetes provided that it is taken as part of a diet low in fat and high in dietary fibre and is substituted for other foods in the diet of an equal energy value[26]. Even so, care must be taken in how this message is presented to people with diabetes since many of the general population currently have higher than recommended sucrose intakes.

Fructose is a sweet-tasting monosaccharide found in fruit, vegetables and honey. It produces a smaller rise in blood glucose than does an isocaloric amount of sucrose and so has traditionally been used as a sucrose substitute in diabetic diets. With the relaxation of the sucrose restriction there is now no reason to recommend fructose in place of sucrose. Other nutritive sweeteners include sugar alcohols (polyols) such as sorbitol, which also produce a lower glycaemic response than sucrose. Again, there would seem to be no advantage of the sugar alcohols over sucrose, and excessive amounts may have a laxative effect. Non-nutritive sweeteners (such as saccharin, aspartame and acesulfame K) are commonly consumed by people with diabetes, especially in 'low-calorie' soft drinks and for sweetening beverages. Acceptable daily limits for intakes of these individual compounds are determined, and although it is unlikely that an individual would approach these daily limits, people who consume a lot should use a mixture[26]. Women will frequently enquire as to the safety of non-nutritive sweeteners during pregnancy. Current scientific evidence suggests that consumption of these compounds within the acceptable daily limits has no harmful effects on mother or fetus[27].

PROTEIN

A restriction of dietary protein has been shown to reduce albuminuria and maintain glomerular filtration rate in early diabetic nephropathy[39]. However, despite considerable research interest, the question of the possible effects of dietary protein intake on the development of diabetic nephropathy remains uncertain. Although the evidence for a beneficial effect of a general protein restriction for people with diabetes is weak, it would seem sensible to recommend that they avoid a higher than average intake of protein. As discussed earlier, the protein requirements of pregnancy are easily met by a mixed diet with an average protein intake.

METHODS OF DIETARY PRESCRIPTION

For all people with diabetes it is important to have a regular meal pattern with total food intake distributed throughout the day. For those treated with insulin (and some oral hypoglycaemic agents) a regular eating pattern is essential to prevent hypoglycaemia. Regular meals and snacks containing complex carbohydrate are required to balance the peak action of extrinsic insulin to minimize the risk of hypoglycaemia.

Specific advice about the total amount and type of carbohydrate and its distribution across the daily meals should be tailored for each individual according to nutritional requirements and metabolic control. People must have some understanding of the relative amounts of carbohydrate contained in different foods if they are to adapt their diets to eat approximately the same amount of carbohydrate at the same time each day. Simple meal planning advice based on household measures of food is usually sufficient to ensure an appropriate distribution of carbohydrate foods across meals and snacks. People taking insulin should be taught how to adapt their insulin doses and/or food intake according to different circumstances, such as planned changes from their normal exercise pattern.

Multiple daily insulin injections allow for greater flexibility in food intake and exercise patterns. People can be taught to adjust pre-meal insulin doses to compensate for the effects of exercise or deviations from their usual food intake, and to delay pre-meal insulin to cope with meals that are late.

CURRENT APPROACHES TO THE DIETARY MANAGEMENT OF DIFFERENT TYPES OF DIABETES IN PREGNANCY

The general dietary principles for diabetes are applicable to women who already have, or who develop, insulin-dependent diabetes during pregnancy, to those who are known to have non-insulin-dependent diabetes before pregnancy, and to those who develop gestational diabetes. In each case the dietary management needs to be adapted to the different metabolic changes that are characteristic of the different type of diabetes during pregnancy. Some of the special dietary considerations and different points of emphasis for the different types of diabetes in pregnancy are described below.

INSULIN-DEPENDENT DIABETES

Within the first weeks of pregnancy, often before a woman realizes that she is pregnant, a previously well-controlled woman with insulin-dependent diabetes may note uncharacteristically low blood glucose values and even symptoms of hypoglycaemia. This signifies the early metabolic change to pregnancy causing increased tissue sensitivity to insulin.

By the middle of the first trimester women may experience increased excursions in blood glucose levels, and mild to severe episodes of hypoglycaemia. This problem may be further compounded by the nausea characteristic of early pregnancy, with or without vomiting. Even mild nausea and changes in appetite may decrease food intake and affect the timing of meals. During this period women are recommended to take small, frequent meals throughout the day, selecting foods that they find acceptable. Early pregnancy is also often characterized by an extreme feeling of tiredness leading to reduced physical activity. These deviations from normal daily routine and food intake must be taken into account and insulin doses adjusted accordingly.

For most women a daily meal pattern of three meals with a snack between meals is the most satisfactory. A bedtime snack is recommended to decrease the risk of overnight hypoglycaemia and fasting ketosis. A consistent meal pattern with frequent self-monitoring of blood glucose will aid judgement when making fine adjustments to the insulin regimen.

NON-INSULIN-DEPENDENT DIABETES

Women who are known to have non-insulin-dependent diabetes before pregnancy, whether treated by diet alone or with oral hypoglycaemic agents, will normally receive insulin treatment for the course of pregnancy. The US Institute of Medicine recommendation of a lower weight gain for women who start their pregnancy overweight includes overweight women with diabetes[10]. Since most of these women are overweight at conception particular attention should be paid to prevent excessive weight gain.

GESTATIONAL DIABETES

Obesity is a recognized risk factor for the development of gestational diabetes. In practice, because gestational diabetes is most often detected beyond 20 weeks gestation, some women will have already gained in excess of the total recommended weight gain before they come to the attention of the diabetes team. The policy of some diabetes centres to advocate an energy restriction for women with gestational diabetes is discussed below.

There is some controversy about the dietary management of women with gestational diabetes. This controversy has probably arisen because there is no one 'best' dietary strategy. Gestational diabetes has been described as a heterogeneous syndrome, with thin women being insulin deficient relative to the metabolic stress of pregnancy, while overweight women may have normal, elevated, or decreased plasma levels of insulin and varying degrees of insulin resistance. This heterogeneity has been offered as an explanation for the differing metabolic responses of women with gestational diabetes to test meals[40]. A study has shown a high correlation between the percentage of carbohydrate (33–55%) in a mixed meal and postprandial glycaemic response in women with gestational diabetes, which varied between individuals and according to the time of the day that the meal was eaten[41]. These results emphasize the potential hazard of giving a standard dietary prescription to women with gestational diabetes and the need to validate any dietary prescription with blood glucose monitoring. The diet should be regularly reviewed and adjusted as pregnancy progresses.

Energy Restriction and Gestational Diabetes

Energy-restricted diets are used in the treatment of gestational diabetes[42], although this line of treatment is controversial, with some authorities expressing the previously described concerns about the safety of energy restriction in pregnancy. Furthermore, there is no general agreement on how severely energy should be restricted, or how this treatment regimen compares to treatment with insulin[17].

Dornhorst and colleagues used a dietary energy intake of 5.02–7.52 MJ per day; 80–130 kJ/kg (1200–1800 kcal per day; 20–30 kcal/kg) in women with gestational diabetes, discouraging weight gain after 28 weeks gestation, to reduce the incidence of macrosomia to that of the non-diabetic population. This level of energy restriction did not result in babies small for gestational age even though mean weight gains after 28 weeks gestation were less than 2 kg[42].

Investigation of the metabolic effects of 6.92 MJ per day and 5.02 MJ per day (1655 kcal per day and 1200 kcal per day) diets in obese women with gestational diabetes found a greater improvement in glycaemic control associated with both levels of energy restriction compared with women treated with insulin. The energy-restricted groups, but not the insulin-treated group, showed reductions in plasma triglyceride concentrations. Plasma triglycerides are elevated in gestational diabetes and are strongly associated with fetal macrosomia[17].

The level of energy restriction imposed is important in the avoidance of maternal ketosis. The above trial of a 5.02 MJ per day (1200 kcal per day) diet in obese pregnant women with gestational diabetes showed an improvement in glycaemic control but this was accompanied by a significant increase in ketonaemia and ketonuria[43]. In contrast, the 6.92 MJ per day (1655 kcal per day) diet was effective in improving maternal metabolic parameters without marked ketonuria[17]. There remain unresolved concerns about the possible teratogenic effects of maternal ketosis. The report of the association of maternal third trimester ketonaemia with reduced intelligence scores of their offspring in early childhood underlines the need for further research into the optimal dietary treatment of gestational diabetes[16]

Women who develop gestational diabetes are known to be at increased risk of developing non-insulin-dependent diabetes later in life[44]. There may be particular benefit to these women of continuing to follow the dietary advice given during pregnancy to maintain a healthy body weight which may delay the later onset of diabetes[45].

Exercise and Gestational Diabetes

Physical exercise is associated with lower plasma insulin concentrations and increased sensitivity to insulin in skeletal muscle and adipose tissue of people with non-insulin-dependent diabetes. To maintain these changes individuals are required to exercise at least every other day. When no exercise is performed for 24 h glucose tolerance shows a significant decline[46].

Recent research has investigated whether exercise is a useful treatment for women wiith gestational diabetes. Supervised exercise programmes have been shown to improve maternal glucose tolerance when used as an adjunct to dietary treatment and have the potential to obviate the need for insulin treatment[47]. On the basis of this research, women with gestational diabetes can be recommended to undertake supervised exercise programmes provided that they have no medical or obstetric contraindications[27].

High-fibre Diets and Gestational Diabetes

Whilst pregnant women in the Western world have a worsening glucose tolerance during pregnancy, this effect is not seen in African women who traditionally obtain a greater proportion of their dietary energy from carbohydrate and have a higher fibre intake[48]. This observation prompted trials to discover the metabolic effects of high-fibre diets in pregnant women with and without diabetes. Some studies have shown that very high fibre intakes prevent the loss of insulin sensitivity in the third trimester of pregnancy and so improve glucose tolerance[49,50]. However, not all studies have shown an improvement in glucose tolerance with very high fibre intakes. A recent study that used a commercially available fibre drink to supplement the fibre intake of women with gestational diabetes showed no improvement in glucose control[51].

The general recommendation for all people with diabetes is that they should consume about half of their dietary energy from carbohydrate foods, especially complex carbohydrates rich in dietary fibre. Achievement of this recommendation means a considerable change in eating habits for many people. Whilst women with gestational diabetes are to be encouraged to choose foods rich in dietary fibre, it is unrealistic to expect women to comply with the very high fibre intakes prescribed to some research subjects.

REFERENCES

1 Hytten FE, Leitch I. *The Physiology of Human Pregnancy*, 2nd edn. Blackwell Scientific, Oxford, 1971.
2 FAO/WHO/UNU (Food and Agriculture Organization/World Health Organization/United Nations University) Expert Consultation. *Energy and Protein Requirements*. Technical Report Series No. 724. World Health Organization, Geneva, 1985.

3 Durnin JVGA. Energy requirements of pregnancy. *Diabetes* 1991; 40 (Suppl. 2): 152–6.
4 Durnin JVGA. Energy requirements of pregnancy: an integration of the longitudinal data from the five-country study. *Lancet* 1987; **ii**: 1131–3.
5 Durnin JVGA, Grant S, McKillop FM, Fitzgerald G. Maternal and child health. *Lancet* 1985; **ii**: 823–5.
6 de Groot LCPGM, Boekholt HA, Spaaiji CJK *et al.* Energy balances of healthy Dutch women before and during pregnancy. Limited scope for metabolic adaptations in pregnancy. *Am J Clin Nutr* 1994; **59**: 827–32.
7 Prentice AM, Goldberg GR, Davies HL *et al.* Energy sparing adaptations in human pregnancy assessed by whole body calorimetry. *Br J Nutr* 1989; **62**: 5–22.
8 Poppit SA, Prentice AM, Jequier *et al.* Evidence of energy sparing in Gambian women during pregnancy: a longitudinal study using whole-body calorimetry. *Am J Clin Nutr* 1993; **57**: 353–64.
9 Department of Health. *Dietary Reference Values for Food Energy and Nutrients for the United Kingdom.* Report on Health and Social Subjects 41. HMSO, London, 1991.
10 Institute of Medicine. *Nutrition During Pregnancy.* National Academy Press, Washington, 1990.
11 Naeye RL. Weight gain and outcome of pregnancy. *Am J Obstet Gynecol* 1979; **135**: 3–9.
12 Boyd ME, Usher RH, McLean FH. Fetal macrosomia: prediction risks, proposed management. *Obstet Gynecol* 1983; **61**: 715–22.
13 Hytten FE. Weight gain in pregnancy. In: Hytten FE, Chamberlain GVP (eds), *Clinical Physiology in Obstetrics.* 2nd edn. Blackwell Scientific, Oxford, 1991; 173–203.
14 King JC, Butte NF, Bronstein MN *et al.* Energy metabolism during pregnancy: influence of maternal energy status. *Am J Clin Nutr* 1994; **59** (Suppl.): 439s–45s.
15 Barker DJP (ed.). *Fetal and Infant Origins of Adult Disease.* British Medical Journal, London, 1992.
16 Rizzo T, Metzger BE, Burns WJ, Burns K. Correlations between antepartum maternal metabolism and intelligence of offspring. *N Engl J Med* 1991; **325**: 911–16.
17 Knopp RH, Magee MS, Raisys V, Benedetti T. Metabolic effects of hypocaloric diets in management of gestational diabetes. *Diabetes* 1991; **40** (Suppl. 2): 165–71.
18 Taffel SM, Keppel KG, Jones GK. Medical advice on maternal weight gain and actual weight gain: results from the 1988 National Maternal and Infant Health Survey. *Ann NY Acad Sci* 1993; **678**: 293–316.
19 Black AE, Wiles SJ, Paul AA. The nutrient intakes of pregnant and lactating mothers of good socio-economic status in Cambridge, UK: some implications for recommended daily allowances of minor nutrients. *Br J Nutr* 1986; **56**: 59–72.
20 Doyle W, Crawford MA, Laurance BM, Drury P. Dietary survey during pregnancy in a low socio-economic group. *Hum Nutr Appl Nutr* 1982; **36A**: 95–106.
21 Anderson AS, Lean MEJ. Dietary intake in pregnancy: a comparison between 49 Cambridge women and current recommended intake. *Hum Nutr Appl Nutr* 1986: **40A**: 40–8.
22 Naismith DJ. Protein metabolism in pregnancy. In: Philipp EE, Barnes J, Newton M (eds), *Scientific Foundations of Obstetrics and Gynaecology.* Heinemann, London, 1977; 503–27.
23 Hytten FE. Nutrition. In: Hytten FE, Chamberlain GVP (eds), *Clinical Physiology in Obstetrics.* 2nd edn. Blackwell Scientific, Oxford, 1991; 150–72.
24 British Diabetic Association: Nutrition Subcommittee. Dietary recommendations for diabetics for the 1980s. *Hum Nutr Appl Nutr* 1982; **36A**: 378–94.
25 American Diabetes Association. Principles of nutrition and dietary recommendations for individuals with diabetes mellitus. *Diabetes* 1979; **28**: 1027–50.
26 British Diabetic Association: Nutrition Subcommittee. *Dietary Recommendations for People with Diabetes: An Update for the 1990s.* Diabet Med 1992; **9**: 189–202.
27 American Diabetes Association. Nutritional principles for the management of diabetes and related complications. *Diabetes Care* 1994; **17**: 490–518.
28 European Association for the Study of Diabetes, Nutrition Study Group. Nutritional recommendations for individuals with diabetes mellitus. *Diabetes Nutr Metab* 1988; **1**: 145–9.
29 Lean MEJ, Powrie JK, Anderson AS, Garthwaite PH. Obesity, weight loss and prognosis in type 2 diabetes. *Diabetic Med* 1990; **7**: 228–33.

30 Salans LB. Obesity and non-insulin-dependent diabetes mellitus. In: Berry EM, Blondheim SH, Eliahou HE, Shafrir E (eds), *Recent Advances in Obesity Research*, Vol. V. John Libby, London, 1987; 26–32.

31 Baumann WA, Schwartz E, Rose HG *et al.* Early and long-term effects of acute caloric deprivation in obese diabetic subjects. *Am J Med* 1988; **85**: 38–46.

32 Vinik AI, Jenkins DJA. Dietary fibre in the management of diabetes. *Diabetes Care* 1988; **11**: 160–73.

33 Frost G, Wilding J, Beecham J. Dietary advice based on the glycaemic index improves dietary profile and metabolic control in Type 2 diabetes. *Diabet Med* 1994; **11**: 297–301.

34 James WPT, Ferro-Luzzi A, Izaksson B, Szostak WB. *Healthy Nutrition*. WHO Regional Publications No. 24. World Health Organization, Copenhagen, 1988.

35 Expert Panel on Detection, Evaluation and Treatment of High Blood Cholesterol in Adults. Summary of the second report of the national cholesterol education program (NCEP) expert panel on detection, evaluation and treatment of high blood cholesterol in adults. *JAMA* 1993; **269**: 3015–23.

36 Coulston AM, Hollenbeck CB, Swislocki ALM *et al.* Deleterious metabolic affects of high carbohydrate containing diets in patients with non insulin dependent diabetes. *Am J Med* 1987; **82**: 213–20.

37 Reaven G. Dietary therapy for non-insulin-dependent diabetes mellitus. *N Engl J Med* 1988; **319**: 862–4.

38 Stringer MD, Gorog PG, Freeman A, Kakkar VV. Lipid peroxides and atherosclerosis. *Br Med J* 1989; **298**: 281–98.

39 Viberti GC. Low-protein diet and progression of diabetic kidney disease. *Nephrol Dial Transplant* 1988; **3**: 334–9.

40 Hollingsworth DR, Ney DM. The dietary management of diabetes during pregnancy. In: Reece EA, Coustan DR (eds), *Diabetes Mellitus in Pregnancy: Principles and Practice*. Churchill Livingstone, Edinburgh, 1988; 285–311.

41 Peterson CM, Jovanovic-Peterson L. Percentage of carbohydrate and glycemic response to breakfast, lunch, and dinner in women with gestational diabetes. *Diabetes* 1991; **40** (Suppl. 2): 172–4.

42 Dornhorst A, Nicholls JSD, Probst F *et al.* Calorie restriction for treatment of gestational diabetes. *Diabetes* 1991; **40** (Suppl. 2): 161–4.

43 Magee MS, Knopp RH, Benedetti TJ. Metabolic effects of 1200-kcal diet in obese pregnant women with gestational diabetes. *Diabetes* 1990; **39**: 234–40.

44 Dornhorst A, Bailey PC, Anyaoku V *et al.* Abnormalities of glucose tolerance following gestational diabetes. *Q J Med* 1990; **284**: 1219–28.

45 O'Sullivan JB. Body weight and subsequent diabetes mellitus. *JAMA* 1982; **248**: 947–52.

46 Miller WJ, Sherman WM, Ivy JL. Effect of strength training on glucose tolerance and post-glucose insulin response. *Med Sci Sprots Exerc* 1984; **16**: 539–43.

47 Jovanovic-Peterson L, Peterson CM. Is exercise safe or useful for gestational diabetic women? *Diabetes* 1991; **40** (Suppl. 2): 179–81.

48 Fraser RB. The effect of pregnancy on the normal range of the glucose tolerance test in Africans. *E Afr Med J* 1985; **58**: 90–5.

49 Fraser RB, Ford FA, Lawrence GF. Insulin sensitivity in the third trimester of pregnancy: a randomised study of dietary effects. *Br J Obstet Gynaecol* 1988; **95**: 223–9.

50 Fraser RB. Nutrition in pregnancy. *Practitioner* 1990; **234**: 586–90.

51 Reece EA, Hagay Z, Caseria D *et al.* Do fibre-enriched diets have glucose-lowering effects in pregnancy? *Am J Perinatol* 1993; **10**: 272–4.

9

Diabetic Retinopathy in Pregnancy

EVA M. KOHNER

St Thomas' Hospital, London, UK

As recently as 1971 White[1] advised termination of pregnancy in patients with progressive proliferative retinopathy. But in the following year Martin and Taft[2] showed that termination was not absolutely necessary, as pituitary ablation was possible during the course of pregnancy, with favourable outcome of the pregnancy as well as for the diabetic retinopathy. The results of the Diabetic Retinopathy Research Group's report in 1976 clearly indicated that proliferative diabetic retinopathy is treatable by photocoagulation[3], and shortly after that the first report on effective photocoagulation of diabetic retinopathy during pregnancy appeared[4].

It is now clearly established that retinopathy is not a contraindication to pregnancy; however, the effect of pregnancy on retinopathy is less clear. Nor are there clear rules about the management of retinopathy in pregnancy. In addition pregnancy is thought by many to be a risk factor for both development and progression of diabetic retinopathy. This chapter will therefore address the following questions:

1. What is the evidence for diabetic retinopathy deteriorating during pregnancy?
2. What are the possible mechanisms which lead to deterioration of the retinopathy?
3. How should diabetic retinopathy be managed before and during the pregnancy and in the immediate postpartum period?

Diabetes and Pregnancy: An International Approach to Diagnosis and Management.
Edited by A. Dornhorst and D. R. Hadden.
© 1996 John Wiley & Sons Ltd.

EVIDENCE FOR RETINOPATHY DETERIORATING DURING PREGNANCY

Until the 1980s no adequate study was performed, which could have clearly indicated the relationship between pregnancy and retinopathy. The reports available depend on observations which vary considerably in quality. In addition no adequate data on the patients' diabetic control was available. Not unexpectedly therefore the results are variable. Thus Dibble found retinopathy deteriorating in three out of 19 patients[5], and Rodman reported that as many as 85% of his patients with background retinopathy deteriorated[6].

The first careful study which compared pregnant diabetic patients with a control group of patients of similar age and duration of diabetes who were not pregnant came from Dublin[7]. In this study by Maloney and Drury 53 pregnant and 39 non-pregnant diabetic patients were followed carefully with frequent observation and retinal photographs, which were analysed quantitatively. The initial visit in all patients was within the first trimester of pregnancy. More pregnant than non-pregnant patients had retinopathy at the initial examination (62.3% vs 46.2%). Only one of the non-pregnant patients who had proliferative retinopathy deteriorated during the follow-up period. Among the pregnant patients one with background retinopathy deteriorated to proliferative level, and most others with background retinopathy showed advance of their lesions. Eight patients developed retinopathy for the first time. There was a remarkable improvement in the postpartum period, so that by six months postpartum only 29 patients still had retinopathy. Dramatic regression also occurred in the one patient who developed proliferative retinopathy. This careful study therefore clearly indicated worsening of retinopathy during pregnancy, with regression of lesions postpartum.

In a detailed study using fluorescein angiograms (which most people would consider contraindicated during pregnancy) Soubrane and co-workers noted that microaneurysm numbers (indicating severity of background retinopathy) increased during pregnancy, and reduced after delivery, though the numbers remained higher than they were at entry into the study[8].

In the Wisconsin epidemiological study Klein looked at the progression of retinopathy related to pregnancy[9]. She too looked at a control group of non-pregnant diabetic patients. At their first visit there was no difference in the retinopathy status between the two groups. Because of the importance of diabetic control and blood pressure for the progression of diabetic retinopathy Klein also subdivided the patients according to quartiles of glycated haemoglobin, and of blood pressure. For each increasing quartile of glycated haemoglobin, pregnant diabetic patients had an increased tendency for deterioration, and non-pregnant patients an increased tendency for improvement. The findings were similar for diastolic blood pressure.

Interestingly, the number of pregnancies did not relate to the severity of retinopathy when duration of diabetes was taken into account[10]. This suggests that indeed there is a marked improvement of retinopathy in the postpartum period, though this is difficult to assess from the Klein study, as the patients had only two sets of photographs: during pregnancy and as soon as possible after delivery[9].

Thus both the descriptive reports and the controlled studies indicate that retinopathy tends to deteriorate during pregnancy, with many improving in the postpartum period. It must, however, be emphasized that not all patients deteriorate, and the experience of the author is that many with mild lesions stay mild throughout pregnancy. In contrast, not all patients will regress following pregnancy, and careful follow-up is essential (Figure 9.1).

WHAT ARE THE MECHANISMS THAT LEAD TO DETERIORATION OF RETINOPATHY?

There are three well-recognized pathogenic mechanisms in diabetic retinopathy: hormonal, metabolic and haemodynamic. How do these three affect retinopathy in pregnancy?

HORMONAL CHANGES

Pregnancy is associated with a number of hormonal changes, and some of these are exaggerated in diabetic patients. In normal pregnancies there is a rise of oestrogens, progesterone, placental lactogen and placental growth hormone. The growth hormone stimulates insulin-like growth factor 1 (IGF-I) production, which results in a switch-off of pituitary growth hormone secretion. Prolactin levels rise, as the cells normally producing growth hormone will now secrete prolactin. In a study of hormonal changes from Finland by Larinkari *et al.*[11] oestradiol levels were similar in diabetic and non-diabetic patients, but progesterone and placental lactogen were significantly increased during the last trimester of pregnancy in diabetes. Those with retinopathy already had increased levels during the second trimester. Prolactin levels declined in the diabetic pregnancies, not only in this study but also in that reported by Sadovsky *et al.*[12]. The fact that prolactin levels in diabetic patients are not elevated suggests the possibility that in diabetic patients the pituitary growth hormone secretion is not switched off. As growth hormone is thought to be of importance, at least as a permissive factor in proliferative retinopathy, its presence may result in worsening of retinopathy. The elevated levels of IGF-I could also result in increased angiogenesis.

METABOLIC CHANGES

The beneficial effect of strict diabetic control on the fetus has been recognized for a long time. Thus in diabetic clinics considerable effort is put

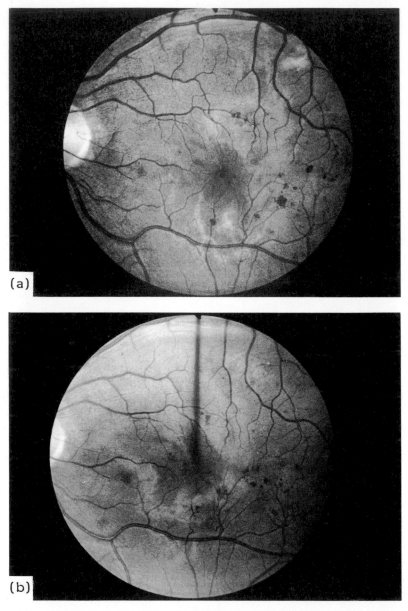

Figure 9.1. (a) Left macular region during the second trimester of pregnancy. There is one cotton wool spot and multiple haemorrhages and microaneurysms. (b) Same as (a), but four months post partum. Although the cotton wool spot has disappeared, there are now intraretinal microvascular abnormalities and early new vessels

into achieving normalization of blood glucose in the pregnant woman. In most diabetic patients this is achievable, since they do want healthy and normal babies. Could it be that rapid normalization of blood glucose in previously poorly controlled diabetic patients is actually detrimental to retinopathy? When insulin pumps and multiple injections were first introduced in the early 1980s diabetic control was improved to a remarkable degree. However, in the controlled studies of the Steno Hospital[13], the Kroc study[14] and the Oslo study[15], it was noted that during the first few months following introduction of good or even excellent blood glucose control retinopathy deteriorated in some, though not all patients. In a few patients proliferative lesions developed; in others features of diabetic retinopathy such as microaneurysms and haemorrhages deteriorated, while retinal cotton wool spots appeared, often in large numbers. These lesions tended to regress, or at least not advance, after the first few months. Indeed in the two-year follow-up of both the Kroc and the Steno studies[16,17] the strictly controlled patients ultimately fared better than the conventionally treated patients. These studies suggest that the rapid improvement of control of diabetes in pregnancy may precipitate deterioration of retinopathy (Figure 9.2). In this context it is interesting to note that in the paper by Maloney and Drury[7] microaneurysms and dot haemorrhages were increased throughout pregnancy, while larger blot and streak haemorrhages increased after the 20th week. Cotton wool spots, which indicate retinal ischaemia, were highest in the first part of pregnancy. The time course of the appearance of these lesions is similar to that observed in the insulin pump studies. In a detailed study by Phelps *et al.*[18], 35 diabetic pregnancies were monitored for diabetic control and retinopathy. They aimed at strict control, which was achieved by the time of delivery in all patients. In over 50% of their patients retinopathy deteriorated during the pregnancy. This deterioration correlated significantly not only with the level of blood glucose at entry into the study, but also with the magnitude of improvement of the control between the sixth and 14th week after introduction of strict diabetic control.

The deterioration of retinopathy with improved control in pregnancy does not militate against introduction of such control, but emphasizes the importance of good control even before pregnancy, and suggests that in patients where control was poor prior to pregnancy retinal surveillance should be more frequent.

HAEMODYNAMIC CHANGES

Pregnancy is associated with marked physiological changes. The most important of these is the increase in blood volume, increased heart rate and contractility of the heart and reduced peripheral resistance. These result in an increase in cardiac output by some 40% in an average patient. It could also result in an increase in retinal blood flow, which could damage diabetic vessels.

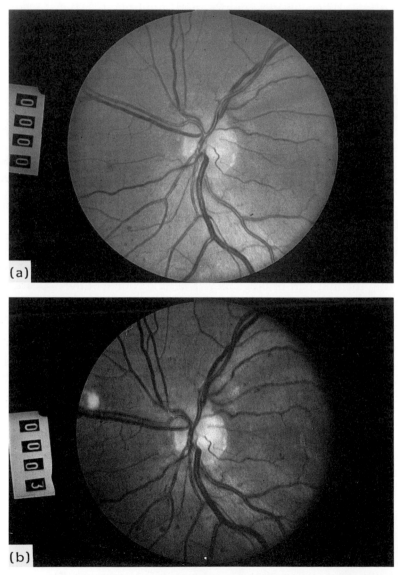

Figure 9.2. (a) Left disc region of a poorly controlled patient, before instituting tight control. Note multiple microaneurysms and few haemorrhages only. (b) Same as (a), but three months after establishing tight control of diabetes. Note increased number of haemorrhages and appearance of multiple cotton wool spots

To test this possibility Chen and co-workers[19] measured retinal blood flow in 19 non-diabetic and 22 diabetic pregnancies using laser Doppler velocimetry, a non-invasive method for the measurement of red cell velocity. Together with vessel diameter measurement this enables calculation of volumetric blood flow. In neither the diabetic nor the non-diabetic patients was there an increase in perfusion pressure. In the non-diabetic patients there was no signficant change in volumetric blood flow between any of the trimesters and the four-month postpartum measurements. In the diabetic patients blood flow increased during the last two trimesters of pregnancy compared with the postpartum measurements. When the diabetic patients were subdivided according to whether their retinopathy deteriorated or remained stable the results diverged. In those with stable retinopathy blood flow did not change significantly in any of the three trimesters, while in those who showed deterioration blood flow was significantly higher in the first and third trimesters of pregnancy than post partum (in the second trimester the trend was similar but did not reach statistical significance). When diabetic control was taken into account, while diabetic control improved in all patients during pregnancy, with an average drop of haemoglobin A_1 (HbA_1) of 2%, those who deteriorated had higher HbA_1 levels prior to the pregnancy and remained with a higher level throughout the pregnancy. Thus it is not clear whether the somewhat worse control resulted in an impaired autoregulation, with worsening of the retinopathy, or whether the increased blood flow alone could have accounted for the deterioration of the retinal lesions. These findings were similar to those observed by Ogasawara[20] in a much smaller group of patients.

That increased blood flow is associated with increased severity of retinopathy has been shown by Patel *et al.*[21]. The increased blood flow which in diabetics could be due to high blood glucose, elevated blood pressure or impaired autoregulation associated with pericyte loss (an early, pre-clinical change in the diabetic retina) is itself detrimental to diabetic retinopathy, as it increases shear stress, which damages the vessel wall, and leads to worsening of retinopathy[22].

In pregnancy all the known pathogenic mechanisms for deterioration of diabetic retinopathy are involved and worsened, and it is therefore not astonishing that in many patients the retinopathy deteriorates more rapidly.

MANAGEMENT OF DIABETIC RETINOPATHY IN PREGNANCY

There is a generally good consensus on the management of retinopathy in pregnancy, and I refer mostly to my own clinical experience.

Management of retinopathy should really start in the pre-conception period. Patients should be counselled and advised to improve their diabetic control at a time when this can be done gradually, so that deterioration of retinopathy associated with rapid improvement of control does not occur. At this stage they should also have their eyes examined, so that if there are any lesions needing photocoagulation this can be done.

Pregnant patients should have an eye examination at their first antenatal visit. If there is no retinopathy it is probably sufficient to see them again at the beginning of each trimester. If there is any retinopathy, however mild, eye examination should be repeated not more than six weeks later. If there is no deterioration two-monthly examinations will suffice. If the retinopathy is more severe, with extensive microaneurysms and blot haemorrhages, or if there is deterioration between the first and second examination, especially if cotton wool spots are developing, at least four-weekly examinations are mandatory.

Patients with proliferative retinopathy, however early, should have photocoagulation. If the new vessels occur late in the pregnancy some will say they can be left, as there is a possibility of reversal in the postpartum period. I do not advise this, as the new vessels may bleed or form a fibrous tissue covering, making their management much more difficult, and not all retinopathy regresses after delivery. If there are complications of new vessels during pregnancy, such as haemorrhage or detachment, vitrectomy can be carried out (Figure 9.3). It is probably safer for the fetus to have the vitrectomy later rather than earlier, and the assistance of an experienced anaesthetist is essential. Vitrectomy can be carried out under local anaesthetic, if necessary. Patients who still have active proliferative retinopathy at the time of labour should have caesarean section and since this is now carried out mostly under epidural anaesthetic the danger to the fetus is negligible.

Retinal photocoagulation for new vessels is similar in its effect in pregnant and non-pregnant diabetic patients (Figure 9.4), though Sinclair *et al.*[23] thought that proliferative lesions occurring early in pregnancy tended to be resistant to treatment.

Macular oedema is not a common complication of diabetic retinopathy in pregnancy, but may occur and is often associated with quite marked loss of vision. The oedema is usually cystoid or diffuse, and does not respond well to photocoagulation. It will occasionally improve with heavy diuretic treatment, which is best tried in hospital. If it occurs towards the end of pregnancy one or two doses of steroids may dramatically remove the fluid. Macular oedema usually disappears following pregnancy, provided there are no other complications, such as renal failure or very severe retinopathy.

While in most patients there is considerable regression of the retinopathy in the postpartum period, this is not invariable. Patients with retinopathy should be followed carefully in this period, especially if they have proliferative changes, and if the mother relaxes her diabetic control to a marked degree.

There is only one group of patients which is relatively safe as far as retinopathy is concerned during pregnancy, and that is the group who have

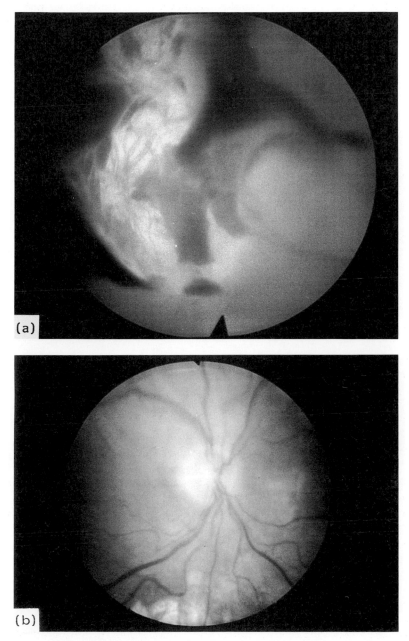

Figure 9.3. (a) Fundus of right eye of patient during the 20th week of pregnancy with intravitreal haemorrhage and retinal detachment. (b) Same as (a), but during the 23rd week of pregnancy, two weeks after vitrectomy, retinal detail still clouded

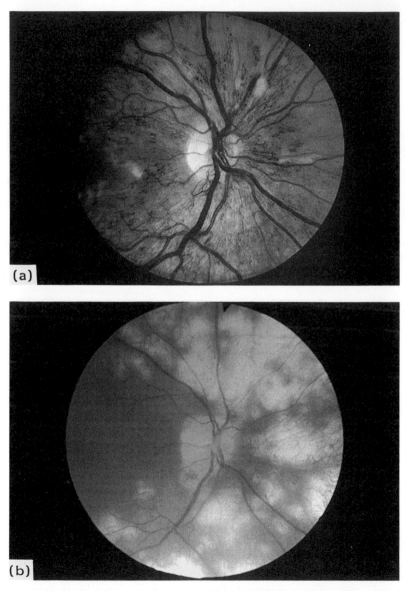

Figure 9.4. (a) Right disc area of patient with proliferative retinopathy at the end of the first trimester of pregnancy. (b) Same as (a), but a few weeks prior to delivery. Extensive photocoagulation scars, no new vessels

had effective and extensive panretinal photocoagulation in a previous pregnancy, or before conception. In contrast, the patient most ar risk is one with a long duration of poorly controlled diabetes, especially if associated with renal impairment and elevated blood pressure. Careful examination and follow-up of the eyes of all pregnant diabetic patients, with early treatment if required, will result in normal vision following pregnancy.

REFERENCES

1 White P. Pregnancy and diabetes. In: Marble A, White P, Bradley RF (eds), *Joslins Diabetes Mellitus*. Lea & Febiger, Philadelphia, 1971, pp 581–98.
2 Martin FR, Taft P. Hypophysectomy for diabetic retinopathy during pregnancy. *Diabetes* 1972; **21**: 972–5.
3 The Diabetic Retinopathy Study Research Group. Preliminary report on effects of photocoagulation. *Am J Ophthalmol* 1976; **81**: 383–90.
4 Cassar J, Kohner EM, Hamilton AM. Diabetic retinopathy and pregnancy. *Diabetologia* 1978; **15**: 105–11.
5 Dibble CM, Kochenour NK, Worley RJ *et al*. Effect of pregnancy on diabetic retinopathy. *Obstet Gynecol* 1982; **59**: 699–704.
6 Rodman HM, Singerman LJ, Aiello LM. Diabetic retinopathy: effects of pregnancy and laser therapy. *Diabetes* 1980; **29**: 1A.
7 Maloney JBM, Drury MI. Diabetic retinopathy during pregnancy. *Am J Ophthalmol* 1982; **93**: 745–756.
8 Soubrane G, Canivet J, Coscas G. Influence of pregnancy on the evolution of background retinopathy. *Int Ophthalmol* 1985; **8**: 249–55.
9 Klein BEK, Moss SE, Klein R. Effect of pregnancy on progression of diabetic retinopathy. *Diabetes Care* 1990; **13**: 34–40.
10 Klein BEK, Klein R. Gravidity and diabetic retinopathy. *Am J Epidemiol* 1984; **119**: 564–9.
11 Larinkari J, Laatikainen L, Ranta R *et al*. Metabolic control and serum hormone levels in relation to retinopathy in diabetic pregnancy. *Diabetologia* 1982; **22**: 327–32.
12 Sadovsky E, Weinstein D, Ben-David M, Polishuk WZ. Serum prolactin in normal and pathologic pregnancies. *Obstet Gynecol* 1977; **50**: 559–61.
13 Lauritzen T, Larsen KF, Larsen H-W *et al*. Effect of one year near normal blood glucose on retinopathy in insulin dependent diabetics. *Lancet* 1983; **i**: 200–3.
14 The Kroc Collaborative Study Group. Blood glucose control and the evolution of diabetic retinopathy and albuminuria. *N Engl J Med* 1984; **311**: 365–72.
15 Brinchmann-Hansen O, Dahl-Jorgensen K, Hanssen KF. Effects of intensified insulin treatment on various lesions of diabetic retinopathy. *Am J Ophthalmol* 1985; **100**: 644–53.
16 The Kroc Collaborative Study Group. Diabetic retinopathy after two years of intensified insulin therapy. *JAMA* 1988; **260**: 37–41.
17 Lauritzen T, Frost-Larsen K, Larsen H-W *et al*. Two years experience with continuous subcutaneous insulin infusion in relation to retinopathy and neuropathy. *Diabetes* 1986; Suppl. 3: 74–9.
18 Phelps RL, Sakol P, Metzger BE *et al*. Changes in diabetic retinopathy during pregnancy: correlation with regulation of hyperglycaemia. *Arch Ophthalmol* 1986; **104**: 1806–10.
19 Chen HC, Newsom RSB, Patel V *et al*. Retinal blood flow changes during pregnancy in women with diabetes. *Invest Ophthalmol Vis Sci* 1994; **35**: 3199–208.
20 Ogasawara II, Feke GT, Goger DG *et al*. Retinal blood flow increases during pregnancy in normal and diabetic subjects. *Invest Ophthalmol Vis Sci Suppl* 1991; **32**: 364 (Abstract).
21 Patel V, Rassam SMB, Newsome RSB *et al*. Retinal blood flow in diabetic retinopathy. *Br Med J* 1992; **230**: 221–5.
22 Kohner EM, Patel V, Rassam SMB. The role of retinal blood flow and autoregulation in the evolution of diabetic retinopathy. *Diabetes* 1995; **44**: 603–7.
23 Sinclair SH, Nesler CL, Schwartz SS. Retinopathy in the pregnant diabetic. *Clin Obstet Gynecol* 1985; **28**: 536–52.

10

Management and Outcome of Pregnancies Complicated by Diabetic Nephropathy

JOHN L. KITZMILLER and C. ANDREW COMBS

Good Samaritan Health System, San Jose, California, USA

Diabetic nephropathy is the leading cause of end-stage renal disease in the Western world, and is also linked to cardiovascular disease as the major cause of deaths related to diabetes mellitus[1,2]. In pregnancy, diabetic nephropathy can strongly influence the outcome of gestation via increased risks of fetal growth retardation, stillbirth, and preterm delivery with associated neonatal disorders. The maternal hazards of diabetic nephropathy include renal failure during or after pregnancy, superimposed pre-eclampsia, and the risk of eventual morbidity or death from macrovascular disease. In spite of these possible complications, women with diabetic nephropathy and their partners often desire to have a child. Careful management using a multidisciplinary team approach will usually produce a good outcome, although concerns persist about preservation of maternal heatlh. Rational management is based on new information on the development and pathogenesis of diabetic nephropathy[3-9] as well as on the published clinical studies of the course and outcome of pregnancy. Both topics are reviewed in this chapter.

COURSE AND DEVELOPMENT OF DIABETIC NEPHROPATHY

Overt clinical diabetic nephropathy is characterized by proteinuria, (total protein excretion > 0.5 g/24 h) or urinary albumin excretion > 200 μg/min or > 300 mg/24 h[10], hypertension, declining glomerular filtration rate (~ 12 ml/min per year), and eventual end-stage renal failure with uremia[11]. In

Diabetes and Pregnancy: An International Approach to Diagnosis and Management.
Edited by A. Dornhorst and D. R. Hadden.
© 1996 John Wiley & Sons Ltd.

recent years, investigators have focused on early changes in renal function and structure which could predict advanced diabetic nephropathy and identify subjects for preventive treatment. Incipient diabetic nephropathy is indicated by repetitive subclinical increases in urinary excretion of albumin, known as microalbuminuria (two or three samples 20–200 μg/min, 30–300 mg/24 h)[7,10,11].

The prevalence of microalbuminuria in insulin-dependent diabetes of > 10 years duration has been 15–30%[8] and is highest with poor glycemic control marked by even modestly elevated glycohemoglobin[12,13], hypertension[14–16], elevated low-density lipoprotein cholesterol[16] and smoking[17]. Studies conducted before aids to self-management of diabetes were available (use of glycohemoglobin assays and self-monitoring of blood glucose) indicated that 85% of diabetic women with microalbuminuria ultimately progressed to diabetic nephropathy[7,10,18–21]. In a clinical setting devoted to strict metabolic control in 1985–1991, in which glucose test strips were free of charge, only 31% of 79 patients with persistent microalbuminuria progressed to diabetic nephropathy after five years of follow-up, compared to 2% of normoalbuminuric patients[20]. Elevated glycohemoglobin and blood pressure levels predicted progression. In this study, calculation of the annual increase in urinary albumin excretion (progression > 5% per year) was a more specific method of identifying patients who will develop diabetic nephropathy[22]. Until recently, proteinuria developed gradually over 20–30 years of diabetes in 30–50% of women, and ~ 60% progressed to renal failure by 10 years of clinical proteinuria[11,23,24]. However, for cases of insulin-dependent diabetes diagnosed in the 1960s in Scandinavia and exposed to modern diabetes management, the cumulative incidence of nephropathy was only 9–16% after a 20-year duration of diabetes[25–27]. On the other hand, a recent prospective study from Copenhagen still revealed a prevalence of nephropathy of 32%, and 27% persistent microalbuminuria, in 233 insulin-dependent patients with diabetes of onset in 1965–1974 who were followed from 1984 to 1991[2]. The authors attributed the higher rates to persistently elevated glycohemoglobin levels and a 64% frequency of smoking in the group.

Factors which may influence the susceptibility to diabetic nephropathy include genetic predisposition[28], such as differences in the angiotensin converting enzyme gene[29], or familial clustering of other influences, such as poor glycemic control, hyperlipidemia or hypertension[28]. According to the Steno hypothesis diabetic nephropathy reflects widespread vascular damage, and thus represents genetic susceptibility to the deleterious effects of hyperglycemia[30]. The concept was expanded to consider common genetic susceptibility factors for both nephropathy and macrovascular disease (premature atherosclerosis), based on epidemiological links and the possible common pathogenesis of albuminuria and atherosclerosis[8].

A variety of renal lesions are described in patients with diabetes. The information in Table 10.1 summarizes studies of renal function and structure in subjects with diabetes of variable duration, and differentiates the early and advanced stages of the development of diabetic nephropathy[11,31,32]. Early in the course of diabetes there is usually increased kidney size and glomerular volume[33], glomerular hypertrophy with an enlarged capillary surface area and presumed increased intraglomerular pressure[11,34], and generalized hyperfiltration marked by glomerular filtration rate > 150 ml/min[11,34–36]. In these early years of diabetes, there is a gradual increase in the thickness of the glomerular basement membrane, often followed by mesangial expansion[37–40].

In addition to microalbuminuria[10], incipient diabetic nephropathy is characterized by glomeruli with increased capillary surface area, with the glomerular filtration rate often remaining above normal[36–38,41]. As noted, progression of microalbuminuria is related to glycemic control[42] and is followed by modest increases in diastolic blood pressure[14,38,41].

In overt clinical diabetic nephropathy characterized by increasing proteinuria, and by progressive decline in the glomerular filtration rate by 1.0–1.2 ml/min per month[38,41], hypertension is common and the rate of decline of glomerular filtration is related to the diastolic blood pressure[38]. The glomerular pathology shows further increase in basement membrane thickness and arteriolar hyalinosis, and a continuing increase in the total mesangium (cells and matrix), enlarging from 33% to 57% of the glomerular tuft[1,5,40,43]. Mesangial expansion interfaces with endothelial capillaries and decreases the peripheral capillary filtration surface (Figure 10.1)[3,5,40,44,45]. A

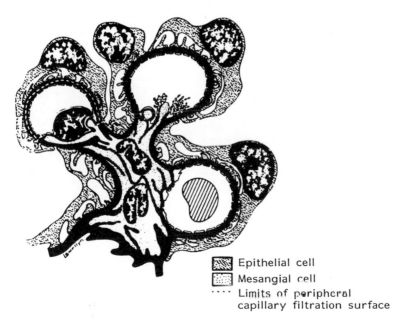

Epithelial cell
Mesangial cell
···· Limits of peripheral
capillary filtration surface

Figure 10.1. Schematic representation of the glomerular tuft illustrating the limits of the peripheral capillary filtration surface related to mesangial expansion. From Mauer SM, Steffes MW, Ellis EN *et al*. Structural functional relationship in diabetic nephropathy. *J Clin Invest*. 1984; **74**: 1143–55. Used with permission

Table 10.1. Stages in renal involvement in insulin-dependent diabetes mellitus

Stage and time sequence	Designation	Main characteristics	Main structural changes	GFR (ml/min)	Albumin excretion (mg/24 h)	Blood pressure	Suggested main pathophysiological change
Stage I — At clinical diagnosis	Hyperfunction and hypertrophy stage	Large kidneys and glomerular hyperfiltration	Glomerular hypertrophy; normal BM and mesangium	150	May be increased but readily reversible	Normal	Glomerular volume expansion and increased intraglomerular pressure
Stage II — In short-term diabetes (1–15 years)	'Silent' stage with normal urinary albumin excretion, but structural lesion present		Increasing BM thickness and mesangial expansion	With or without hyperfiltration[a,b]	Nl (often increased in stress situations)	Normal	Changes as indicated above but quite variable (dependent on metabolic control)? In addition, increased accumulation of BM and BM-like material
In long-term diabetes (>15 years)		Normal urinary albumin excretion	No or few studies	With or without hyperfiltration[a,b]	Nl (often increased in stress situations)	Normal or slightly elevated	
Stage III — Early	Incipient diabetic nephropathy (microalbuminuria)	Persistently elevated urinary albumin excretion	Severity probably in between II and IV	160	30–105	Often elevated compared with	Glomerular closure probably starts in this stage.
Late				130	105–300 (considerable range)	healthy subjects; also elevated during exercise	
Stage IV — Early	Overt diabetic nephropathy	Clinical proteinura	Further increase in BM thickening and mesangial expansion.	130–70	>300	Often frank hypertension	High rate of glomerular closure and advancing mesangial expansion.
Intermediate			Increasing rate of glomerular closure.	70–30	Increasing clinical proteinura	Hypertension in almost all patients	Hyperfiltration in remaining glomeruli (deleterious?)
Advanced			Hypertrophy of remaining glomeruli	30–10		Hypertension in almost all patients	
Stage V	Uremia	End-stage renal failure	Generalized glomerular closure	0–10	Decreasing (due to nephron closure)	High but often controlled by dialysis treatment	Advanced lesions and glomerular closure

GFR, glomerular filtration rate; BM, basement membrane.
[a]Changes probably present in all stages when glycemic control imperfect.
[b]Possible marker of future nephropathy (if GFR >150 ml/min).
Modified from Mogensen and Schmitz, *Medical Clinics of North America* 1988; 72: 1470–6. Used with permission.

compensatory enlargement of open glomeruli may temporarily preserve the filtration surface[43,46], but as this process becomes limited and there is an increase in hyalinized, obliterated glomeruli[40,43], glomerular filtration declines markedly[5].

End-stage renal failure is characterized by generalized glomerular closure, marked decrease in glomerular filtration (creatinine clearance < 10 ml/min), and rising plasma creatinine and blood urea. The percentage of occluded sclerotic glomeruli relates to the degree of azotemia and there is also capillary closure within non-sclerotic glomeruli[43,46]. Worsening hypertension accompanies the renal failure.

PATHOGENESIS OF DIABETIC NEPHROPATHY

Approaches to the prevention and amelioration of early diabetic nephropathy before and during pregnancy are based on experimental studies of pathogenesis.

EFFECTS OF HYPERGLYCEMIA ON THE GLOMERULUS

Hyperglycemia induces the compositional changes of the glomerular basement membrane and mesangial extracellular matrix which are related to increasing albuminuria and the later decrease in glomerular filtration. In cultured endothelial and mesangial cells excess glucose leads to increased expression of collagen IV, laminin and fibronectin, and decreased heparan sulfate[50,55] proteoglycan (HS-PG)[47–49], which is also found in the glomerular basement membrane of diabetic subjects. There is a relative loss of sulfate anions[55], which normally form an electronegative barrier to filtration of negatively charged albumin[56–58]. Mesangial expansion may also be facilitated by the decreased density of HS-PG[59].

In glomerular disease, hyperglycemia also causes non-enzymatic glycosylation of collagen IV, fibronectin and laminin, which decreases their affinity to binding HS-PG[60], and decreases the turnover of glycosylated collagen IV[61]. These mechanisms can lead to the reduced density of anionic HS-PG compared to collagen IV in the glomerular extracellular matrix[8]. The early glycation products formed by adducting glucose to proteins undergo a complex series of rearrangements to form advanced glycation end products[61–63]. Endothelial, vascular smooth muscle and mesangial cells contain advanced glycation end product-specific receptors[63,64]. *In vitro*, advanced glycation end products stimulate mesangial cell production of fibronectin, laminin and collagen IV[65,66]. *In vivo*, their deposition within the glomerulus is associated with the pathological changes of diabetic nephropathy (thickening of the glomerular basement membrane, mesangial matrix expansion[64] and increased endothelial permeability[67]). These effects can be blocked by the advanced glycation end product inhibitor aminoguanidine[68,69].

Another process possibly leading to the glomerular and vascular damage of diabetes is glucose autooxidation[70], which is catalyzed by metal ions and yields reactive oxygen species: free radicals, hydrogen peroxide, and hydroxyl radicals[71]. The reactive oxygen species, if not neutralized by antioxidants such as vitamin E and C, glutathione or lipoic acid, can cause peroxidation of membrane lipids and induce oxidation of low-density lipoproteins, with cytotoxic effects on endothelium, and increased permeability[72]. In diabetic rats, impaired degradation of hydrogen peroxide was found in isolated glomeruli compared to controls[73]. The rate of free radical production is also markedly enhanced by early glycation products[74]; and reactive oxygen species may amplify the toxic effects of advanced glycosylated end products on endothelium[72].

Excess glucose also activates the family of protein kinase C enzymes in glomerular endothelial and messangial cells via the formation of diacylglycerol[75,76]. Protein kinase C activation has been associated with increased endothelial permeability to albumin[77], and with increased mesangial cell contraction, proliferation and matrix protein synthesis[76,78].

HYPERFILTRATION

The observation of increased renal size and filtration in early diabetes led to the hypothesis that renal hypertrophy and hyperfiltration contributed to the development of clinical nephropathy[79,80]. Proteinuria is more likely to develop when glomerular filtration has been elevated[20], but recent studies correlating renal volume with histopathology or with changes in the glomerular filtration rate have not entirely supported the necessity for renal hypertrophy in the pathogenesis of nephropathy[81–83]. The hyperfiltration hypothesis is supported by experimental studies in which renal ablation resulted in single-nephron hyperfiltration in the remaining kidney, hypertension and glomerular lesions similar to those of diabetes (increased mesangial area and decreased peripheral capillary surface) and ultimately glomerulosclerosis[84,85]. The increased glomerular filtration rate is associated with enhanced renal flow, elevated glomerular transcapillary hydraulic pressure, and with a four-fold increase in protein excretion due to impaired charge and size selective permeability of the glomerulus to plasma proteins[84,85]. A model of streptozotocin-induced diabetes in rats also produced hyperfiltration; a 40% increase in glomerular filtration rate was secondary to increased renal plasma flow due to vasodilatation, and to increased transcapillary pressure difference[84].

Hyperglycemia may induce glomerular hyperfiltration. Intravenous glucose infusions raise the glomerular filtration rate in normal controls, and produce larger increases in glomerular filtration and renal plasma flow in diabetic subjects[86]. To exclude the systemic hormonal changes which accompany hyperglycemia, Kasiske and colleagues studied the isolated perfused rat kidney from control and diabetic animals[87]. Increased glucose in the perfusate caused vasodilatation and increased glomerular filtration measured by increased inulin clearance. Mannitol was used as a control for the osmotic effects of glucose, and it produced vasoconstriction. The hyperfiltration produced by glucose was blocked when prostaglandin synthetase inhibitors were administered. The authors reviewed other evidence that prostaglandin metabolism is altered in the glomerulus in diabetes and that hyperglycemia increases vascular production of prostaglandins[87].

Hypertension is also an important factor in the progression of clinical diabetic nephropathy, and Parving[80] and Hostetter[84] link hypertension to hemodynamic changes that could be associated with increased glomerular filtration of macromolecules and the structural endothelial–mesangial abnormalities of diabetes. Thus, there is evidence that hyperglycemic and hemodynamic changes lead to hyperfiltration in the glomeruli[88] and this predisposes to development of the lesions of clinical diabetic nephropathy. However, not all diabetic subjects with early hyperfiltration go on to develop nephropathy; hyperfiltration may be a predisposing process, but is not a sufficient explanation of the pathogenesis of diabetic nephropathy.

MANAGEMENT OF DIABETIC NEPHROPATHY BEFORE AND DURING PREGNANCY

CONTROL OF HYPERGLYCEMIA AND THE COURSE OF DIABETIC NEPHROPATHY AND PREGNANCY

Development of diabetic nephropathy is related to poor glycemic control in both insulin-dependent and non-insulin-dependent diabetes, as consistently demonstrated by several large epidemiological studies[89-93]. Higher levels of glycosylated hemoglobin were found in groups of patients with both incipient and overt diabetic nephropathy compared to diabetic controls, and the association persisted in multivariate analyses that controlled for other factors such as age, duration of diabetes, blood pressure control and dietary protein intake[89-93].

Short-term trials of intensive insulin therapy to achieve normoglycemia for a few weeks to one year generally showed improvements in several of the indirect markers of the severity of early diabetic nephropathy, including microalbuminuria, kidney volume and amino acid-stimulated rise in glomerular filtration[94-96]. Three recent long-term controlled trials of intensified insulin therapy demonstrated that good metabolic control can prevent or delay the progression from incipient to overt nephropathy[42,97-99]. In studies from the Steno Hospital, Denmark, 70 insulin-dependent diabetic patients without clinical diabetic nephropathy were randomized to conventional subcutaneous insulin therapy or intensive therapy with insulin pumps and frequent adjustment of insulin dosage based on self-monitoring of blood glucose[97]. Intensive therapy for three to five years resulted in a reduction in the number of patients who progressed from incipient nephropathy to overt nephropathy (two of nine in the intensive group (22%) vs 10 of 10 in the conventional group ($p < 0.01$)[97]. Similar results were obtained in the Stockholm Diabetes Intervention Study conducted for seven years[98,99]. Nephropathy developed more commonly in those with standard treatment (nine of 54, 17%) than in those with intensified treatment (one of 48, 2%, $p=0.01$)[99]. The much larger North American Diabetes Control and Complications Trial (DCCT), involving 1441 insulin-dependent diabetic subjects from 29 centers, demonstrated that intensive treatment for six to nine years, with maintenance of glycohemoglobin near the normal levels and postprandial blood glucose less than 10 mM (180 mg/dl), reduced the appearance of incipient diabetic nephropathy by 34% and overt nephropathy by 54%[42].

Thus, all trials are consistent in showing that good metabolic control can often prevent the progression from incipient to overt nephropathy. Further, the DCCT showed that such control can also prevent or delay the onset of incipient nephropathy. Unfortunately, these studies do not address the question as to whether intensified diabetes treatment can prevent the progression from overt nephropathy to end-stage renal disease. Older studies suggested that glycemic control alone is inadequate to prevent progression once overt nephropathy is established[100,101]. This does not imply, however, that strict control is not of value for patients with overt diabetic nephropathy. The Steno study, the Stockholm study and the DCCT all showed that good glycemic control also prevented the progression of diabetic retinopathy and neuropathy[42,97-99]. Thus, intensive therapy aiming for near-normoglycemia should now be considered the standard of appropriate care of all patients with diabetes, with careful consideration of risks and prevention of insulin-induced hypoglycemia[102].

The maternal and perinatal benefits of intensified diabetes treatment before and during pregnancy are reviewed elsewhere in this volume. Instituting a program of strict glycemic control before pregnancy is attempted, with maintenance of glycohemoglobin within four standard deviations of the normal mean[103] and peak postprandial blood glucose less than 8.9 mM (160 mg/dl)[104], can prevent excess major congenital malformations and spontaneous abortions in diabetic women[104-107]. After initial controversy[108-110], the evidence from clinical studies indicates that pre-conception glycemic control continued in early pregnancy also reduces major congenital anomalies in babies of women with diabetic vascular disease (Table 10.2)[104-107]. Throughout pregnancy, strict glycemic control should be maintained in women with diabetic nephropathy (fasting and pre-meal blood glucose 3.9–5.6 mM (70–100 mg/dl), peak postprandial blood glucose 6.1–7.2 mM (110–130 mg/dl)) in order to prevent fetal hyperinsulinemia[111,112] and its deleterious effects on fetal growth[113,114] and the neonatal hazards of prematurity[115-117]. In women with diabetic

Table 10.2. The importance of pre-conception counseling in diabetic vascular disease. Ratio of major congenital anomalies to total pregnancy outcomes for White classes B, C and classes D, R, F

| Author | Onset of intensified care | | | |
| | Pre-conception | | Post-conception | |
	B, C	D, R, F	B, C	D, R, F
Fuhrmann *et al.*[105]	1/71	0/57	11/171	11/121
Steel[107]	0/64	2/79	5/51	5/45
Kitzmiller *et al.*[104]	1/53	0/31	8/79	4/31
	2/188	2/167	24/301	20/197
	(1.1%)	(1.2%)	(8.0%)	(10.2%)

nephropathy and reduced renal clearance of creatinine and insulin, physicians should be aware that doses of insulin lower than usual can often maintain euglycemia.

ANTIHYPERTENSIVE TREATMENT

Longitudinal studies show that hypertension usually appears after there is already evidence of incipient diabetic nephropathy, suggesting that hypertension is a consequence of the processes of early renal disease rather than the cause of it[14,118,119]. Nonetheless, there is widespread agreement that uncontrolled hypertension accelerates the progression from incipient to overt nephropathy and from overt nephropathy to end-stage renal disease[36,38]. Modest blood pressure elevations that are often considered 'high normal' are believed to cause worsening of diabetic nephropathy[120], and antihypertensive therapy has been extensively investigated to determine if strict control of arterial pressure might slow the progression of the nephropathy.

Kasiske *et al.* presented a meta-regression analysis of 100 studies of various antihypertensive agents for diabetic nephropathy[121]. Regardless of the agent used, the analysis indicated that reduction of arterial pressure resulted in both a decrease in urinary protein excretion and a sparing of glomerular filtration ($p<0.001$ for both effects). Angiotensin converting enzyme (ACE) inhibitors appeared to be especially beneficial because these agents were associated with an additional decrease in proteinuria that was independent of their blood pressure lowering effect ($p<0.0001$). The authors noted that: 'the salutary effect of ACE inhibitors on proteinuria was seen whether or not the patient had hypertension, whether or not the patient had microalbuminuria or clinically apparent proteinuria, and whether the patient had type I or type II diabetes'[121]. It may be that ACE inhibitors have a favorable local effect on intrarenal hemodynamics, in addition to their systemic action, at least when low sodium intake is used by treated subjects[122,123].

Although the value of ACE inhibitors in slowing the progression from incipient to overt diabetic nephropathy[124] and from overt nephropathy to end-stage renal disease[125] has been confirmed in double-blind randomized controlled trials, use of this class of compounds is contraindicated in pregnancy due to the possibility of fetal and neonatal renal failure[126,127]. Thus, in preparing for pregnancy in women with incipient or overt diabetic nephropathy, it is prudent to try to achieve control of hypertension and stable renal function with other pharmacological agents.

For diabetic women in general, a 1989 consensus statement recommended such therapy if systolic pressure rises by 20 mmHg or more, or if diastolic pressure rises by 10 mmHg or more above baseline over two years[128]. Mogensen and colleagues recommend initiating therapy if mean arterial pressure exceeds 90–95 mmHg (roughly 120/80)[129]. A 1993 consensus statement stated that the goal of therapy is to keep systolic pressure below 130 mmHg and diastolic pressure below 85 mmHg[130]. The latter statement also recommends treatment of isolated systolic hypertension, defined as a systolic pressure of ≥ 140 mmHg. The value of ambulatory blood pressure measurements in monitoring antihypertensive treatment and the progression of diabetic nephropathy is emphasized[131–134].

There is a wide choice of agents to use in addition to ACE inhibitors. The 1993 consensus statement on treatment of hypertension in diabetes concludes that α_1-receptor blockers, calcium antagonists and low-dose thiazide diuretics may be especially useful[130]. The statement also classifies several agents that should be used 'with caution' because of potential adverse effects on glycemic control and lipid balance, interference with hypoglycemia awareness, or other complications. These include β-adrenergic blockers, combined α- and β-adrenergic blockers, centrally acting α_2-agonists, potassium-sparing agents and sympatholytics[130]. Drugs we find to be useful and relatively safe before and during pregnancy include methyldopa, diltiazem, clonidine and prazosin. Methyldopa is little used outside of pregnancy due to poor compliance associated with drowsiness and refractoriness after six to nine months of use, associated with increased plasma volume[135]. However, this drug has been widely used during pregnancy[136,137] and follow-up studies of the offspring show normal child development up to age 10 years[138]. We restrict diuretic therapy to cases of severe fluid retention, since even chronic thiazide therapy restricts the expected expansion of plasma volume in pregnant women with essential hypertension[139]. Whether these data apply to hypertensive women with diabetic nephropathy is unknown[140,141].

Studies of Bakris and colleagues[142,143] indicate that certain calcium antagonists (diltiazem), as well as converting enzyme inhibitors (lisinopril), 'attenuate the rise in glomerular capillary pressure, glomerular hypertrophy, and mesangial matrix expansion in diabetic animal models'[123].

In a randomized, prospective, parallel group study, these agents resulted in a slower rate of decline of glomerular filtration, lower urinary albumin excretion, and a better overall metabolic profile in hypertensive patients with non-insulin-dependent diabetes and overt nephropathy, compared to the combination of a loop diuretic (furosemide) and β-adrenoreceptor antagonist (atenolol), even given a similar level of arterial pressure control in all treatment groups1[23]. Diltiazem seems to have a greater effect on lowering proteinuria in diabetic subjects than other calcium antagonists, such as nifedipine[142-144]. Although α_1-receptor blockers (prazosin) and calcium antagonists (diltiazem) may be preferred in pregnancy because of their potential beneficial effect on the long-term course of nephropathy, there are inadequate data at this time about potential teratogenicity[145], so alternative agents should be used in the first trimester. Therefore, we prefer α-methyldopa as a first-line agent and add clonidine and/or β-blockers if additional therapy is needed at the beginning of pregnancy. Diltiazem can be added at the end of the first trimester if needed, to replace the β-blocker, due to a possible association of fetal growth retardation with continued use of β-blockers during pregnancy[137].

LOW-PROTEIN DIET AND NEPHROPATHY

In experimental renal diseases, diets high in protein accelerate disease progression[145]. In diabetic rats, high protein intake was found to dilate the glomerular afferent arterioles, and increase glomerular pressure, blood flow, proteinuria and glomerular scarring[146]. These observations led to speculation that dietary protein restriction in diabetic nephropathy might be beneficial.

The authors of five studies reported that a low protein diet (0.6–0.8 g/kg body weight) maintained for a few years in diabetic subjects with nephropathy led to decreased proteinuria and a slowing of the fall in glomerular filtration. In the first four of these studies, the patients served as their own controls during sequential observation periods[146-150]. While the results were suggestive of benefit, the best evidence comes from the randomized trial by Zeller *et al.*[151]. In this study, 35 insulin-dependent diabetic patients were randomized to a diet containing 0.6 g/kg protein, 0.5–1 g phosphorus and 2 g sodium per day versus their usual diet containing at least 1 g/kg protein and 1 g phosphorus. After a mean follow-up of three years, the glomerular filtration rate had declined by 37 ml/min in the control group and only 9.5 ml/min in the low-protein diet group ($p < 0.05$)[151].

The suggestion that protein restriction in the 0.6 mg/kg range would result in protein undernutrition[152] was not confirmed by other studies[153,154]. Therefore, we conclude that dietary protein should be restricted to 0.6–0.8 mg/kg per day in women with overt nephropathy in the non-pregnant state. Further investigation is needed to determine whether similar restriction is beneficial for patients with incipient diabetic nephropathy. During pregnancy, we restrict dietary protein intake to 60–80 g per day in patients with clinical diabetic nephropathy. Although lower values may be beneficial for the long-term course of nephropathy, we believe that this amount is probably the minimum acceptable for fetal development[155].

PRE-CONCEPTION EVALUATION OF WOMEN WITH DIABETIC NEPHROPATHY

Pre-conception care of women with diabetic nephropathy should include careful assessment of maternal health. Evaluation of renal function and staging of nephropathy should be a part of the management of every diabetic woman. Possibly due to the physiological plasma flow-dependent glomerular hyperfiltration state of pregnancy[150], plus a decrease in tubular reabsorption of low molecular weight proteins[157], total proteinuria increases during pregnancy[158,159]. Therefore it may be difficult to determine whether incipient or overt diabetic nephropathy is present if the initial renal evaluation is done during gestation. A 24 h urine specimen should be collected for determination of albumin excretion and creatinine clearance. The albumin assay should be performed by a reference laboratory because numerous technical problems can cause invalid results in laboratories that do not run such assays routinely. A 24 h collection is preferred to a shorter timed collection because protein excretion follows a diurnal rhythm. Use of a protein/creatinine ratio in a single voided spot urine can lead to large errors[160].

Evaluation for heart disease should be carried out before conception in patients with overt diabetic nephropathy because these patients have a high risk of significant coronary disease[161,162]. A careful history and physical examination should be supplemented with an electrocardiograph. Manske *et al.* found virtually no significant coronary disease among diabetic patients with end-stage renal disease if age was less than 45 years, diabetes duration was less than 25 years, and there were no ST–T wave changes[163]. If any of these risk factors are present, evaluation by a cardiologist is indicated. Although reports appearing in 1953–1977 indicated a high maternal mortality in diabetic women with a history of myocardial infarction[164,165], subsequent reports on pregnancies in a few diabetic women with signs of coronary artery disease without myocardial infarction, or with prior coronary artery bypass grafts, are more optimistic[165–167].

Ophthalmological evaluation is necessary in preparing for pregnancy because almost all women with diabetic nephropathy have some degree of retinopathy. Pregnancy and the level of glycemia, and diastolic pressure to a lesser extent, are associated with the progression of diabetic retinopathy[168]. In a prospective study of 155 diabetic women with gradable fundus photographs in early pregnancy and post partum, 140 did not have proliferative retinopathy at baseline[169]. In this study, proliferative retinopathy developed during pregnancy in 6.3% with mild, and in 29%

with moderate-to-severe background retinopathy. Elevated glycohemoglobin at baseline and the magnitude of improvement of glucose control in early pregnancy were associated with a higher risk of progression of retinopathy[169]. These data provide more support for the importance of excellent metabolic control before conception. If proliferative retinopathy is identified, it should be in spontaneous remission or treated by laser photocoagulation prior to pregnancy because this substantially reduces the chances of recurrence during pregnancy[170].

COURSE OF PREGNANCY IN WOMEN WITH DIABETIC NEPHROPATHY

CHARACTERISTICS OF PATIENTS

In the past, diabetic nephropathy was associated with poor fetal and maternal outcome. In the large series at the Joslin Diabetes Center, Hare and White reported only 62% viable fetal survival for 179 pregnancies delivered in 1924–1962, compared to 79% for 89 pregnancies in 1963–1975[164], and 22% of the mothers had died by 10 years after the last pregnancy in a follow-up study done in 1963[171]. In 1974 Pedersen *et al.* reported similar figures from a large retrospective survey of the diabetic pregnant population in Copenhagen[172]. In the 1977 edition of his landmark book on diabetes and pregnancy, Pedersen stated that pregnancy should be discouraged and therapeutic abortion offered to patients with nephropathy, 'in particular those with renal failure and preexisting hypertension, [since] the prognosis for the baby is poor; the perinatal mortality rate is extraordinarily high, as is the rate of congenital malformations, and the "quality" of the few surviving babies is below standard'[173]. However, in the subsequent era (1975–1992) of improved treatment of diabetes and hypertension and of the development of perinatology and neonatology, perinatal outcome improved dramatically[117], and most women with diabetic nephropathy have chosen to continue their pregnancies.

In the period 1981–1995, seven groups of authors[174–180] reported clinical studies of 129 continuing pregnancies in women with overt diabetic nephropathy in sufficient detail for metanalysis. The pregnancies included in the analysis were studied in the years 1975–1992 and data were available for the first half of pregnancy (Table 10.3). The authors diagnosed diabetic nephropathy on sustained clinical proteinuria (total urinary protein ≥ 300 mg[178] or ≥ 400 mg/24 h[174,175,177,179,180] or dipstick positive[176]), which was present before or during early pregnancy. Renal biopsies were not performed during pregnancy, but Grenfell's series included two diabetic women with glomerulonephritis diagnosed on prior biopsies[176]. All authors employed intensified insulin treatment of diabetes[115,181,182], but self-monitoring of blood glucose was universal only in the four studies

Table 10.3. Characteristics of patients in clinical studies of pregnant women with diabetic nephropathy

Author	Years of study	Pregs	Self-Monit. of blood glucose	Proliferative retinopathy	HCT <28	Hypertension		24 h protein (g)			Creatinine clearance (ml/min)			Serum creatinine	
														≥106 ≥1.2	>134 μM >1.5 mg/dl
						Systolic	Diastolic	<1.0	1.0–2.9	≥3	<60	60–79	≥80		
Kitzmiller et al.[174]	1975–8	24	None	8(33%)	11(42%)	16(67%)	8(33%)	9	13	2	8	7	9	7(29%)	4(17%)
Jovanovic and Jovanovic[175]	1980–3	8	All	7(87%)	NA	4	4(50%)	3	3	2	0	3	5	NA	NA
Grenfell et al.[176b]	1974–84	22	NA	8(36%)	NA	NA	(14%)	NA	NA	NA	NA	NA	NA	1/10	0/10
Dicker et al.[177]	1981–4	4	All	2(50%)	NA	1	1(25%)	1	3	0	1	2	1	2	0
Reece et al.[178]	1975–84	30	Some	20(67%)	13(43%)	11(37%)	8(26%)	10	12	8	6	4	20	1(3%)	3(10%)
Biesenbach et al.[179]	1982–7	5	All	5(100%)	NA	4	1(30%)	0	2	3	1	4	0	3	1
Kimmerle et al.[180]	1982–92	36	All	32(89%)	NA	NA	19(53%)	10	21	5	3	7	26	7(19%)	5(16%)
Totals		129		82(64%)			44(34%)	33/107 (30.8%)	54/107 (50.5%)	20/107 (18.7%)	19/107 (17.8%)	27/107 (25.2%)	61/107 (57%)	21/121 (17.4%)	13/121 (10.7%)

Header spanning columns: "Data obtained in first half of pregnancy[a]"

NA, not available.
[a]Kimmerle et al. included two patients without pregnancy data prior to 20 weeks gestation.
[b]Grenfell et al. included two diabetic women with glomerulonephritis on renal biopsy and two diabetic women with persistent proteinuria 'not classified as having diabetic nephropathy as retinopathy was not present.'

conducted in 1980–1992[175,177–179]. All groups employed antihypertensive therapy using multiple agents if arterial pressure exceeded 140/90[174–180]. One-third of the patients had diastolic hypertension in the first half of pregnancy (Table 10.3). Kitzmiller[174] and Reece[178] reported individual data on 54 patients, of whom 27 (50%) had systolic hypertension in early pregnancy compared to 16 (30%) with diastolic hypertension.

A history of proliferative retinopathy was obtained in 64% of the pregnant women with diabetic nephropathy (range 33–100% in the seven individual studies; Table 10.3)[174–180]. Five authors[174,175,177,179,180] provided information on the course of retinopathy in 77 pregnancies; of these, 11 women (15.3%) required laser photocoagulation for neovascularization and three suffered vitreous hemorrhage during pregnancy (3.9%)[174,180] all in association with accelerated hypertension. Reece[178] reported two patients who developed congestive heart failure during pregnancy and Kimmerle[180] noted a stable course in one woman who had two myocardial infarctions prior to pregnancy.

Anemia is common in pregnancy with diabetic nephropathy (Table 10.3), probably resulting from the combination of decreased erythropoietin production in the kidney and the physiological hemodilution of gestation. The degree of anemia is related to the degree of renal dysfunction as reflected by lower creatinine clearance and is not generally associated with abnormal serum iron studies[174]. In severe cases, synthetic erythropoietin can be used[183]. The dosage should be kept low, with a goal to correct the anemia over several weeks, in order to avoid hypertensive reactions or hyperviscosity syndromes.

RENAL FUNCTION DURING PREGNANCY IN DIABETIC NEPHROPATHY

It is important to consider the physiological changes in renal function in normal pregnancy before discussing patients with abnormal renal function. Notwithstanding some variation in early studies of normal pregnant women, it is now generally accepted that effective renal plasma flow (measured by clearance of *para*-aminohippurate) increases by 60–80% in pregnancy, with a significant fall in the third trimester, and glomerular filtration rate (measured by inulin or iohexol clearance) is increased by approximately 50% throughout pregnancy (Table 10.4)[158,184,185]. Twenty-four-hour creatinine clearance is a non-invasive index of glomerular filtration[184], and there is a mean increment of 45% by the second trimester in normal pregnancy[158,185,186], with a consistent decrease to non-pregnant values in the last weeks of gestation[187]. Urinary total protein excretion (Table 10.4)[159,186] and urinary β_2-microglobulin and light chain excretion[188] increase in normotensive pregnant control subjects, suggesting a reduction in tubular reabsorption of protein[157,188], since urinary excretion of albumin, a function of glomerular barrier selectivity[157], increases only slightly or not at all during pregnancy (Table 10.4)[159,188–191], a finding duplicated in timed

Table 10.4. Glomerular filtration rate (GFR) measured by iohexol clearance, 24 h creatinine clearance (CCr), and urinary total protein and albumin excretion in normotensive pregnant control subjects and diabetic pregnant women

Measure	Author	Subjects	Trimester of pregnancy			Before or >5 weeks after pregnancy
			First	Second	Third	
GFR (ml/min per 1.79 m²)[a]	Krutzen et al.[185]	13 controls	–	138 ± 15	143 ± 18	101 ± 8
		16 DM	–	139 ± 15	130 ± 15	111 ± 21
24 h CCr (ml/min)[a]	Davison[158]	10 controls	128 ± 21	144 ± 31	128 ± 22	91 ± 11
Urinary total protein (mg/24 h)[a]	Davison[158]	10 controls	103 ± 49	151 ± 40	180 ± 50	97 ± 52
	Higby et al.[159]	270 controls	80 ± 61	117 ± 69	115 ± 69	–
24 h Urinary albumin (mg/24 h)[a]	Higby et al.[159]	270 controls	9.9 ± 5.3	10.8 ± 6.9	12.8 ± 9.5	–
(mg/24 h)[b]	Lopez-Espinoza et al.[189]	14 controls	–	6.8 (1.8–15)	11.7 (4.9–31.8)	–
(mg/24 h)[b]	Pedersen et al.[188]	13 controls	5.7 (3.0–12.2)	3.7 (1.9–5.8)	5.5 (1.4–12.3)	5.0 (1.9–19)
Timed overnight collection Urinary albumin (μg/l)[b]	McCance et al.[190]	25 controls	–	2.5 (0.1–5.7)	4.0 (0.2–14.7)	3.0 (0.9–212)
		14 DM	–	2.9 (0.6–8.4)	6.7 (0.8–123)	3.7 (1.1–12.8)
	MacRury et al.[191]	22 controls	5.8 (3.7–10.7)	5.1 (3.6–10.4)	4.9 (2.9–7.3)	–
		22 DM	5.0 (3.0–14)	6.0 (5.0–12)	7.5 (3.5–16)	–

[a]Mean + SD.
[b]Median (range).

overnight urine collections at sequential stages of pregnancy in 38 insulin-dependent diabetic pregnant women without microalbuminuria prior to gestation[190,191].

With diabetic nephropathy, the physiological changes of pregnancy are superimposed upon a progressive glomerular disease. The pathophysiological consequences during pregnancy depend on the stage of nephropathy and probably also on such factors as blood pressure, glycemic control and protein intake. Regarding the renal characteristics of 107 pooled pregnant subjects with diabetic nephropathy at initial evaluation in early pregnancy (excepting Grenfell *et al.*[176]), proteinuria exceeded 3 g/24 h in 19% and creatinine clearance was preserved above 79 ml/min in 57% and reduced to less than 60 ml/min in 18% (Table 10.3)[174–180]. 'Baseline' renal function was considered to be impaired on the basis of elevated serum creatinine levels in 34 of 121 subjects (28.1%). Davison has reviewed the reasons that evaluation of renal function in pregnancy must be based on the clearance of creatinine rather than on its plasma concentration[184].

The normal pregnancy-induced rise in glomerular filtration observed in women with insulin-dependent diabetes[185,192] is found in the third trimester in only about one-third of patients with overt diabetic nephropathy (Table 10.5)[174,178]. In another third, the glomerular filtration rate remains stable, and in the final third it decreases. In the pooled series of women with diabetic nephropathy, late pregnancy creatinine clearance was preserved above 79 ml/min in 45%, and was less than 60 ml/min in 38% (Table 10.6). The decrease may reflect the underlying natural history of the progression of diabetic nephropathy which averages about 10 ml/min per year in non-pregnant subjects without intervention[11]. Reece[178] and Biesenbach[179] attribute the decline in creatinine clearance to the development or worsening of pre-existing hypertension. Jovanovic reported that a decrease in creatinine clearance during pregnancy could be prevented in a small group of women with diabetic nephropathy by strictly controlling blood pressure and blood glucose[175].

Table 10.5. Changes in creatinine clearance (CCr) in 44 women with diabetic nephropathy (measurements in both first and third trimesters of pregnancy[a])

First trimester		Third trimester		
CCr	*n* (%)	Increased > 25%	Stable	Decreased > 15%
> 90 ml/min	14 (32%)	3 (21%)	5 (36%)	6 (43%)
60–89 ml/min	20 (45.5%)	9 (45%)	6 (30%)	5 (25%)
< 60 ml/min	10 (22.5%)	2 (20%)	6 (60%)	2 (20%)
Total	44	14 (32%)	17 (30%)	13 (29%)

[a]Data stratified by CCr in first trimester: normal, moderate reduction and severe reduction.
Data pooled from Kitzmiller *et al.*[174], Jovanovic and Jovanovic[175] and Reece *et al.*[178].

184

Table 10.6. Late pregnancy renal function in clinical studies of women with diabetic nephropathy

Author	Years of study	Preg.	Hypertension		24 h proteinuria (g)			Creatinine clearance (ml/min)			Serum creatinine	
			Systolic ≥140	Diastolic ≥90	<1.0	1.0–2.9	≥3	<60	60–70	≥80 (ml/min)	≥106 ≥1.2	≥134 μm ≥1.5 mg/dl
Kitzmiller[165]	1975–8	24	18(75%)	18(75%)	0	7	17(71%)	10(42%)	4(16%)	10(42%)	5(21%)	8(33%)
Jovanovic[166]	1980–3	8	4	4(50%)	3	3	2(25%)	1	1	6(75%)	2/19(10.5%)	4/19(21%)
Grenfell[167]	1974–84	22	NA	16(72%)	NA	NA	NA	NA	NA	NA	NA	NA
Dicker[168]	1981–4	4	3	3(75%)	0	1	3(75%)	1	3	0	1(25%)	1(25%)
Reece[169]	1975–84	30	21(70%)	18(60%)	5	3	22(73%)	11(37%)	4	15(50%)	5(17%)	8(27%)
Biesenbach[170]	1982–7	5	5	5(100%)	0	0	5(100%)	4		1	NA	NA
Kimmerle[171]	1982–92	36	NA	35(97%)	5	12	19(53%)	NA	NA	NA	6(17%)	8(22%)
		129		100 (77.5%)	13/107 (12.1%)	26/107 (24.3%)	68/107 (63.6%)	27/71 (38%)	12/71 (17%)	32/71 (45%)	19/113 (17%)	29/113 (26%)

NA, not available.

Total proteinuria typically increases greatly during pregnancy in patients with diabetic nephropathy (Figure 10.2)[174–180]. In the pooled series, 24 h proteinuria exceeded 3 g in 64% of patients (Table 10.6). Although some of this increase may be due to the underlying progression of nephropathy, or to the glomerular endotheliosis of superimposed pre-eclampsia, much of the increase may be caused by the physiological hyperfiltration and reduced proximal tubular reabsorption of pregnancy[156,157,188], since the proteinuria generally subsides after delivery. Regarding the increased rate of protein excretion as pregnancy progresses, Reece and co-authors wrote:

> This pregnancy-related, transient increase in protein excretion in patients with preexisting proteinuria parallels in an amplified manner the changes in

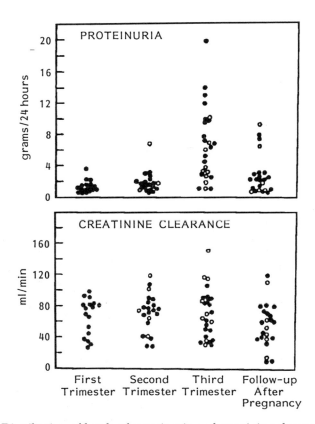

Figure 10.2. Distribution of levels of proteinuria and creatinine clearance in women with diabetic nephropathy in each trimester of pregnancy and at a follow-up visit 9–35 months after delivery. Closed circles indicate women studied in each trimester; open circles indicate women not seen in the first trimester. From Kitzmiller JL, Brown ER, Phillippe M *et al.* Diabetic nephropathy and perinatal outcome. *Am J Obst Gynecol* 1981; **141**: 174. Used with permission

protein excretion observed in normal pregnancy, and could represent an increase in the amount of filtered protein, a decrease in tubular reabsorption of filtered protein, or both. It seems likely that a decrease in proximal tubular transport processes, including reabsorption of filtered protein, plays an important role in amplifying protein excretion during pregnancy in patients with preexisting alterations in filtered protein because of glomerular injury[178].

Truly massive proteinuria developed in 44% of 107 pregnant women with diabetic nephropathy[174,175,177–180], reaching levels of 5–9 g/24 h in 27.1% and exceeding 10 g/24 h in 16.8% (Table 10.7). Excessive proteinuria often leads to hypoalbuminemia, decreased plasma oncotic pressure and generalized edema. Optimal treatment is problematic. Dietary protein supplementation or albumin infusions may be temporarily helpful, but they can also further increase renal blood flow and protein excretion. Diuretics may be helpful, but they must be used judiciously during pregnancy because excessive lowering of plasma volume can adversely affect uteroplacental perfusion. Kimmerle *et al.*[180] point out the importance of starting antihypertensive treatment at levels lower than 100–105 diastolic (which is the threshold suggested for non-diabetic pregnant women)[136,137,193], in order to prevent a massive loss of protein and hypoalbuminemia. Hypoalbuminemia causing a further decrease in intravascular volume might contribute to decreased uteroplacental blood flow which is believed to be one of the causes of pre-eclampsia[11,180].

The percentage of patients with a significant decline in renal function during pregnancy (Table 10.7) is somewhat greater in women with diabetic nephropathy[174–180] than in women with non-diabetic glomerular diseases[194–196], especially when subjects are grouped by whether initial renal function was preserved or impaired (Table 10.8). Katz and colleagues found that renal function decreased in 16% of 121 pregnancies in 89 women with various renal disorders, and signficant hypertension occurred in 23%[194]. Hou *et al.* reported data on 25 pregnancies in 23 women with moderate renal insufficiency (serum creatinine ≥ 1.4 mg/dl at onset of pregnancy)[195]. Twelve women had primary glomerular diseases, five had interstitial diseases, and six had other renal disease. In seven women with baseline serum creatinine ranging from 1.7 to 2.7 mg/dl, 'pregnancy was accompanied by a decline in renal function that was believed to be greater than expected from the natural history of the disease'[195]. Of the 12 women with glomerular disease, six developed accelerated hypertension. Abe *et al.* studied 105 pregnancies in 72 women with non-diabetic glomerulopathies, and in 11 cases (10.5%) renal function decreased during pregnancy or after delivery[196]. 'Most of these cases showed good renal function before pregnancy but had either marked tubulointerstitial changes or high blood pressure or both'[196]. Comparing these studies to the pooled series of women with diabetic nephropathy, accelerated hypertension and decline in renal function during pregnancy is more common in the diabetic women (Tables 10.6–10.8).

Table 10.7. Course of renal parameters[a] during and after pregnancy in clinical studies of women with diabetic nephropathy

Author	Years of study	Pregs.	Initial renal function[b]		Accel. HTN	Massive proteinuria		Decrease in CCr	Rise in serum creat.	Follow-up after pregnancy						
			Preserved	Impaired		5-9 g/d	≥10 g/d			N	Years (median)	Massive Proteinuria ≥5 g/d	Decline[c] rate CrCl ml/min per month	Serum creat. ≥134	Renal failure[d]	Died
Kitzmiller et al.[174]	1975-8	24	9	15	8	8	6	5	12	23	1-3(1.7)	4	-0.39	10	3	0
Jovanovic and Jovanovic[175]	1980-3	8	5	3	2	1	2	1	NA	(8)	6 weeks	0	NA	NA	NA	NA
Grenfell et al.[176]	1974-4	22	21	1	16	NA	NA	NA	4	17	0.5-10(2.0)	NA	NA	4	2	1
Dicker et al.[177]	1981-4	4	2	2	3	2	0	0	1	4	0.5-1.0	0	NA	1	0	0
Reece et al.[178e]	1975-4	30	20	10	9	10	3	11	10	26	0.5-9(1.0)	7/16	NA	11/21	6	0
Biesenbach et al.[179]	1982-7	5	0	5	5	2	2	4	4	5	1-3.5(2.4)	NA	1.69	5	5	0
Kimmerle et al.[180]	1982-92	36	26	10	23	6	5	14/28	14	29	0.3-9	NA	0.65	NA	8	4
Totals		129	83	46 (35.7%)	66 (51.2%)	29/107 (27.1%)	18/107 (16.8%)	35/99 (35.4%)	45/121 (37.2%)	104 (81%)				31/70 (44%)	24 (23.1%)	5 (4%)

[a]Significant change during pregnancy defined as >15% of initial values.
[b]Impaired renal function defined as serum creatinine >106 μM (>1.2 mg/dl) or creatinine clearance (CCr) <80 ml/min in early pregnancy.
[c]Creatinine clearance at >2 months follow-up minus creatinine clearance in early pregnancy divided by months from early pregnancy to follow-up.
[d]Renal failure treated with hemodialysis or renal transplantation.
[e]Of 26 women followed for >2 months post partum, 16 had 24h urine protein measured, 9 had creatinine clearance measured, and 21 had serum creatinine measured.
HTN – hypertension.

Table 10.8. Perinatal outcome and course during pregnancy for diabetic women with and without nephropathy compared to non-diabetic women with glomerular diseases

Source (ref.)	Established diabetes without nephropathy		Diabetic nephropathy [174-180]		Non-diabetic glomerular diseases	
			Initial renal function			
	1975–8	1987–92	Preserved	Impaired[a]	Preserved	Impaired[a]
	Kitzmiller et al.[174]	Kimmerle et al.[180]	[174-180]	[174-180]	Katz et al.[194]	Katz et al.[194] Hou et al.[195]
Pregnancies	232	110	83	46	59	29
Delivery <34 weeks	10 (4.3%)	3 (2.7%)	17 (20.5)	20 (43.5%)	3 (5.1%)	11 (37.9%)
Stillborn	1 (0.4%)	0	2 (2.4%)	2 (4.3%)	3 (5.1%)	2 (6.9%)
Liveborn	231	110	83[b]	44	58[b]	27
SGA	5 (2.2%)	2 (1.8%)	10 (12.3%)[c]	5 (32.6%)	20 (33.9%)[c]	10 (34.5%)
Neonatal death	6 (2.6%)[d]	0	0	4 (9.1%)[d]	2 (3.4%)[d]	3 (1.1%)[d]
Perinatal survival	(97%)	(100%)	(97.6%)	(87.0%)	(91.8%)	(82.8%)
Accelerating hypertension	–	–	36 (43.4%)	30 (65.2%)	13 (22.0%)	(51.7%)
Decline in renal function	–	–	19 (22.9%)	27 (58.7%)	3 (5.1%)	7 (24.1%)

SGA, small for gestational age.
[a]Serum creatinine ≥106 μm (≥1.2 mg/dl) or creatinine clearance <80 ml/min.
[b]Includes twin gestation.
[c]Excluding twin gestation.
[d]Percentage of liveborn infants.

If the creatinine clearance falls below 30 ml/min, the kidneys are on the verge of failure, and consultation with a nephrologist should be sought. Such patients may become candidates for dialysis if the serum potassium rises or uremia ensues. Patients who have been undergoing dialysis before pregnancy often need more frequent dialysis during pregnancy. Since urea, creatinine and other metabolites that accumulate in uremia[197] can cross the placenta[198] and cause a fetal osmotic diuresis[199], close fetal monitoring is essential in maternal renal failure[197]. According to Maikranz and Katz[199], dialysis should be tailored to keep the blood urea < 50 mg/dl. Both hemodialysis and peritoneal dialysis have been used in pregnancy[200–202].

The goals of dialysis are to keep the electrolytes in balance, to prevent metabolic acidosis, and to prevent uremia. Maternal hypercalcemia and increased uterine irritability are considerations[199]. Pregnancy complications are frequent among patients undergoing dialysis, including pre-eclampsia, placental abruption and stillbirth. The latter two probably are related to rapid shifts in maternal intravascular volume and hypotension. It has been suggested that chronic ambulatory peritoneal dialysis may be safer than hemodialysis during pregnancy because such volume shifts can be avoided more easily[18]. For hemodialysis, Maikranz and Katz[199] advise direct-vision catheter placement. With hemodialysis, it is important to use shorter and more frequent (daily) dialysis, avoiding high-flux dialysis, and carefully to adjust heparin dosage to prevent hemorrhagic complications[199].

Davison studied the effect of pregnancy on kidney function in non-diabetic renal allograft recipients[158]. In late pregnancy, mean 24 h creatinine clearance decreased by 34% and total protein excretion increased three times above non-pregnant levels, usually exceeding 300 mg/24 h, but in most patients this did not represent graft deterioration nor lead to permanent impairment[158]. A later case-controlled study of 18 renal allograft recipients who became pregnant and were followed for 4–23 years after pregnancy (mean 12 years) showed no evidence of an adverse effect of pregnancy on long-term renal function or development of hypertension[203].

In the pooled series of 129 pregnant women with diabetic nephropathy, only three pregnancies were included in diabetic women who had a renal transplant[174,180]. Creatinine clearance rose normally during pregnancy in one of these women[174], and remained low at 32–35 ml/min in the other two[180]. Pregnancies in nine other diabetic women 0.5–5 years after renal transplantation were analyzed by Ogburn et al.[204]. Creatinine clearance early in pregnancy was preserved > 80 ml/min in four but declined in the third trimester in two of these patients in association with accelerated hypertension. In the five women with early reduction of creatinine clearance (45–68 ml/min), only one showed an apparent rise of glomerular filtration rate in pregnancy, and four demonstrated accelerated hypertension in the third trimester[204].

ACCELERATED HYPERTENSION DURING PREGNANCY

To establish the limits of normality in a prospective controlled study, Peterson *et al.* examined changes in cholesterol, triglycerides, body weight and blood pressure in 312 diabetic and 356 control women recruited within 21 days after conception[205]. The upper 95% confidence limits in the healthy control group at 28 weeks gestation were 130 mmHg for systolic arterial pressure and 81 mmHg for diastolic pressure. The commonly targeted blood pressure of 140/90 'was 3 SD above the normal mean at any observation point during gestation in the control group'[205]. Systolic blood pressure increased during pregnancy in the diabetic women, whose diastolic pressure was also higher at entry and throughout gestation compared to controls.

The pre-eclampsia syndrome was diagnosed in 12% of 107 women with established diabetes in Ottawa, after exclusion of patients with nephropathy or chronic hypertension[206]. In a Cincinnati study of 88 diabetic women of White classes B–C, 9.1% had an increase in mean arterial pressure ≥ 20 mmHg from baseline, 'regardless of the presence or severity of proteinuria'[207]. The pregnancy-induced hypertension was significantly associated with nulliparity and poor glycemic control in the first and second trimesters. In women with diabetic nephropathy, accelerated hypertension during pregnancy is an alarming finding, since it can be associated with a decline in renal function and worsening retinopathy[174,178,180]. Many women with nephropathy have chronic hypertension antedating pregnancy, as noted previously. In the pooled series of 129 women with diabetic nephropathy[174–180] in late pregnancy, severe blood pressure elevations were noted in 43% of 83 with initially preserved renal function, compared to 59% of 46 with impaired renal function (Table 10.8). Accelerated hypertension was somewhat more common in the women with diabetic nephropathy than in patients with non-diabetic glomerular diseases reported by Katz[194] and Hou[195].

The picture of accelerated hypertension in pregnant women with diabetic nephropathy is clinically indistinguishable from severe pre-eclampsia because these women also typically have increasing proteinuria. In the pooled series of 107 women[174,175,177–180], superimposed pre-eclampsia was diagnosed in 28%. However, it is possible that this is not 'true' pre-eclampsia, but rather a transient, pregnancy-associated worsening of the chronic hypertension and proteinuria. Most authors agree that the definition of pre-eclampsia is rather arbitrary in this setting[174,178,180] although the distinction may be of clinical importance because severe pre-eclampsia is regarded as an indication for prompt delivery, whereas an exacerbation of chronic hypertension may simply be treated with antihypertensive therapy. In a minority of cases, there may be thrombocytopenia or transaminase elevations that would support a diagnosis of pre-eclampsia[178]. However, in most cases there are no definitively distinctive clinical findings. Hyperuricemia is not helpful since it was found in 46% of pregnant women with diabetic nephropathy in one series[174]. Thus, the decision to deliver the infant must be based on a careful assessment that balances the course and severity of the maternal condition, the gestational age, and tests of fetal well-being. Preterm delivery is common among women with overt nephropathy, and most of this is necessitated by pre-eclampsia[208].

Pre-eclampsia may be nearly as common with incipient nephropathy as it is with overt diabetic nephropathy[209,210]. Mogensen and Klebe reported on nine insulin-dependent diabetic women with urinary albumin excretion 20–200 µg/min in early pregnancy ('microalbuminuria'), compared to 14 whose albumin excretion rate did not exceed 20 µg/min until full term[211]. There was one stillbirth in the first and two in the second groups, at 28–31 weeks gestation. There was a distinct rise in mean arterial pressure in the group developing microalbuminuria in late pregnancy, but only one case was diagnosed as pre-eclampsia. Data on glycemic control were not given in reference to the stillbirths. No other adverse outcomes were reported in the 'microalbuminuria' group. Of note, in the case of pre-eclampsia, the increase in proteinuria occurred several weeks before the clinical onset of pre-eclampsia and also occurred several weeks before two of the stillbirths. The authors suggested that microalbuminuria might be a 'sensitive marker of generalized subclinical vascular disturbance and damage' and might be 'useful in the early prediction of complications' of pregnancy in insulin-dependent diabetes[211].

McCance *et al.*[190] followed 14 insulin-dependent diabetic women with serial measures of urinary albumin excretion throughout pregnancy. Three of them developed pre-eclampsia, but the authors stated that there was no evidence for an increase in urinary albumin excretion antedating the pre-eclampsia. Altman reported a normal outcome in three diabetic women with microalbuminuria 58–115 mg/24 h[212]. Winocour *et al.* studied 23 non-azotemic insulin-dependent diabetic women throughout pregnancy[213]. Of the four cases with urinary albumin excretion over 20 µg/min prior to pregnancy or in early pregnancy, four developed pre-eclampsia (75%), compared to three of 19 (15%) with urinary albumin excretion below this level. In a logistic regression analysis, it was found that urinary albumin was the best single predictor of pre-eclampsia in these women, followed by mean arterial pressure in the second trimester.

In our own study of 311 diabetic women from two institutions, we found that the risk of pre-eclampsia was clearly related to the degree of proteinuria in early pregnancy[214]. With total protein excretion rates below 190 mg/24 h, the rate of pre-eclampsia was 10%; with excretion of 190–499 mg/24 h in 45 women, the rate was 40%; and with overt diabetic nephropathy in 62 women, the rate was 47%. On logistic regression analysis, the increased risk of pre-eclampsia associated with elevated total protein excretion persisted after controlling for the effects of chronic hypertension, nulliparity, retinopathy and early pregnancy glycemic control. Patients with total protein excretion rates in the 190–499 μg/24 h range also had an increase in the rate of preterm delivery, most of which was attributable to pre-eclampsia. We speculated that total protein excretion in this range might be a marker for incipient diabetic nephropathy, although we did not perform specific assays for albumin excretion.

Thus we believe that women with incipient nephropathy are likely to be at high risk of pre-eclampsia and its attendant complications. However, further prospective data including pre-pregnancy urinary albumin values are clearly needed to further define the risks of pre-eclampsia and other pregnancy complications. Low-dose aspirin in the second and third trimesters may slightly reduce the rate of pre-eclampsia and resultant preterm delivery in low-risk patients[215,216], and slightly increase the chance of placental abruption[215], although there are no data addressing whether this therapy is effective in women with diabetic nephropathy. An ongoing clinical trial by the National Institutes of Health Maternal–Fetal Medicine Units may help to answer this question. Calcium supplementation may also reduce the risk of superimposed pre-eclampsia[217,218].

OBSTETRICAL MANAGEMENT AND PERINATAL OUTCOME

The formerly high perinatal mortality rates of about 30% in women with diabetic nephropathy, with losses due to major malformations, premature delivery because of pre-eclampsia, and severe growth delay with asphyxia[117], have improved substantially in the past two decades. In series reported in 1981–1994 with pooled data on 129 patients, perinatal mortality was 6.1% (Table 10.9)[174–180]. Improved peri-conception glycemic control has decreased the incidence of major malformations in women with diabetic nephropathy[104–107]. Advances in perinatal care such as fetal surveillance, sonographic recognition of growth delay, and better control of hypertension have reduced the fetal death rate and have improved the condition of those infants who still require preterm delivery. Advances in neonatal care continue to reduce the mortality and morbidity of premature neonates. However, pregnancy in women with diabetic nephropathy still carries a high rate of complications that place the fetus and newborn in jeopardy.

Intrauterine growth retardation still occurs at roughly twice the rate as in the general population (Table 10.9). The incidence of growth retardation (19.8% in the pooled series[174–180]) is related to the severity of nephropathy and hypertension. Intrauterine growth retardation was found in 12.3% of infants of 83 women with diabetic nephropathy with preserved initial renal function, compared to 32.6% of 46 babies of mothers with diabetic nephropathy and impaired renal function in early pregnancy (Table 10.8). In Table 10.10, the three-fold damaging influence of accelerated

Table 10.9. Perinatal outcome in clinical studies of women with diabetic nephropathy

Author	Years of study	Pregs.	Superimp. pre-eclampsia[a]	Acute fetal distress	Gestational age at delivery (weeks from LMP) <30	30-33	34-36	>37	C-sect.	Fetal death	Live born	Twins	Birth weight for gestational age SGA	AGA	LGA	Major congen. malfs	RDS	Neonatal death	Perinatal survival
Kitzmiller et al.[174]	1985-8	24	4 (17%)	5 (19%)	2	6	10	6	20	2	23	1	5	18	2	3	6(24%)	1	22/25 (88%)
Grenfell et al.[176]	1974-84	22	NA	NA	1	5	5	11	16	0	23	1	3	18	2	1	NA	0	23/23
Jovanovic and Jovanovic[175]	1980-3	8	2 (25%)	0	0	0	0	7	NA	0	8	0	0	8	0	0	1	0	8/8
Dicker et al.[177]	1981-4	4	3 (75%)	1	0	0	4	0	3	0	4	0	0	3	1	0	2	0	4/4
Reece et al.[178]	1975-84	30	11 (35%)	7 (23%)	3	4	10	13	21	2	28	0	5	23	3	3	6(19%)	0	28/30 (93%)
Biesenbach et al.[179]	1982-7	5	3 (60%)	2 (40%)	1	3	1	0	3	0	5	0	4	1	0	0	4	3	2/5
Kimmerle et al.[180]	1982-92	36	7 (19%)	NA	1	10	6	9	31	0	36	0	9	24	3	2	9(25%)	0	36/36
Totals		129	30/107 (28%)	15/71 (21%)	8	29	36	46 (36%)	94/121 (78%)	4 (3.1%)	127		26 (19.8%)	95	11 (8.4%)	9 (6.9%)	28 (22%)	4 (3.1%)	123/131 (93.9%)

NA, not available; LMP, last menstrual period; SGA, small for gestational age; AGA, average weight for gestational age; LGA, large for gestational age; RDS, respiratory distress syndrome
[a] Pre-eclampsia-like syndrome defined as 'worsening hypertension and multisystemic involvement usually resulting in coagulopathy and abnormal liver function' by Reece et al.[178], and as 'acute worsening of hypertension (>15% of diastolic blood pressure) in the presence of proteinuria >3 g per day and generalized edema' by Kimmerle et al.[180].

Table 10.10. Influence of accelerated hypertension on the frequency of intrauterine growth retardation in 70 women with diabetic nephropathy with and without impaired renal function in early pregnancy

| | Initial renal function | |
	Preserved	Impaired[a]
N	35	35
40 No accelerated hypertension	1/22 (4.5%)	3/18 (16.7%)
30 Accelerated hypertension	2/13 (15.4%)	8/17 (47.1%)

[a]Serum creatinine $\geq 106\ \mu$m (≥ 1.2 mg/dl) or creatinine clearance < 80 ml/min at the initial assessment during pregnancy.

hypertension during pregnancy on the rate of intrauterine growth retardation is seen in women with diabetic nephropathy both with and without initial impaired renal function. It is hoped that strict control of hypertension will reduce the incidence of growth retardation. Also, we generally advise all women with clinical diabetic nephropathy to rest in bed in the lateral decubitus position for several hours each day in the second half of pregnancy to maximize uteroplacental blood flow, in the hope that this will help prevent excess proteinuria and accelerated hypertension. If intrauterine growth retardation is suspected, we advise nearly complete bedrest.

To prevent excess morbidity from growth retardation, hypoxia and asphyxia, fetal surveillance must be able to identify the problems[219]. There are no controlled trials regarding the optimum method of fetal surveillance in diabetic women. We instruct all diabetic women in fetal movement counting. In women with diabetic nephropathy, serial sonographic assessments of fetal growth should be used in the late second and third trimesters. If there is evidence of growth delay, we begin non-stress testing immediately. Because these tests may have false non-reactivity, it is important to use the contraction stress test and sonographic biophysical profile as backup tests. Even in the absence of intrauterine growth retardation, we start weekly non-stress testing on all women with clinical diabetic nephropathy by 28 weeks of gestation and increase to twice weekly by 36 weeks of gestation. Umbilical artery Doppler velocimetry has been studied in a few women with diabetic nephropathy[220,221]. Growth-retarded fetuses tend to have elevated Doppler S/D ratios. If Doppler studies are abnormal but more traditional indicators of fetal well-being such as fetal heart rate and amniotic fluid volume are normal, immediate preterm delivery is probably not justified, but daily fetal surveillance is indicated. Further, Salvesen *et al.*[221] found that fetal acidemia in diabetic pregnancies was not accompanied by abnormal Doppler studies, which rather suggested a relationship of acidemia to glycemic control[221]. Evidence of fetal distress is common in growth-retarded fetuses and cesarean delivery is frequently required (Table 10.9). The rate of cesarean section was 78% in the pooled series of women with diabetic nephropathy[174-180]. The timing of delivery depends on the gravity of the maternal hypertension and renal failure, gestational age, evidence of fetal lung maturity and severity of fetal condition. Vaginal delivery can generally be attempted at any gestational age as long as the intrapartum fetal heart rate tracing is reassuring and there are no obstetric indications for cesarean delivery.

Preterm delivery remains a significant problem in pregnancies complicated by diabetic nephropathy (Tables 10.8 and 10.9), occurring before 34 weeks gestation in 29% of pregnancies in the pooled series[174-180]. About half of preterm births in women with diabetic nephropathy are attributable to pre-eclampsia or accelerated hypertension[208]. Many of the remainder occur because of fetal distress, with or without growth retardation. Because preterm delivery is so likely, we believe that these patients should receive care at a tertiary center with an intensive care nursery. Although neonatal mortality from prematurity continues to decline, preterm delivery still carries considerable short-term morbidity from respiratory distress, hyperbilirubinemia, apnea/bradycardia, and a host of other expensive complications. All investigators agree[174-180] that the major maternal predictors of perinatal morbidity are the extent of impaired renal function indicated by creatinine clearance and the degree of hypertension.

Regarding the management of pre-eclampsia, recent controlled trials[222,223] demonstrated the superiority of magnesium sulfate therapy over diazepam or phenytoin in prevention of eclampsia and other maternal and neonatal complications. A randomized comparison of regional and general anesthesia for cesarean delivery in pregnancies complicated by severe pre-eclampsia showed that all three techniques were equally acceptable[224]. These data should apply to women with diabetic nephropathy.

There is some controversy about the long-term development of infants of diabetic mothers with clinical nephropathy. Using standardized psychomotor assessments, Kimmerle *et al.* found evidence of psychomotor delay in eight of 34 infants born to mothers in Dusseldorf with nephropathy (21%) (in one case, this was attributed to a major malformation)[180]. All but one of the other cases were associated with preterm delivery, growth retardation, or both. In five of the cases, the delay was classified as 'severe'. While these outcomes were worse than those reported in the prospective follow-up studies of Kitzmiller *et al.*[174] and Reece *et al.*[178], they underscore the importance of preventing growth retardation and prematurity.

MATERNAL OUTCOME AND DIABETIC NEPHROPATHY

Does the worsening of hypertension and proteinuria during pregnancy accelerate the progression of diabetic nephropathy to end-stage renal disease? Investigators reporting long-term follow-up after delivery found that 24 of 104 women with diabetic nephropathy (23%) had progressed to end-stage renal disease within 1–10 years[174,176–180]. The women progressing were in the group of 46 women with impaired renal function in early pregnancy (Table 10.7), representing a 52% risk of this progression after pregnancy. However, it must be borne in mind that nephropathy frequently progresses to end-stage renal disease even in the absence of pregnancy, so these observations do not establish that pregnancy accelerates the process. No case-controlled studies have been conducted in women with diabetic nephropathy with and without pregnancy.

Three groups of investigators studied the fall in creatinine clearance during the years immediately after pregnancy in women with diabetic nephropathy[174,180,225]. All three observed creatinine clearance to decline at an average rate of 8–10 ml/min per year of follow-up. This rate is no different from that reported for diabetic nephropathy patients in general[11], and it does not support the idea that pregnancy accelerates the process of nephropathy. Diabetic nephropathy is a progressive disease, with or without pregnancy. Until recently, the progression from overt nephropathy to end-stage occurred in an average of about 10 years. It remains to be seen what impact interventions such as antihypertensive therapy, strict glycemic control and low-protein diets will have on this rate. Once end-stage disease occurs, the median survival time is only three years, and seven-year survival is only 20%. It has been argued that 'the poor maternal prognosis is an important reason for discouraging pregnancies [in women with nephropathy] despite the good short-term results'[176]. We do not agree with this negative viewpoint, but it emphasizes the importance of thorough counseling prior to pregnancy.

Women bordering on end-stage renal disease (creatinine clearance below 30 ml/min, serum creatinine over 3 mg/dl) should be considered for renal transplantation or dialysis before pregnancy. Patients in whom hypertension cannot be controlled should be advised that there is a low probability of a successful pregnancy. Women with proliferative retinopathy should be in remission or have laser photocoagulation before becoming pregnant because exacerbations are much less frequent under these conditions.

As we have previously written[226]:

Absent these contraindications, the decision to become pregnant or to continue a pregnancy should largely be one of informed consent. A woman with diabetic nephropathy must be counseled about the progressive nature of the disease. It is important to discuss the implications of a chronic disease on her ability to raise a child and to note that she may not survive the child's adolescence. The likely financial burden of pregnancy and neonatal care should be disclosed. After adequate counseling, it is up to the patient and her partner to decide whether to proceed with pregnancy. If this is their wish, with meticulous attention to glycemic control, blood pressure control, diet, bedrest, and fetal surveillance, an excellent outcome can often be obtained[226].

REFERENCES

1 Stephenson JM, Kenny S, Stevens LK *et al.* WHO Multinational Study Group. Proteinuria and mortality in diabetes: the WHO multinational study of vascular disease in diabetes. *Diabetic Med* 1995; **12**: 149–55.
2 Rossing P, Rossing K, Jacobsen P, Parving HH. Unchanged incidence of diabetic nephropathy in IDDM patients. *Diabetes* 1995; **44**: 739–43.
3 Mauer SM, Steffes MW, Ellis EN *et al.* Structural–functional relationship in diabetic nephropathy. *J Clin Invest* 1984; **74**: 1143–55.
4 Osterby R, Parving H-H, Nyberg G *et al.* Morphology of diabetic glomerulopathy and relationship to hypertension. *Diabete Metab* 1989; **15**: 278–83.
5 Osterby R, Parving HH, Hommel E *et al.* Glomerular structure and function in diabetic nephropathy: early to advanced stages. *Diabetes* 1990; **39**: 1057–63.
6 Mogensen CE. Early glomerular hyperfiltration in insulin-dependent diabetes and late nephropathy. *Scand J Clin Lab Invest* 1986; **46**: 201–6.
7 Mogensen CE. Microalbuminuria as a predictor of clinical diabetic nephropathy. *Kidney Int* 1987; **31**: 673–7.
8 Deckert T, Kofoed-Enevoldsen A, Norgaard *et al.* Microalbuminuria: implications for micro- and macrovascular disease. *Diabetes Care* 1992; **15**: 1181–91.
9 Larkins RG, Dunlop ME. The link between hyperglycaemia and diabetic nephropathy. *Diabetologia* 1992; **35**: 499–504.
10 Mogensen CE, Chachati A, Christensen CK *et al.* Microalbuminuria: an early marker of renal involvement in diabetes. *Uremia Invest* 1985–86; **9**: 85–95.
11 Mogensen CE, Schmitz O. The diabetic kidney: from hyperfiltration and microalbuminuria to end-stage renal failure. *Med Clin North Am* 1988; **72**; 1465–92.
12 D'Antonio JA, Ellis D, Doft BH *et al.* Diabetes complications and glycemic control: the Pittsburgh Prospective Insulin-Dependent Diabetes Cohort Study status report after 5 yr of IDDM. *Diabetes Care* 1989; **12**: 694–700.
13 EURODIAB IDDM Complications Study Group: Microvascular and acute complications in IDDM patients: the EURODIAB IDDM Complications Study. *Diabetologia* 1994; **37**: 278–85.
14 Mathiesen ER, Ronn B, Jensen T *et al.* Relationship between blood pressure and urinary albumin excretion in development of microalbuminuria. *Diabetes* 1990; **39**: 245–9.
15 Raal FJ, Kalk WJ, Taylor DR *et al.* The relationship between the development and progression of microalbuminuria and arterial blood pressure in type 1 (insulin-dependent) diabetes mellitus. *Diabetes Res Clin Pract* 1992; **16**: 221–7.
16 Coonrod BA, Ellis D, Becker DJ *et al.* Predictors of microalbuminuria in individuals with IDDM. *Diabetes Care* 1993; **16**: 1376–83.
17 Chase HP, Garg SK, Marshall G *et al.* Cigarette smoking increases the risk of albuminuria among subjects with type 1 diabetes *JAMA* 1991; **254**: 614–17.
18 Parving H-H, Oxenboll B, Svendsen PAA *et al.* Early detection of patients at risk of developing diabetic nephropathy: a longitudinal study of urinary albumin excretion. *Acta Endocrinol* 1982; **100**: 550–5.
19 Viberti GC, Hill RD, Jarrett RJ *et al.* Microalbuminuria as a predictor of clinical nephropathy in insulin-dependent diabetes mellitus. *Lancet* 1982; **i**: 1430–2.
20 Mogensen CE, Christensen CK. Predicting diabetic nephropathy in insulin-dependent patients. *N Engl J Med* 1984; **311**: 89–93.
21 Mathiesen ER, Oxenboll B, Johansen K *et al.* Incipient nephropathy in type 1 (insulin-dependent) diabetes. *Diabetologia* 1984; **26**: 406–10.
22 Almdal T, Feldt-Rasmussen B, Norgaard K, Deckert T. The predictive value of microalbuminuria in IDDM. *Diabetes Care* 1994; **17**: 120–5.
23 Deckert T, Andersen AR, Christiansen JS, Andersen JK. Course of diabetic nephropathy: factors related to development. *Acta Endocrinol* 1981; **97** (Suppl. 242): 14.
24 Andersen AR, Christiansen JS, Andersen JK *et al.* Diabetic nephropathy in type 1 (insulin-dependent) diabetes mellitus. *Diabetologia* 1985; **28**: 590–6.
25 Kofoed-Enevoldsen A, Borch-Johnsen K, Kreiner S *et al.* Declining incidence of persistent proteinuria in type I (insulin-dependent) diabetic patients in Denmark. *Diabetes* 1987; **36**: 205–9.

26 Krolewski AS, Warram JH, Christlieb AR *et al.* The changing natural history of nephropathy in type I diabetes. *Am J Med* 1985; **78**: 785–94.

27 Bojestig M, Arnqvist HJ, Hermansson G *et al.* Declining incidence of nephropathy in insulin-dependent diabetes mellitus. *N Engl J Med* 1994; **330**: 15–18.

28 Seaquist ER, Goetz FC, Rich S, Barbosa J. Familial clustering of diabetic kidney disease: evidence for genetic susceptibility to diabetic nephropathy. *N Engl J Med* 1989; **320**: 1161–5.

29 Doria A, Warram JH, Krolewski AS. Genetic predisposition to diabetic nephropathy: evidence for a role of the angiotensin I-converting enzyme gene. *Diabetes* 1994; **43**: 690–5.

30 Deckert T, Feldt-Rasmussen B, Borch-Johnsen K *et al.* Albuminuria reflects widespread vascular damage: the Steno hypothesis. *Diabetologia* 1989; **32**: 219–26.

31 Mogensen CE. The effect of blood pressure intervention on renal function in insulin-dependent diabetes. *Diabete Metab* 1989; **15**: 343–51.

32 Hirsch IB. Current concepts in diabetic nephropathy. *Clin Diabetes* 1994; **12**: 8–12.

33 Christiansen JS, Gammelgaard J, Tronier B. Kidney function and size in diabetics before and during initial insulin treatment. *Kidney Int* 1982; **21**: 683.

34 Mogensen CE. Glomerular filtration rate and renal plasma flow in short-term juvenile diabetes mellitus. *Scand J Clin Lab Invest* 1971; **28**: 91.

35 Hirose K, Tsuchida H, Osterby R, Gundersen HJG. A strong correlation between glomerular filtration rate and filtration surface in diabetic kidney hyperfunction. *Lab Invest* 1980; **43**: 434.

36 Mogensen CE, Osterby R, Gundersen HJG. Early functional and morphologic vascular renal consequences of the diabetic state. *Diabetologia* 1979; **17**: 71.

37 Osterby R, Gundersen HJG. Glomerular size and structure in diabetes mellitus. I. Early abnormalities. *Diabetologia* 1975; **11**: 225.

38 Mogensen CE, Christensen CK, Vittinghus E. The stages in diabetic renal disease, with emphasis on the stage of incipient diabetic nephropathy. *Diabetes* 1983; **32** (Suppl. 2): 64.

39 Chavers BM, Bilous RW, Ellis EN *et al.* Glomerular lesions and urinary albumin excretion in type I diabetes without overt proteinuria. *N Engl J Med* 1989; **320**: 966–70.

40 Steffes MW, Osterby R, Chavers B, Mauer M. Mesangial expansion as a central mechanism for loss of kidney function in diabetic patients. *Diabetes* 1989; **38**: 1077–81.

41 Viberti GC, Bilous RW, Mackintosh D, Keen H. Monitoring glomerular function in diabetic nephropathy: a prospective study. *Am J Med* 1983; **74**: 256.

42 Diabetes Control and Complications Trial Research Group. The effect of intensive treatment of diabetes on the development and progression of long-term complications in insulin-dependent diabetes mellitus. 1993; *N Engl J Med* **329**: 977–86.

43 Osterby R, Gundersen HJG, Nyberg G, Aurell M. Advanced diabetic glomerulopathy: quantitative structural characterization of non-occluded glomeruli. *Diabetes* 1987; **36**: 612–19.

44 Ellis EN, Steffes MW, Goetz FC *et al.* Glomerular filtration surface in type I diabetes mellitus. *Kidney Int* 1986; **29**: 889–94.

45 Osterby R, Parving HH, Nyberg G *et al.* A strong correlation between glomerular filtration rate and filtration surface in diabetic nephropathy. *Diabetologia* 1988; **31**: 265–70.

46 Osterby R, Gundersen HJG, Horlyck A *et al.* Diabetic glomerulopathy: structural characteristics of the early and advanced stages. *Diabetes* 1983; **32** (Suppl. 2): 79.

47 Cagliero E, Roth T, Roy S, Lorenzi M. Characteristics and mechanisms of high-glucose-induced overexpression of basement membrane components in cultured human endothelial cells. *Diabetes* 1991; **40**: 102–10.

48 Haneda M, Kikkawa R, Horide N *et al.* Glucose enhances type IV collagen production in cultured rat glomerular mesangial cells. *Diabetologia* 1991; **34**: 198–200.

49 Pugliese G, Pricci F, Pugliese F *et al.* Mechanisms of glucose-enhanced extracellular matrix accumulation in rat glomerular mesangial cells. *Diabetes* 1994; **43**: 478–90.

50 Vernier RL, Steffes MW, Sisson-Ross S, Mauer SM. Heparan sulfate proteoglycan in the glomerular basement membrane in type 1 diabetes mellitus. *Kidney Int* 1992; **41**: 1070–80.

51 Falk RJ, Scheinman JI, Mauer SM, Michael AF. Polyantigenic expansion of basement membrane constituents in diabetic nephropathy. *Diabetes* 1983; **32** (Suppl. 22): 34–9.

52 Shimomura H, Spiro RG. Studies on macromolecular components of human glomerular

basement membrane and alterations in diabetes: decreased levels of heparan sulfate proteoglycan and laminin. *Diabetes* 1987; **36**: 374–81.

53 Tamsma JT, Van Den Born J, Bruin JA *et al.* Expression of glomerular extracellular matrix components in human diabetic nephropathy: decrease of heparan sulphate in the glomerular basement membrane. *Diabetologia* 1994; **37**: 313–20.

54 Rohrbach DH, Wagner CW, Star VL *et al.* Reduced synthesis of basement membrane heparan sulphate proteoglycan in streptozotocin-induced diabetic mice. *J Biol Chem*; **258**: 11672–11677.

55 Cohen MP, Klepser H, Wu VY. Undersulfation of glomerular basement membrane heparan sulfate in experimental diabetes and lack of correction with aldose reductase inhibition. *Diabetes* 1988; **37**: 1324–7.

56 Viberti G, Mackintosh D, Keen H. Determinants of the penetration of proteins through the glomerular barrier in insulin-dependent diabetes mellitus. *Diabetes* 1983; **32** (Suppl. 2): 92.

57 Nakamura Y, Myers BD. Charge selectivity of proteinuria in diabetic glomerulopathy. *Diabetes* 1988; **37**: 1202–11.

58 Kanwar YS, Liu ZZ, Kashihara N, Wallner EI. Current status of the structural and functional basis of glomerular filtration and proteinuria. *Semin Nephrol* 1991; **11**: 390–413.

59 Groggel GC, Marinides GN, Hovingh P *et al.* Inhibition of rat mesangial cell growth by heparan sulfate. *Am J Physiol* 1990; **258**: F259–65.

60 Tarsio FJ, Reger LA, Furcht LT. Molecular mechanisms in basement membrane complications of diabetes: alterations in heparin, laminin and type IV collagen association. *Diabetes* 1988; **37**: 532–9.

61 Brownlee M, Cerami A, Vlassar H. Advanced glycosylation end products in tissue and the biochemical basis of diabetic complications. *N Engl J Med* 1988; **318**: 1315–21.

62 Brownlee M. Glycation and diabetic complications. *Diabetes* 1994; **43**: 836–41.

63 Vlassara H, Bucala R, Striker L. Pathogenic effects of advanced glycosylation: biochemical, biologic, and clinical implications for diabetes and aging. *Lab Invest* 1994; **70**: 138–51.

64 Skolnik EY, Yang Z, Makita Z *et al.* Human and rat mesangial cell receptors for glucose-modified proteins: potential role in kidney tissue remodelling and diabetic nephropathy. *J Exp Med* 1994; **174**: 515–24.

65 Doi T, Vlassara H, Kirstein M *et al.* Receptor specific increase in extracellular matrix production in mouse mesangial cells by advanced glycosylation end products is mediated via platelet derived growth factor. *Proc Natl Acad Sci USA* 1992; **89**: 2873–7.

66 Striker LJ, Peten EP, Elliot SJ *et al.* Mesangial cell turnover: effect of heparin and peptide growth factors. *Lab Invest* 1991; **64**: 446–56.

67 Esposito C, Gerlach H, Brett J *et al.* Endothelial receptor-mediated binding of glucose-modified albumin is associated with increased monolayer permeability and modulation of cell surface coagulant properties. *J Exp Med* 1989; **170**: 1387–1407.

68 Edelstein D, Brownlee M. Aminoguanidine ameliorates albuminuria in diabetic hypertensive rats. 1992; **35**: 96–7.

69 Ellis EN, Good BH. Prevention of glomerular basement membrane thickening by amnioguanidine in experimental diabetes mellitus. *Metabolism* 1991; **40**: 1016–19.

70 Shah SV. Role of reactive oxygen metabolites in experimental glomerular disease. *Kidney Int* 1989; **35**: 1093–106.

71 Wolff SP, Dean RT. Glucose autoxidation and protein modification: the potential role of autoxidation glycosylation in diabetes. *Biochem J* 1987; **245**: 243–50.

72 Packer L. The role of anti-oxidative treatment in diabetes mellitus. *Diabetologia* 1993; **36**: 1212–13.

73 Tada H, Kuboki K, Ishii H *et al.* Impaired degradation of hydrogen peroxide in isolated glomeruli of streptozocin-induced diabetes. *Diabetes* 1994; **43** (Suppl. 1): 105A.

74 Mullarkey CJ, Edelstein D, Brownlee M. Free radical generation by early glycation products: a mechanism for accelerated atherogenesis in diabetes. *Biochem Biophys Res Commun* 1990; **173**: 932–9.

75 Ayo SH, Radnik R, Garoni J *et al.* High glucose increases diacylglycerol mass and activates protein kinase C in mesangial cell cultures. *Am J Physiol* 1990; **260**: F185–91.

76 Derubertis FR, Craven PA. Activation of protein kinase C in glomeruli cells in diabetes.

Diabetes 1994; **43**: 1–8.

77 Lynch JJ, Ferro TJ, Blumenstock FA *et al*. Increased endothelial albumin permeability mediated by protein kinase C activation. *J Clin Invest* 1990; **85**: 1991–8.

78 Studer RK, Craven PA, DeRubertis FR. Thromboxane stimulation of mesangial cell fibronectin synthesis is signaled by activation of protein kinase C and is modulated by cGMP. *J Am Soc Nephrol* 1993; **4**: 458.

79 Brenner BM. Hemodynamically mediated glomerular injury and the progressive nature of kidney disease. *Kidney Int* 1983; **23**: 647.

80 Parving H-H, Viberti GC, Keen H *et al*. Hemodynamic factors in genesis of diabetic microangiopathy. *Metabolism* 1983; **32**: 943–9.

81 Wiseman M, Viberti GC. Kidney size and glomerular filtration rate in type I (insulin-dependent) diabetes mellitus revisited. *Diabetologia* 1983; **25**: 530.

82 Ellis EN, Steffes MW, Goetz FC *et al*. Relationship of renal size to nephropathy in type I (insulin-dependent) diabetes. *Diabetologia* 1985; **28**: 12.

83 Wiseman MJ, Saunders AJ, Keen H, Viberti G. Effect of blood glucose control on increased glomerular filtration rate and kidney size in insulin-dependent diabetes. *N Engl J Med* 1985; **3112**: 617.

84 Hostetter TH, Renneke HG, Brenner BM. The case for intrarenal hypertension in the initiation and progression of diabetic and other glomerulopathies. *Am J Med* 1982; **72**: 375.

85 Steffes MW, Brown DM, Mauer SM. Diabetic glomerulopathy following unilateral nephrectomy in the rat. *Diabetes* 1978; **27**: 35.

86 Christiansen JS, Frandsen M, Parving H-H. Effect of intravenous glucose infusion on renal function in normal man and insulin-dependent diabetics. *Diabetologia* 1981; **21**: 368.

87 Kasiske BL, O'Donnell MP, Keane WF. Glucose-induced increases in renal hemodynamic function: possible modulation by renal prostaglandins. *Diabetes* 1985; **34**: 360.

88 Bank N. Mechanisms of diabetic hyperfiltration. *Kidney Int* 1991; **40**: 792–807.

89 Jerums G, Cooper ME, Seeman E *et al*. Comparison of early renal dysfunction in type I and type II diabetes: differing associations with blood pressure and glycaemic control. *Diabetes Res Clin Pract* 1988; **4**: 133–41.

90 McNally PG, Burden AC, Swift PFG *et al*. The prevalence and risk factors associated with the onset of diabetic nephropathy in juvenile-onset (insulin-dependent) diabetics diagnosed under the age of 17 years in Leicestershire 1930–1985. *Q J Med* 1990; **76**: 831–44.

91 Kalk WJ, Osler C, Taylor D, Panz VR. Prior long-term glycaemic control and insulin therapy in insulin-dependent diabetic adolescents with microalbuminuria. *Diabetes Res Clin Pract* 1990; **9**: 83–8.

92 Watts F, Harris R, Shaw KM. The determinants of early nephropathy in insulin-dependent diabetes mellitus: a prospective study based on the urinary excretion of albumin. *Q J Med* 1991; **79**: 365–78.

93 McCance DR, Hadden DR, Atkinson AB *et al*. The relationship between long-term glycaemic control and diabetic nephropathy. *Q J Med* 1992; **82**: 53–61.

94 Feldt-Rasmussen B, Mathiesen ER, Hegedus L, Deckert T. Kidney function during 12 months of strict metabolic control in insulin-dependent diabetic patients with incipient nephropathy. *N Engl J Med* 1986; **314**: 665–70.

95 Tuttle KR, Bruton JL, Perusek MC *et al*. Effect of strict glycemic control on renal hemodynamic response to amino acids and renal enlargement in insulin-dependent diabetes mellitus. *N Engl J Med* 1991; **324**: 1626–32.

96 Tuttle KR, DeFronzo RA, Stein JH. Treatment of diabetic nephropathy. a rational approach based on its pathophysiology. *Semin Nephrol* 1991; **11**: 220–35.

97 Feldt-Rasmussen B, Mathiesen ER, Jensen T *et al*. Effect of improved metabolic control on loss of kidney function in type 1 (insulin-dependent) diabetic patients: an update of the Steno studies. *Diabetologia* 1991; **34**: 164–70.

98 Reichard P, Rosenqvist U. Nephropathy is delayed by intensified insulin treatment in patients with insulin-dependent diabetes mellitus and retinopathy. *J Intern Med* 1989; **226**: 81–7.

99 Reichard P, Nilsson B-Y, Rosenqvist U. The effect of long-term insulin treatment on the development of microvascular complication of diabetes mellitus. *N Engl J Med* 1993; **329**: 304–9.

100 Viberti GC, Bilous RW, Mackintosh D. Long-term correction of hyperglycemia and progression of renal failure in insulin-dependent diabetes. *Br Med J* 1983; **286**: 598–602.

101 Tamborlane WV, Puklin JE, Bergman M. Long-term improvement of metabolic control with the insulin pump does not reverse microangiopathy. *Diabetes Care* 1982; **5** (Suppl. 1): 58.

102 American Diabetes Association. Standards of medical care for patients with diabetes mellitus. *Diabetes Care* 1995; **18** (Suppl. 1): 8–15.

103 Kitzmiller JL, Buchanan T, Kjos S, Combs CA. Technical review: preconception care of diabetes, congenital malformations, and spontaneous abortions. *Diabetes Care* 1996; **19**.

104 Kitzmiller JL, Gavin LA, Gin GD *et al.* Preconception care of diabetes: glycemic control prevents congenital anomalies. *JAMA* 1991; **265**: 731–6.

105 Fuhrmann K, Reiher H, Semmler K, Glockner E. The effect of intensified conventional insulin therapy before and during pregnancy on the malformation rate in offspring of diabetic mothers. *Exp Clin Endocrinol* 1984; **83**: 173–7.

106 Damm P, Molsted-Pedersen L. Significant decrease in congenital malformations in newborn infants of an unselected population of diabetic women. *Am J Obstet Gynecol* 1989; **161**: 1163–7.

107 Steel JM, Johnstone FD, Hepburn DA, Smith A. Can pre-pregnancy care of diabetic women reduce the risk of abnormal babies? *Br Med J* 1990; **301**: 1070–4.

108 Miller E, Hare JW, Cloherty JP *et al.* Elevated maternal hemoglobin A1c in early pregnancy and major congenital anomalies in infants of diabetic mothers. *N Engl J Med* 1981; **304**: 1331–4.

109 Miodovnik M, Mimouni F, Dignam PS. Major malformations in infants of IDDM women: vasculopathy and early first-trimester poor glycemic control. *Diabetes Care* 1988; **11**: 713–18.

110 Molsted Pedersen L, Tygstrups I, Pedersen J. Congenital malformations in newborn infants of diabetes women: correlation with maternal diabetic vascular complications. *Lancet* 1964; **i**: 1124–6.

111 Sosenko IR, Kitzmiller JL, Loo SW *et al.* The infant of the diabetic mother: correlation of increased cord C-peptide levels with macrosomia and hypoglycemia. *N Engl J Med* 1979; **301**: 859–62.

112 Weiss PAM, Winter R, Purstner P. Insulin levels in amniotic fluid: management of pregnancy in diabetes. *Obstet Gynecol* 1978; **51**: 292–5.

113 Jovanovic-Peterson L, Peterson C, Reed G *et al.* Institute of Child Health and Human Development. Diabetes in Early Pregnancy Study. Maternal postprandial glucose levels and infant birth weight: the diabetes in early pregnancy study. *Am J Obstet Gynecol* 1991; **164**: 103–11.

114 Combs CA, Gunderson E, Kitzmiller JL *et al.* Relationship of fetal macrosomia to maternal postprandial glucose control during pregnancy. *Diabetes Care* 1992; **15**: 1251–7.

115 Jovanovic L, Druzin M, Peterson C. Effect of euglycemia on the outcome of pregnancy in insulin-dependent diabetic women as compared with normal control subjects. *Am J Med* 1981; **71**: 921–7.

116 Greene MF, Hare JW, Krache M *et al.* Prematurity among insulin-requiring diabetic gravid women. *Am J Obstet Gynecol* 1989; **161**: 106–11.

117 Kitzmiller JL. Sweet success with diabetes: the development of insulin therapy and glycemic control for pregnancy. *Diabetes Care* 1993; **16** (Suppl. 3): 107–21.

118 Feldt-Rasmussen B, Norgaard K, Jensen T *et al.* The role of hypertension in the development of nephropathy in type 1 (insulin-dependent) diabetes mellitus. *Acta Diabetol Lat* 1990; **27**: 173–9.

119 Mogensen CE, Hansen KW, Osterby R, Damsgaard EM. Blood pressure elevation versus abnormal albuminuria in the genesis and prediction of renal disease in diabetes. *Diabetes Care* 1992; **15**: 1192–204.

120 Chase HP, Garg SK, Harris S *et al.* High-normal blood pressure and early diabetic nephropathy. *Arch Intern Med* 1990; **150**: 639–41.

121 Kasiske BL, Kalil RSN, Ma JZ *et al.* Effect of antihypertensive therapy on the kidney in patients with diabetes: a meta-regression analysis. *Ann Intern Med* 1993; **118**: 129–38.

122 Heeg JE, de Jong PE, Van der Hem GK, de Zeuuw D. Efficacy and variability of the

antiproteinuric effect of ACE inhibitors by lisinopril. *Kidney Int* 1989; **36**: 272–9.
123 Slataper R, Vicknair N, Sadler R, Bakris L. Comparative effects of different antihypertensive treatments on progression of diabetic renal disease. *Arch Intern Med* 1993; **153**: 973–80.
124 Viberti B, Mogensen CE, Groop LC, Pauls JF, for the European Microalbuminuria Captopril Study Group. Effect of captopril on progression to clinical proteinuria in patients with insulin-dependent diabetes mellitus and microalbuminuria. *JAMA* 1994; **271**: 275–9.
125 Lewis EJ, Hunsicker LG, Bain RP, Rohde RD, for the Collaborative Study Group. The effect of angiotensin-converting-enzyme inhibition on diabetic nephropathy. *N Engl J Med* 1993; **329**: 1456–62.
126 Rosa FW, Bosco LA, Graham CF *et al*. Neonatal anuria with maternal angiotensin-converting enzyme inhibition. *Obstet Gynecol* 1989; **74**: 371.
127 Hanssens M, Keirse MJNC, Vankelecom F, Assche FAV. Fetal and neonatal effects of treatment with angiotensin-converting enzyme inhibitors in pregnancy. *Obstet Gynecol* 1991; **78**: 128–35.
128 Consensus Statement. Diabetic nephropathy. *Am J Kidney Dis* 1989; **13**: 2–6.
129 Mogensen CE, Hansen KW, Pederson MM, Christensen CK. Renal factors influencing blood pressure threshold and choice of treatment for hypertension in IDDM. *Diabetes Care* 1991; **14** (Suppl. 4): 13–26.
130 Consensus Statement. Treatment of hypertension in diabetes. *Diabetes Care* 1993; **16**: 1394–401.
131 Coats AJS, Conway J, Sommers VK. Ambulatory pressure monitoring in the assessment of antihypertensive therapy. *Cardiovasc Drugs Res* 1989; **3**: 303–11.
132 Benhamou PY, Halimi S, De Gaudemaris R *et al*. Early disturbances of ambulatory blood pressure load in normotensive type I diabetic patients with microalbuminuria. *Diabetes Care* 1992; **15**: 1614–19.
133 Moore WV, Donaldson DL, Chonko AM *et al*. Ambulatory blood pressure in type I diabetes mellitus: comparison to presence of incipient nephropathy in adolescents and young adults. *Diabetes* 1992; **41**: 1035–41.
134 Poulsen L, Hansen KW, Mogensen CE. Ambulatory blood pressure in the transition from normo- to microalbuminuria. *Diabetes* 1994; **43**: 1248–53.
135 Fairlie FM, Sibai BM. Hypertensive diseases in pregnancy. In: Reece EA, Hobbins JC, Mahoney MJ, Petrie RH (eds), *Medicine of the Fetus and Mother*. Lippincott, Philadelphia, 1992; 938–9.
136 National High Blood Pressure Education Program Working Group. Report on high blood pressure in pregnancy. *Am J Obstet Gynecol* 1990; **163**: 1689–712.
137 Cunningham FG, Lindheimer MD. Hypertension in pregnancy. *N Engl J Med* 1992; **326**: 927–32.
138 Cockburn J, Ounsted M, Moar VA, Redman CWG. Final report of study on hypertension during pregnancy: the effects of specific treatment on the growth and development of the children. *Lancet* 1982; **i**: 647–51.
139 Sibai BM, Grossman RA, Grossman HG. Effects of diuretics on plasma volume in pregnancies with longterm hypertension. *Am J Obstet Gynecol* 1984; **150**: 831–5.
140 Soffronoff EC, Kaufmann BM, Connaughton JF. Intravascular volume determinations and fetal outcome in hypertensive diseases of pregnancy. *Am J Obstet Gynecol* 1977; **127**: 4–8.
141 Mulec H, Blohme G, Kullenberg K *et al*. Latent overhydration and nocturnal hypertension in diabetic nephropathy. *Diabetologia* 1995; **38**: 216–20.
142 Bakris GL. The effects of calcium antagonists on renal hemodynamics, urinary protein excretion and glomerular morphology in diabetic states. *J Am Soc Nephrol* 1991; 2 (Suppl. I): 21–29.
143 Bakris GL, Barnhill BW, Sadler R. Treatment of arterial hypertension in diabetic man: importance of therapeutic selection. *Kidney Int* 1992; **41**: 898–906.
144 Demarie B, Bakris GL. Effects of different calcium antagonists on proteinuria associated with diabetes mellitus. *Ann Intern Med* 1990; **113**: 987–8.
145 Magee LA, Conover B, Schick B *et al*. Exposure to calcium channel blockers in human pregnancy: a prospective, controlled, multicentre cohort study. *Teratology* 1994; **49**: 372–6.

146 Zatz R, Meyer TW, Rennke HG *et al.* Predominance of hemodynamic rather than metabolic factors in the pathogenesis of diabetic glomerulopathy. *Proc Natl Acad Sci USA* 1985; **82**: 5963–7.

147 Barsotti G, Ciardella F, Morelli E *et al.* Nutritional treatment of renal failure in type 1 diabetic nephropathy. *Clin Nephrol* 1988; **29**: 280–7.

148 Evanoff G, Thomspon C, Brown J, Weinman E. Prolonged dietary protein restriction in diabetic nephropathy. *Arch Intern Med* 1989; **149**: 1129–33.

149 Walker JD, Dodds RA, Murrells TJ *et al.* Restriction of dietary protein and progression of renal failure in diabetic nephropathy. *Lancet* 1989; **ii**: 1411–15.

150 Dodds RA, Keen H. Low protein diet and conservation of renal function in diabetic nephropathy. *Diabete Metab* 1990; **16**: 464–9.

151 Zeller K, Whittaker E, Sullivan L *et al.* Effect of restricting dietary protein on the progression of renal failure in patients with insulin-dependent diabetes mellitus. *N Engl J Med* 1991; **324**: 78–84.

152 Brodsky IG, Robbins DC, Hiser E *et al.* Effects of low-protein diets on protein metabolism in insulin-dependent diabetes mellitus patients with early nephropathy. *J Clin Endocrinol Metab* 1992; **75**: 351–7.

153 Levine SE, D'Elia JA, Bistrian B *et al.* Protein-restricted diets in diabetic nephropathy. *Nephron* 1989; **52**: 55–61.

154 Shichiri M, Hishio Y, Ogura M, Marumo F. Effect of low-protein, very-low-phosphorus diet on diabetic renal insufficiency with proteinuria. *Am J Kidney Dis* 1991; **18**: 26–32.

155 Committee on Nutritional Status During Pregnancy and Lactation, Institute of Medicine, National Academy of Sciences. Estimated requirements of protein and amino acids. In: *Nutrition During Pregnancy Part II. Dietary Intake and Nutrient Supplements.* National Academy Press, Washington, DC, 1990; 382–4.

156 Baylis C. Renal disease in gravid animal models. *Am J Kidney Dis* 1987; **9**: 350–3.

157 Bernard A, Thielemans N, Lauwerys R, Van Lierde M. Selective increase in the urinary excretion of protein 1 (Clara cell protein) and other low molecular weight proteins during normal pregnancy. *Scand J Clin Lab Invest* 1992; **52**: 871–8.

158 Davison JM. The effect of pregnancy on kidney function in renal allograft recipients. *Kidney In* 1985; **27**: 74–9.

159 Higby K, Suiter CR, Phelps JY *et al.* Normal values of urinary albumin and total protein excretion during pregnancy. *Am J Obstet Gynecol* 1994; **171**: 984–9.

160 Combs CA, Wheeler BC, Kitzmiller JL. Urinary protein/creatinine ratio before and during pregnancy in women with diabetes mellitus. *Am J Obstet Gynecol* 1991; **165**: 920–3.

161 Jensen T, Borch-Johnson K, Kofoed-Enevoldsen A, Deckert T. Coronary heart disease in young type 1 (insulin dependent) diabetic patients with and without diabetic nephropathy: incidence and risk factors. *Diabetologia* 1987; **30**: 144–8.

162 Valdorf-Hanson F, Jensen T, Borch-Johnsen K, Deckert T. Cardiovascular risk factors in type 1 (insulin-dependent) diabetic patients with and without proteinuria. *Acta Med Scand* 1987; **222**: 439–44.

163 Manske CL, Thomas W, Wang Y, Wilson RF. Screening diabetic transplant candidates for coronary artery disease: identification of a low risk subgroup. *Kidney Int* 1993; **44**: 617–21.

164 Hare JW, White P. Pregnancy in diabetes complicated by vascular disease. *Diabetes* 1977; **26**: 953–5.

165 Reece EA, Egan JFX, Coustan DR *et al.* Coronary artery disease in diabetic pregnancies. *Am J Obstet Gynecol* 1986; **154**: 150–1.

166 Kitzmiller JL, Aiello LM, Kaldany A, Younger MD. Diabetic vascular disease complicating pregnancy. *Clin Obstet Gynecol* 1981; **24**: 107–23.

167 Salomon NW, Page US, Okies JE *et al.* Diabetes mellitus and coronary artery bypass: short-term risk and long-term prognosis. *J Thorac Cardiovasc Surg* 1983; **85**: 264.

168 Klein BEK, Moss SE, Klein R. Effect of pregnancy on progression of diabetic retinopathy. *Diabetes Care* 1990; **13**: 34–40.

169 Chew EY, Mills JL, Metzger BE *et al.* Metabolic control and progression of retinopathy. *Diabetes Care* 1995; **18**: 631–7.

170 Kitzmiller JL, Gavin LA, Gin G *et al.* Managing diabetes and pregnancy (monograph). In: *Current Problems in Obstetrics, Gynecology, and Fertility.* Yearbook, July–August 1988.

171 White P. Pregnancy in diabetes. In: *Joslin's Diabetes Mellitus*, 11th ed. Lea & Febiger, Philadelphia, 1971; 581–98.

172 Pedersen J, Molsted-Pedersen L, Andersen B. Assessors of fetal perinatal mortality in diabetic pregnancy. *Diabetes* 1974; **23**: 302–5.

173 Pedersen J. *The pregnant diabetic and her newborn*, 2nd edn. Williams & Wilkins, Baltimore, 1977; 9.

174 Kitzmiller JL, Brown ER, Phillippe M *et al*. Diabetic nephropathy and perinatal outcome. *Am J Obstet Gynecol* 1981; **141**: 741–51.

175 Jovanovic R, Jovanovic L. Obstetric management when normoglycemia is maintained in diabetic pregnant women with vascular compromise. *Am J Obstet Gynecol* 1984; **149**: 617–23.

176 Grenfell A, Brudenell JM, Doddridge MC, Watkins PJ. Pregnancy in diabetic women who have proteinuria. *Q J Med* 1986; **228**: 379–86.

177 Dicker D, Feldberg D, Peleg D *et al*. Pregnancy complicated by diabetic nephropathy. *J Perinat Med* 1986; **14**: 299–306.

178 Reece E, Coustan DR, Hayslett JP *et al*. Diabetic nephropathy: pregnancy performance and fetomaternal outcome. *Am J Obstet Gynecol* 1988; **159**: 56–66.

179 Biesenbach G, Stoger H, Zazgornik J. Influence of pregnancy on progression of diabetic nephropathy and subsequent requirement of renal replacement therapy in female type I diabetic patients with impaired renal function. *Nephrol Dial Transplant* 1992; **7**: 105–9.

180 Kimmerle R, Zab RP, Cupisti S *et al*. Pregnancies in women with diabetic nephropathy: longterm outcome for mother and child. *Diabetologia* 1995; **38**: 227–35.

181 Coustan DR, Berkowitz RL, Hobbins JC. Tight metabolic control of overt diabetes in pregnancy. *Am J Med* 1980; **68**: 845–52.

182 Muhlhauser I, Bruckner I, Berger M *et al*. Evaluation of an intensified insulin treatment and teaching programme as routine management of Type 1 (insulin-dependent) diabetes. *Diabetologia* 1987; **30**: 681–90.

183 Yankowitz J, Piraino B, Laifer A *et al*. Use of erythropoietin in pregnancies complicated by severe anemia of renal failure. *Obstet Gynceol* 1992; **80**: 485–9.

184 Davison JM. The physiology of the renal tract in pregnancy. *Clin Obstet Gynecol* 1985; **28**: 257–65.

185 Krutzen E, Olofsson P, Back SE, Nilsson-Ehle P. Glomerular filtration rate in pregnancy: a study in normal subjects and in patients with hypertension, preeclampsia and diabetes. *Scand J Clin Lab Invest* 1992; **52**: 387–92.

186 Davison JM, Noble MCB. Serial changes in 24 hour creatinine clearance during normal menstrual cycles and the first trimester of pregnancy. *Br J Obstet Gynaecol* 1981; **88**: 10.

187 Davison JM, Dunlop W, Ezimokhai M. Twenty-four-hour creatinine clearance during the third trimester of normal pregnancy. *Br J Obstet Gynaecol* 1980; **87**: 106.

188 Pedersen EB, Rasmussen AB, Johannesen P *et al*. Urinary excretion of albumin, beta-2-microglobulin and light chains in pre-eclampsia, essential hypertension in pregnancy and normotensive pregnant and non-pregnant control subjects. *Scand J Clin Lab Invest* 1981; **41**: 777–84.

189 Lopez-Espinoza I, Humphreys S, Redman CWG. Urinary albumin excretion in pregnancy. *Br J Obstet Gynaecol* 1986; **93**: 176–81.

190 McCance DR, Traub AI, Harley JMG *et al*. Urinary albumin excretion in diabetic pregnancy. *Diabetologia* 1989; **32**: 236–9.

191 MacRury SM, Pinion S, Quin JD *et al*. Blood rheology and albumin excretion in diabetic pregnancy. *Diabetic Med* 1995; **12**: 51–5.

192 Sims EAH. Serial studies of renal function in pregnancy complicated by diabetes mellitus. *Diabetes* 1961; **10**: 190–7.

193 Redman CWG. Treatment of hypertension in pregnancy. *Kidney Int* 1980; **18**: 267–78.

194 Katz AI, Davison JM, Hayslett JP *et al*. Pregnancy in women with kidney disease. 1980; **18**: 192–206.

195 Hou SH, Grossman SD, Madias NE. Pregnancy in women with renal disease and moderate renal insufficiency. *Am J Med* 1985; **78**: 185–94.

196 Abe S, Amagasaki Y, Konishi K *et al*. The influence of antecedent renal disease on pregnancy. *Am J Obstet Gynecol* 1985; **153**: 508–14.

197 Moya FR, Reece EA, Hobbins JC. Fetal–neonatal uremia in advanced maternal diabetes. *Clin Pediatr* 1984; **23**: 229–31.
198 MacCarthy P, Pollak V. Maternal renal disease: effect on the fetus. *Clin Perinatol* 1981; **8**: 307–19.
199 Maikranz P, Katz AI. Acute renal failure in pregnancy. *Obstet Gynecol Clin North Am* 1991; **18**: 333–43.
200 Trebbin W. Hemodialysis and pregnancy. *JAMA* 1979; **241**: 1811–12.
201 Hou S. Pregnancy in women requiring dialysis for renal failure. *Am J Kidney Dis* 1987; **9**: 368–94.
202 Kioko EM, Shaw KM, Clarke AD, Warren DJ. Successful pregnancy in a diabetic patient treated with continuous ambulatory peritoneal dialysis. *Diabetes Care* 1983; **6**: 298–300.
203 Sturgiss SN, Davison JM. Effect of pregnancy on long-term function of renal allografts. *Am J Kidney Dis* 1992; **19**: 167–72.
204 Ogburn PL, Kitzmiller JL, Hare JW *et al.* Pregnancy following renal transplantation in class T diabetes mellitus. *JAMA* 1986; **255**: 911–15.
205 Peterson CM, Jovanovic-Peterson L, Mills JL *et al.* National Institute of Child Health and Human Development. The Diabetes in Early Pregnancy Study: changes in cholesterol, triglycerides, body weight, and blood pressure. *Am J Obstet Gynecol* 1992; **66**: 513–18.
206 Garner PR, D'Alton ME, Dudley DK *et al.* Preeclampsia in diabetic pregnancies. *Am J Obstet Gynecol* 1990; **163**: 505–8.
207 Siddiqi T, Rosenn B, Mimouni F *et al.* Hypertension during pregnancy in insulin-dependent diabetic women. *Obstet Gynecol* 1991; **77**: 514–18.
208 Greene MF, Hare JW, Krache M *et al.* Prematurity among insulin-requiring diabetic gravid women. *Am J Obstet Gynecol* 1989; **161**: 106–11.
209 Bar J, Hod M, Erman A *et al.* Microalbuminuria: prognostic and therapeutic implications in diabetic and hypertensive pregnancy. *Diabetic Med* 1995; **48**: 649–56.
210 Biesenbach G, Stoger H, Zasgornik J. Changes in proteinuria and renal function in female type I diabetics during and after pregnancy development on the stage of preexisting diabetic nephropathy. *Klin Wochenschr* 1987; **65**: 1048–53.
211 Mogensen CE, Klebe JG. Microalbuminuria and diabetic pregnancy. In: *The Kidney and Hypertension in Diabetes Mellitus*. Martinus Nijhoff, Boston, 1988; 223–9.
212 Altman JJ, Boillot M, Tchobroutsky C. Microabluminuria in normal and diabetic pregnancy. *Diabetologia* 1987; **30**: 493A.
213 Winocour PH, Taylor RJ, Steel JM. Early alterations of renal function in insulin-dependent diabetic pregnancies and their importance in predicting pre-eclamptic toxaemia. *Lancet* 1984; **ii**: 975–6.
214 Combs CA, Rosenn B, Kitzmiller JL *et al.* Early-pregnancy proteinuria in diabetes related to preeclampsia. *Obstet Gynecol* 1993; **82**: 802–7.
215 Sibai BM, Caritis SN, Thom E *et al.* National Institute of Child Health and Human Development Network of Maternal–Fetal Medicine Units. Prevention of preeclampsia with low-dose aspirin in healthy, nulliparous pregnant women. *N Engl J Med* 1993; **329**: 1213–18.
216 CLASP. A randomized trial of low dose aspirin for the prevention and treatment of preeclampsia among 9,364 pregnant women. *Lancet* 1994; **343**: 619–29.
217 Villar J, Repke K, Belizan JM, Pareja G. Calcium supplementation reduces blood pressure during pregnancy: results of a randomized controlled clinical trial. *Obstet Gynecol* 1987; **70**: 317–22.
218 Sanchez-Ramos L, Briones D, Kaunitz AM *et al.* Prevention of pregnancy-induced hypertension by calcium supplementation in angiotensin II-sensitive patients. *Obstet Gynecol* 1994; **84**: 249–53.
219 Landon MD, Langer O, Gabbe SG. Fetal surveillance in pregnancies complicated by insulin-dependent diabetes mellitus. *Am J Obstet Gynecol* 1992; **167**: 617–21.
220 Landon MB, Gabbe SG, Bruner JP, Ludmir J. Doppler umbilical artery velocimetry in pregnancy complicated by insulin-dependent diabetes mellitus. *Obstet Gynecol* 1989; **73**: 961–5.
221 Salvesen DR, Higueras MT, Brudenell JM *et al.* Doppler velocimetry and fetal heart rate studies in nephropathy diabetics. *Am J Obstet Gynecol* 1992; **167**: 1297–1301.

222 Lucas MJ, Leveno KJ, Cunningham FG. A comparison of magnesium sulfate with phenytoin for the prevention of eclampsia. *N Engl J Med* 1995; **333**: 201–5.

223 Eclampsia Trial Collaborative Group. Which anticonvulsant for women with eclampsia? Evidence from the collaborative eclampsia trial. *Lancet* 1995; **345**: 1455–63.

224 Wallace DH, Leveno KJ, Cunningham FG *et al*. Randomized comparison of general and regional anesthesia for cesarean delivery in pregnancies complicated by severe preeclampsia. *Obstet Gynecol* 1995; **86**: 193–9.

225 Reece EA, Winn HN, Hayslett JY *et al*. Does pregnancy alter the rate of progression of diabetic nephropathy? *Am J Perinatol* 1990; **7**: 193–8.

226 Kitzmiller JL, Combs AC. Diabetic nephropathy. In: Reece EA, Coustan DR (eds), Diabetes *Mellitus in Pregnancy*, 2nd edn. Churchill Livingstone, Edinburgh, 1995; 337.

11

Findings from Cordocentesis in Diabetic Pregnancies

DOUGLAS R. SALVESEN[1] and KYPRIANOS H. NICOLAIDES[2]

[1]Queen Charlotte's and Chelsea Hospital, London, UK and
[2]King's College Hospital, London, UK

This chapter examines the consequences of maternal diabetes mellitus on fetal oxygenation and metabolism and offers an explanation for unexplained stillbirth and macrosomia. The data are mainly derived from the study of fetal blood samples obtained by cordocentesis that was carried out within 24 h before delivery.

CORDOCENTESIS

In the 1960s access to the fetal circulation was achieved by exposing the fetus at the time of hysterotomy. In the 1970s with the development of fibre-optics, fetoscopy was used to visualize and sample the vessels of the chorionic plate and umbilical cord. In the 1980s, improvements in imaging by ultrasonography have enabled fetal blood to be obtained by ultrasound guided puncture of an umbilical cord vessel (cordocentesis), and this technique is currently the most widely used method for fetal blood sampling[1,2]. The assessment of fetal oxygenation in blood obtained by cordocentesis is preferable to the study of cord blood at delivery, as the process of delivery itself may alter the parameters being investigated[3,4]. With the use of cordocentesis fetal oxygenation can be investigated under near-physiological conditions.

The maternal risks from cordocentesis are negligible. The risk of fetal loss associated with cordocentesis is about 1%. However, when cordocentesis is performed in the third trimester complications are easily recognizable and fetal loss can be avoided by prompt delivery.

Diabetes and Pregnancy: An International Approach to Diagnosis and Management.
Edited by A. Dornhorst and D. R. Hadden.
© 1996 John Wiley & Sons Ltd.

HYPERGLYCAEMIA AND HYPERINSULINAEMIA

In normal fetuses, the mean umbilical venous blood glucose concentration is higher than in the umbilical artery, indicating that there is fetal glucose consumption[5]. Furthermore, the maternal glucose concentration is higher than the fetal and the levels in the two compartments are significantly correlated, indicating that the major source of fetal glucose is the mother. Fetal glucose is better correlated with maternal glucose than with fetal insulin, suggesting that the main determinant of fetal blood glucose level is the maternal blood glucose concentration. Insulin can be demonstrated in the human fetus from as early as 8–10 weeks gestation and the umbilical plasma insulin concentration and insulin-to-glucose ratio increase with gestation, reflecting normal fetal pancreatic maturation[6].

In pregnancies complicated by diabetes mellitus, there is a significant association between maternal and fetal blood glucose concentration (Figure 11.1)[7]. The maternal–fetal blood glucose gradient is increased and is significantly associated with maternal blood glucose concentration (Figure 11.2)[7]. Additionally, the fetal insulin concentration and insulin-to-glucose ratio are increased (Figures 11.3 and 11.4) and there are significant associations between fetal insulin concentration and both maternal blood glucose concentration and maternal–fetal blood glucose gradient[7].

The association between maternal glucose concentration and maternal–fetal glucose gradient could represent saturation of facilitative transport. However, previous studies in labour have suggested that saturation of facilitative transport occurs only when the maternal glucose

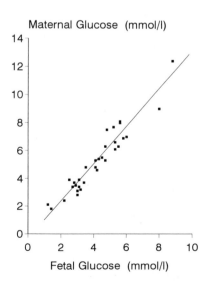

Figure 11.1. Relationship between maternal and fetal blood glucose concentration[7]

concentration exceeds 11 mmol/l and only one of our cases had such a high glucose level[7,8]. Therefore the most likely explanation for the increased maternal–fetal blood glucose gradient and the association with fetal insulin concentration is increased fetal glucose utilization due to the hyperinsulinaemia.

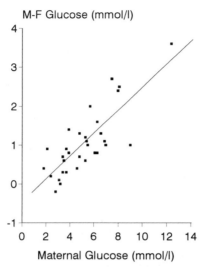

Figure 11.2. Relationship between maternal blood glucose concentration and maternal–fetal blood glucose gradient (M-F Glucose)

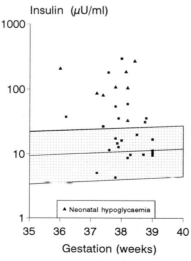

Figure 11.3. Fetal plasma insulin concentration plotted on the reference range with gestation (mean, 5th and 95th centile)[7]

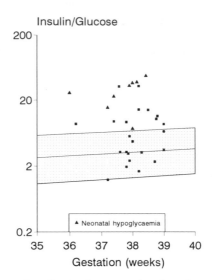

Figure 11.4. Fetal plasma insulin-to-glucose ratio plotted on the refence range with gestation (mean, 5th and 95th centile)[7]

The high fetal insulin concentration and insulin-to-glucose ratio are likely to be due to fetal pancreatic beta cell hyperplasia, which is a well-recognized feature of pregnancies complicated by diabetes mellitus. Supportive evidence for this is provided by the association between fetal insulin-to-glucose ratio and both neonatal hypoglycaemia and macrosomia (Figures 11.4 and 11.5)[7].

These findings provide supportive human evidence for the hypothesis of Pedersen that maternal hyperglycaemia causes fetal hyperglycaemia and hyperinsulinaemia[9]. We have suggested that hyperglycaemia and/or the other metabolic derangements associated with maternal diabetes mellitus during the late second trimester of pregnancy act on the fetal pancreas to cause beta cell hyperplasia[7]. Animal studies have demonstrated that beta cell hyperplasia and precocious pancreatic maturation can be induced by hyperglycaemia and various amino acids. Furthermore, in pregnancies complicated by diabetes mellitus, there are high concentrations of insulin in the amniotic fluid and accelerated growth velocity is evident from at least 28 weeks gestation[10].

Although good diabetic control in the third trimester of pregnancy reduces the incidence of macrosomia, the latter is not always preventable. In pregnant women with diabetes mellitus, despite stringent maternal glycaemic control, the fluctuation in maternal glucose concentration is greater than in non-diabetes and it is possible that during short-lived episodes of hyperglycaemia an already hyperplastic fetal pancreas will

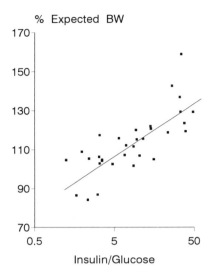

Figure 11.5. Relationship between percentage expected birth weight (BW) and fetal insulin-to-glucose ratio[7]

respond with a disproportionately high release of insulin. Fetal hyperinsulinaemia causes macrosomia either directly through its anabolic effect on nutrient uptake and utilization, or indirectly through related peptides such as insulin-like growth factors[11].

ACIDAEMIA AND HYPERLACTICAEMIA

In normal fetuses, the blood oxygen tension is much lower than in maternal blood, and this may be caused by incomplete venous equilibration of uterine and umbilical circulations or by high placental oxygen consumption[12]. However, the high affinity of fetal haemoglobin for oxygen, together with the high fetal cardiac output in relation to oxygen demand, compensates for the low fetal oxygen tension. The umbilical venous and arterial oxygen tension and pH decrease with gestational age but blood oxygen content does not change because the fetal haemoglobin concentration rises with advancing gestation[12]. Fetal blood lactate concentration does not change with gestation and is higher than in maternal blood, suggesting that there is a common source of lactate which is likely to be the placenta.

In diabetic pregnancies analysis of blood samples obtained by cordocentesis has demonstrated significant acidaemia and hyperlacticaemia in the absence of hypoxaemia (Figures 11.6–11.8)[3,13–15]. This finding of fetal acidaemia may offer an explanation for the unexplained stillbirth of diabetic pregnancies. Possible causes of fetal acidaemia include increased oxygen affinity of maternal haemoglobin, decreased uteroplacental perfusion, decreased placental transfer, increased oxygen affinity of fetal haemoglobin and increased fetal metabolism.

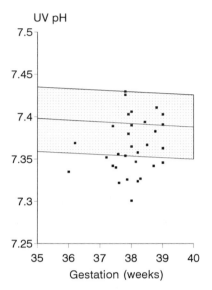

Figure 11.6. Umbilical venous (UV) blood pH plotted on the reference range with gestation (mean, 5th and 95th centiles)[14]

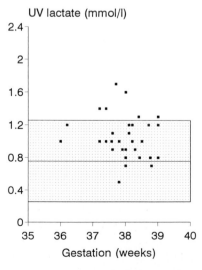

Figure 11.7. Umbilical venous (UV) blood lactate concentration plotted on the reference range with gestation (mean, 5th and 95th centiles)

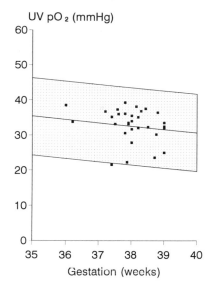

Figure 11.8. Umbilical venous (UV) blood pO_2 concentration plotted on the reference range with gestation (mean, 5th and 95th centiles)[14]

OXYGEN AFFINITY OF MATERNAL BLOOD

Increased maternal glycosylated haemoglobin concentration is associated with an increased oxygen affinity, causing a left shift of the blood oxygen dissociation curve. However, in diabetic pregnancy there is a compensatory increase in the red cell 2,3-diphosphoglycerate (2,3-DPG), which is associated with decreased haemoglobin oxygen affinity and a right shift of the oxygen dissociation curve. Consequently, in pregnancies complicated by maternal diabetes mellitus the p_{50} of the maternal oxygen dissociation curve is not different from normal.

PLACENTAL PERFUSION AND TRANSFER

Radioisotope studies in the 1970s suggested that in pregnancies complicated by diabetes mellitus there may be reduced placental perfusion. Additionally, histological studies have reported decreased villous surface area, villous oedema and thickening of the basement membrane[16]. However, recent studies using Doppler ultrasound have shown that in diabetic pregnancies the uteroplacental circulation is essentially normal, except in those cases complicated by pre-eclampsia and/or intrauterine growth retardation[15]. Furthermore, the finding that acidaemia is not accompanied by hypoxaemia suggests that the acidaemia is unlikely to be due to impaired placental function. In pregnancies complicated by intrauterine growth retardation due to uteroplacental insufficiency, impedance to flow in the uterine and umbilical arteries is increased, acidaemia is accompanied by hypoxaemia and there are significant associations between impedance to flow and the degree of acid base disturbance[17].

OXYGEN AFFINITY OF FETAL BLOOD

As in maternal blood there are opposing effects of increased red cell 2,3-DPG concentration and glycosylation on the haemoglobin oxygen dissociation curve that are unlikely to have a significant influence on fetal oxygenation.

INCREASED FETAL METABOLISM

In pregnant sheep chronic hyperglycaemia results in increased aerobic and anaerobic glucose metabolism with consequent increased oxygen consumption, lactate production and fall in pH and oxygen tension[18-23]. Glucose oxidation and oxygen consumption are also increased by hyperinsulinaemia, and this effect is independent of that caused by hyperglycaemia[22]. Hyperlacticaemia occurs because the fetus has a reduced capacity for oxidative metabolism and low pyruvate dehydrogenase activity. Severe hyperglycaemia is characterized by acidaemia and hypoxaemia, but minor degrees of hyperglycaemia are associated with acidaemia in the absence of hypoxaemia[18]. However, in the presence of mild fetal hypoxaemia, minor degrees of fetal hyperglycaemia do result in severe acidosis and even fetal death[23].

Further evidence to support the hypothesis that fetal acidaemia in diabetic pregnancy is the consequence of increased glucose metabolism is provided by the results of cordocentesis studies. Salvesen *et al.* performed cordocentesis in 32 diabetic pregnancies and reported significant associations between both maternal blood glucose and fetal plasma insulin concentrations and the degree of fetal acidaemia (Figures 11.9 and 11.10)[7].

POLYCYTHAEMIA, ERYTHROBLASTAEMIA, ERYTHROPOIETINAEMIA

Erythropoiesis in the embryo and fetus is achieved in three overlapping anatomical and functional stages. Yolk sac haemopoiesis, in the first 10 weeks of life, is associated with extremely large nucleated red cells (megaloblasts). Hepatic erythropoiesis, which is associated with erythroid differentiation from megaloblasts to macrocytes, extends from the 10th to the 24th gestational week, although the liver continues to produce red cells into the first week of postnatal life. From the 16th week onwards there is a decrease in extramedullary and an increase in medullary erythropoiesis, with a parallel switch of erythroid differentiation from macrocytes to normocytes. In normal pregnancy the fetal erythroblast count decreases exponentially with gestation, whereas the erythrocyte count and haemoglobin concentration increase linearly with gestation[24]. These

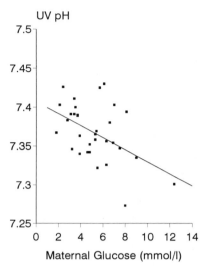

Figure 11.9. Relationship between umbilical venous (UV) blood pH and maternal venous blood glucose concentration

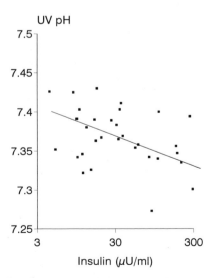

Figure 11.10. Relationship between umbilical venous blood pH and plasma insulin concentration[7]

changes presumably reflect the progressive maturation of the haematopoietic system and the declining contribution of extramedullary erythropoiesis with gestation. In hepatic erythropoiesis, erythroblasts enter the peripheral circulation freely, whereas with marrow erythropoiesis the nucleated erythroid precursors are confined to the parenchyma in which haematopoiesis takes place.

In pregnancies complicated by maternal diabetes mellitus there is fetal polycythaemia, erythroblastosis and increased erythropoietin concentration (Figures 11.11–11.13)[7,14]. However, there was no significant association between fetal erythropoietin and either haematocrit, insulin or pH[14].

The increased fetal erythroblast count suggests that the fetal polycythaemia is at least partly a consequence of recruitment of hepatic erythropoiesis. Although there was a significant association between erythropoietin concentration and erythroblast count, the former explained only 20% of the variance in the latter, suggesting the presence of additional erythrogenic stimulants[14].

Widness *et al.* considered increased erythropoietin concentration to be synonymous with fetal hypoxaemia[25,26]. It is tempting to suggest that maternal hyperglycaemia leads to fetal tissue hypoxia, which in turn causes release of erythropoietin with consequent stimulation of erythropoiesis and compensatory polycythaemia. However, in our study of 31 cases in which erythropoietin was measured, the umbilical venous blood oxygen tension was below the 5th centile in only one case, and despite the presence of

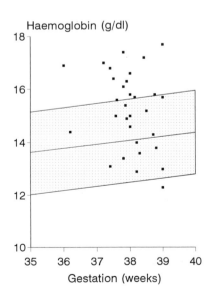

Figure 11.11. Fetal haemoglobin concentration plotted on the reference range with gestation (mean, 5th and 95th centiles)[14]

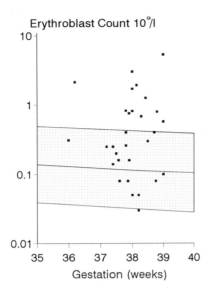

Figure 11.12. Fetal erythroblast count plotted on the reference range with gestation (mean, 5th and 95th centiles)[14]

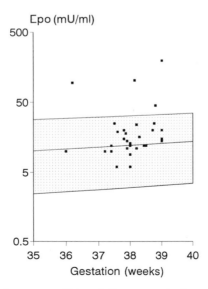

Figure 11.13. Fetal plasma erythropoietin concentration (Epo) plotted on the reference range with gestation (mean, 5th and 95th centiles)[14]

signficant fetal acidaemia fetal erythropoietin was not significantly related to measurable parameters of either short-term or long-term maternal glycaemic control and/or fetal oxygenation[14].

The lack of a significant association between fetal erythropoietin and pH suggests that in diabetes mellitus umbilical venous blood pH may be a poor indicator of tissue oxygenation. Alternatively, acidaemia reflects tissue hypoxia, but blood pH is liable to acute fluctuations dependent on changes in maternal glucose concentration; the lack of a significant association between blood pH and plasma erythropoietin concentration is because the latter increases after medium-term (4–5 h) tissue hypoxia. Similarly, the relationship between maternal glycosylated haemoglobin percentage and fetal haematocrit, but the lack of significant association between fetal erythropoietin and the increased haematocrit, is presumably because the latter is an index of long-term maternal hyperglycaemia and fetal hypoxia[14].

In contrast to maternal diabetes mellitus, in fetal growth retardation due to uteroplacental insufficiency, there are high correlations between fetal blood pH and erythropoietin, presumably because tissue hypoxia is the consequence of chronic impairment of placental perfusion[27]. In pregnancies complicated by diabetes mellitus, decreased fetal blood pH may therefore be considered a short-term measure of tissue hypoxia, whereas increased erythropoietin and haematocrit are medium- and long-term measures respectively.

An alternative explanation for increased fetal erythropoietin and haematocrit, but no significant association between them, is that in maternal diabetes mellitus there is a direct and variable effect of fetal insulin on both erythropoietin production and erythropoiesis. *In vitro* studies have shown that insulin has erythrogenic properties, and both animal and human studies have demonstrated that erythropoietin is increased in association with hyperinsulinaemia in the absence of hypoxaemia[25,26,28].

CONCLUSION

On the basis of currently available data it appears that maternal hyperglycaemia causes fetal hyperglycaemia and hyperinsulinaemia with consequent increased aerobic and anaerobic glucose metabolism, fetal acidaemia and tissue hypoxia (Figure 11.14). Increased fetal erythropoietin is likely to be the consequence of the tissue hypoxia and increased fetal haematocrit is presumably due to increased erythropoiesis, mediated either by erythropoietin and/or hyperinsulinaemia. Furthermore, fetal hyper-glycaemia and/or the other metabolic derangements associated with diabetes mellitus induce fetal beta cell hyperplasia before the third trimester of pregnancy. Fetal beta cell hyperplasia is then the likely cause of fetal macrosomia either directly through the anabolic effects of insulin or indirectly through related peptides.

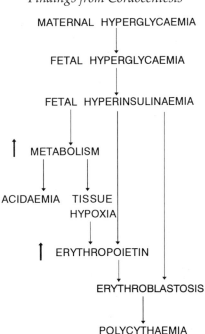

Figure 11.14. Proposed hypothesis to explain the pathogenesis of fetal acidaemia and polycythaemia in pregnancies complicated by maternal diabetes mellitus[14]

REFERENCES

1 Daffos F, Cappella-Pavlovsky M, Forestier F. Fetal blood sampling via the umbilical cord using a needle guided by ultrasound: report of 66 cases. *Prenat Diagn* 1983; **3**: 271–7.
2 Nicolaides KH, Soothill PW, Rodeck CH, Campbell S. Ultrasound guided sampling of umbilical cord and placental blood to assess fetal well-being. *Lancet* 1986; **i**: 1065.
3 Salvesen DR, Brudenell JM, Nicolaides KH. Fetal polycythemia and thrombocytopenia in pregnancies complicated by maternal diabetes mellitus. *Am J Obstet Gynecol* 1992; **166**: 1287–92.
4 Salvesen DR, Brudenell JM, Snijders R, Nicolaides KH. Effect of delivery on fetal erythropoietin and blood gases in pregnancies complicated by maternal diabetes. *Fetal Diagn Ther* 1995; **10**: 141–6.
5 Economides DL, Nicolaides KH. Blood glucose and oxygen tension in small for gestational age fetuses. *Am J Obstet Gynecol* 1989; **160**: 385–9.
6 Economides DL, Proudler A, Nicolaides KH. Plasma insulin in appropriate- and small-for-gestational age fetuses. *Am J Obstet Gynecol* 1989; **160**: 1091–4.
7 Salvesen DR, Brudenell JM, Proudler A *et al.* Fetal pancreatic β-cell function in pregnancies complicated by maternal diabetes mellitus. *Am J Obstet Gynecol* 1993; **168**: 1363–9.
8 Oakley NW, Beard RW, Turner RC. The effect of sustained maternal hyperglycaemia on the fetus in normal and diabetic pregnancies. *Br Med J* 1972; **i**: 466–9.
9 Pedersen J. *The Pregnant Diabetic and her Newborn*, 2nd edn. Williams & Wilkins, Baltimore, 1977; 211–20.
10 Hofman HMH, Weiss PAM, Purstner P *et al.* Serum fructosamine and amniotic fluid insulin levels in patients with gestational diabetes and healthy controls. *Am J Obstet Gynecol* 1990;

162: 1174–7.

11 Wang HS, Chard T. The role of insulin-like growth factor-I and insulin-like growth factor-binding protein-1 in the control of human fetal growth. *J Endocrinol* 1992; **132**: 11–19.

12 Nicolaides KH, Economides DL, Soothill PW. Blood gases, pH and lactate in appropriate and small for gestational age fetuses. *Am J Obstet Gynecol* 1989; **161**: 996–1001.

13 Bradley RJ, Brudenell JM, Nicolaides KH. Fetal acidosis and hyperlacticaemia diagnosed by cordocentesis in pregnancies complicated by maternal diabetes mellitus. *Diabetic Med* 1991; **8**: 464–8.

14 Salvesen DR, Brudenell JM, Nicolaides KH. Fetal plasma erythropoietin in pregnancies complicated by maternal diabetes. *Am J Obstet Gynecol* 1993; **168**: 88–94.

15 Salvesen DR, Brudenell JM, Nicolaides KH. Uteroplacental and fetal Doppler bloodflow studies in pregnancies complicated by maternal diabetes. *Am J Obstet Gynecol* 1993; **168**: 645–52.

16 Fox H. Pathology of the placenta in maternal diabetes mellitus. *Obstet Gynecol* 1969; **34**: 792–8.

17 Bilardo C, Nicolaides KH, Campbell S. Doppler measurements of fetal and uteroplacental circulations: relationship with umbilical venous blood gases at cordocentesis. *Am J Obstet Gynecol* 1990; **162**: 115–20.

18 Robillard JE, Sessions C, Kennedy RL, Smith FG. Metabolic effect of constant hypertonic glucose infusion in well oxygenated fetuses. *Am J Obstet Gynecol* 1978; **130**: 199–203.

19 Phillips AF, Dubin JW, Matty PJ, Raye JR. Arterial hypoxemia and hyperinsulinemia in the chronically hyperglycemic fetal lamb. *Pediatr Res* 1982; **16**: 653–8.

20 Phillips AF, Porte PJ, Stabinsky S *et al.* Effects of chronic fetal hyperglycemia upon oxygen consumption in the ovine uterus and conceptus. *J Clin Invest* 1984; **74**: 279–86.

21 Phillips AF, Rosenkrantz TS, Porte PJ, Raye JR. The effect of chronic fetal hyperglycemia on substrate uptake by the ovine fetus and conceptus. *Pediatr Res* 1985; **19**: 659–66.

22 Hay WW, DiGiacomo JE, Meznarich HK, Zerbe G. Effects of glucose and insulin on fetal glucose oxidation and oxygen consumption. *Am J Physiol* 1989; **256**: E704–13.

23 Shelly HJ, Bassett JM, Milner RDG. Control of carbohydrate metabolism in the fetus and newborn. *Br Med Bull* 1975; **31**: 37–43.

24 Nicolaides KH, Thilaganathen B, Mibashan RS. Cordocentesis in the investigation of fetal erythropoiesis. *Am J Obstet Gynecol* 1989; **161**: 1197–200.

25 Widness JA, Susa JB, Garcia JF *et al.* Increased erythropoiesis and elevated erythropoietin in infants born to diabetic mothers and in hyperinsulinemic rhesus fetuses. *J Clin Invest* 1981; **67**: 637–42.

26 Widness JA, Teramo KA, Clemons GK *et al.* Direct relationship of antepartum glucose control and fetal erythropoietin in human type I (insulin-dependent) diabetic pregnancy. *Diabetologia* 1990; **33**: 378–83.

27 Snijders RJM, Abbas A, Meylbye O *et al.* Fetal erythropoietin concentration in severe growth retardation. *Am J Obstet Gynecol* 1993; **168**: 615–19.

28 Perine SP, Greene MP, Lee PDK *et al.* Insulin stimulates cord blood progenitor growth: evidence for an aetiological role in neonatal polycythemia. *Br J Haematol* 1986; **64**: 503–11.

12

Diabetes in Pregnancy: Lessons from the Fetus

PETER A.M. WEISS

University Clinic of Graz, Austria

The extensive Graz experience with amniotic fluid insulin measurements over a number of years has allowed the fetus to teach us a number of lessons on the pathophysiology of diabetes in pregnancy. These studies are unique and provide very relevant confirmation of many concepts which have arisen from the original hyperglycaemia–hyperinsulinaemia hypothesis.

According to the Pedersen hypothesis[1] fetal and neonatal complications of gestational diabetes are due to fetal hyperinsulinism. Maternal hyperglycemia induces fetal hyperglycemia and consequently fetal hyperinsulinism through fetal beta cell hyperplasia (Figure 12.1). Fetal hyperinsulinism causes macrosomia and hypoglycaemia of the neonate. The immaturity of the organs causes complications in the neonatal period such as respiratory problems, hyperbilirubinaemia, polycythaemia and hypocalcaemia[2].

RISKS OF FETAL HYPERINSULINISM

In 764 offspring of metabolically healthy mothers studied in Graz the mean cord blood insulin level at delivery was 6.9 μU/ml ($\pm$ SD 5.0). Premature birth had no marked influence on the cord blood insulin level, and there was no difference between males and females. The 97th centile for cord blood insulin was 17.4 μU/ml, and less than 1% of the offspring of metabolically healthy mothers showed cord blood insulin levels above 20 μU/ml, the maximum being 26 μU/ml. For gestational diabetic pregnancy 21% of cord blood insulin values were $\geq$ 20 μU/ml (maximum 200 μU/ml),

Diabetes and Pregnancy: An International Approach to Diagnosis and Management.
Edited by A. Dornhorst and D. R. Hadden.
© 1996 John Wiley & Sons Ltd.

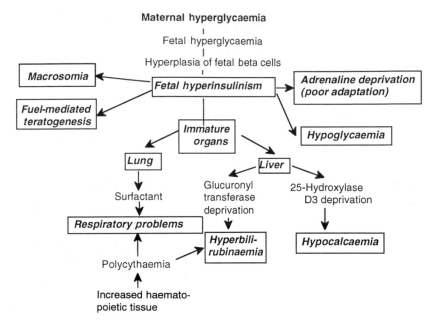

Figure 12.1. Fetal disturbances due to maternal hyperglycaemia (The Pedersen Hypothesis)

and for insulin-dependent diabetic pregnancy 49% were $\geq 20\ \mu U/ml$ (maximum $504\ \mu U/ml$).

The classic diabetogenic complications in newborns of diabetic mothers correlate with the insulin level in cord blood. In three groups of 63 newborns matched according to White classes but with different cord blood insulin levels, the perinatal outcome was distinctly different. Comparing infants with a cord blood insulin $< 20\ \mu U/ml$ with those $> 50\ \mu U/ml$, there was an eight-fold difference in macrosomia, a 15-fold difference in premature delivery, a 2.3-fold difference in caesarean delivery, and a 4.3-fold difference in hypoglycaemia of the newborn (Figure 12.2).

The incidence of respiratory distress syndrome in hyperinsulinaemia infants was exaggerated due to the increased number of premature deliveries, but there was still a five-fold increase in this complication when the cord blood insulin was $> 50\ \mu U/ml$.

One of the most important consequences of fetal hyperinsulinism on the further development of the child is a non-genetically caused inclination to diabetes as early as adolescence or later in life. This has been called 'fuel-mediated teratogenesis' by Freinkel and his group[3]. It comprises damage to and malconditioning of fetal beta cells by glucose oversupply. This subsequently causes obesity and a prediabetic glucose–insulin homeostasis

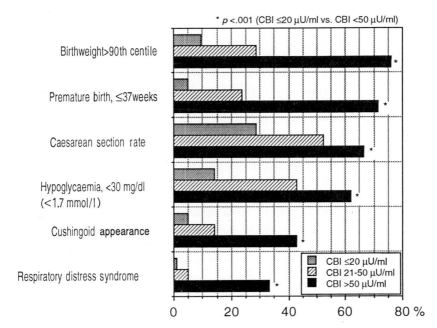

Figure 12.2. Correlation of cord blood insulin (CBI) levels and fetal outcome in three groups of diabetic mothers matched according to White classes but with different cord blood insulin levels ($n=63$)

such as elevated and delayed insulin response to glucose stimuli or impaired glucose tolerance as early as school age. Metzger and co-workers[4] further demonstrated that variations in anthropometric development correlated with amniotic fluid insulin levels at the 32nd to 38th weeks of gestation.

The first lesson from the fetus shows us that fetal hyperinsulinism has short- and long-term risks and consequences for the child and thus must be prevented.

AMNIOCENTESIS

Amniocentesis is a routine in obstetrics and is done on an out-clinic basis at our institution. The most common indications for amniocentesis are genetic analyses in women with an age over 35 years, analyses in fetal hemolytic disease, in suspicion of fetal malformation, and for the determination of fetal lung maturation. In most publications of the last decades repeated amniocenteses for the determination of fetal lung maturation are suggested in diabetic patients. A recent survey in the USA showed that 77–85% of 471 obstetricians take amniotic fluid for determination of fetal lung maturation prior to onset of labour[5], but in cases of insulin measurement there seems to be concern about risks of amniocentesis. Fraser[5a] has commented on the Graz method: 'Why amniocentesis should be a problem in these days of chorionic villus or placental biopsy and cordocentesis is a mystery'. We fully agree with this statement.

There is a detectable risk in early amniocentesis. Follow up of 2000 amniocenteses during the early second trimester showed a total fetal loss of 2.7% in cases versus 2.2% in controls. However, birth weight < 2500 g was evident in 3.6% versus 3.7%, respiratory distress syndrome in 0.8% versus 0.7% and malformations in 1.6% versus 1.9%, respectively[6].

The risk of amniocentesis during the third trimester is lower than that of the second trimester and is not any longer detectable. A recent study on a large series of third trimester amniocenteses in gestational diabetic patients at our clinic showed practically no short-term complications and a very positive attitude of the informed pregnant women to amniocentesis (Haeusler *et al.*, 1996, in preparation). Also long-term follow-up showed no adverse effect of amniocentesis. As long as 7–18 years after amniocenteses there were no related handicaps in the offspring[7].

We started amniotic fluid insulin measurement in the early 1970s. For basal research we first analysed a stock of several hundred deep-frozen amniotic fluid samples. Next we additionally measured insulin in any amniotic fluid from diabetic and non-diabetic mothers with an amniocentesis for fetal hemolytic disease, for determination of fetal lung maturation or for other indications. After we had identified and set up rules of fetomaternal glucose–insulin homeostasis in the course of normal and diabetic pregnancy we finally introduced amniotic fluid insulin measurement in diabetic mothers as an indication for third trimester amniocentesis in the late 1970s.

HOW TO DIAGNOSE FETAL HYPERINSULINISM

AMNIOTIC FLUID INSULIN: EARLY STUDIES

We investigated the correlation of cord blood insulin levels and insulin levels of the first portion of fetal urine collected by a self-adhesive plastic container immediately after birth[8]. There was a significant correlation between the insulin level in the cord blood and in fetal urine as shown in Figure 12.3. Since more than 90% of amniotic fluid in the third trimester consists of fetal urine, the amniotic fluid insulin level also reflects the fetal metabolic situation.

In previous studies in Graz we found that considerable fetal hyperinsulinism developed in conventionally treated (and thus poorly controlled) diabetic mothers in the 1970s, who had a mean blood glucose over 130 mg/dl (7.2 mmol/l)[9,10]. Measurement of amniotic fluid insulin in 84 insulin-dependent diabetic patients showed an increase during the pregnancy, up to about 300 μU/ml at the 37th week[11] (Figure 12.4). The highest amniotic fluid insulin level, more than 600 μU/ml, was measured in a gestational diabetic pregnancy. This is equivalent to the daily insulin production of a 120 kg adult. A considerable decrease of maternal blood glucose by the fetal 'glucose steal' phenomenon[12,13] often puzzled the doctor. Amniotic fluid insulin does not rise significantly before the 26th week of gestation in insulin-dependent diabetic pregnancy or the 28th week of gestation in gestational diabetes.

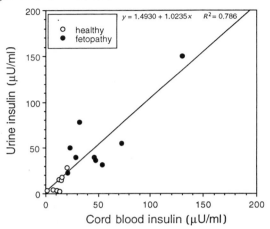

Figure 12.3. Correlation between cord blood insulin and insulin in the first portion of fetal urine. Open circles: metabolically healthy offspring; closed circles: offspring of gestational diabetic mothers with diabetic fetopathy

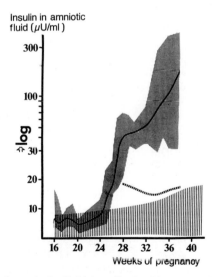

Figure 12.4. Pattern of amniotic fluid insulin in 84 conventionally treated diabetic mothers with a mean blood glucose > 130 mg/dl (7.2 mmol/l). Hatched zone: normal range in metabolically healthy pregnancies*. Broken line: mean amniotic fluid levels during tocolytic treatment with β-mimetic drugs. (*The normal range was higher in early investigations due to a higher unspecific insulin binding in the radioimmunoassay)

These investigations lead to the second lesson from the fetus: amniotic fluid insulin levels reflect the fetal metabolic situation from the 26th week onward in insulin-dependent diabetes and from the 28th week onward in gestational diabetes.

AMNIOTIC FLUID INSULIN: LATER STUDIES

Figure 12.5 shows more than 1800 amniotic fluid insulin levels in metabolically healthy controls and in intensively treated and controlled

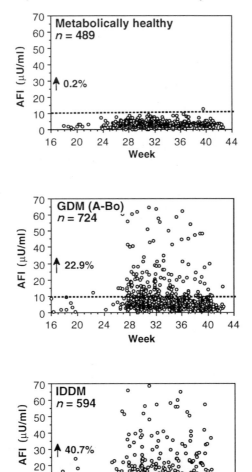

Figure 12.5. Amniotic fluid insulin (AFI) levels in metabolically healthy women, in gestational diabetes and in strictly treated insulin-dependent diabetes. Dotted line: upper limit of normal (10 μU/ml)

diabetic patients from 1980 to 1990 studied in Graz. In healthy controls with a normal oral glucose tolerance test, without tocolytic or glucocorticoid treatment and with a healthy offspring, only 0.2% of amniotic fluid insulin levels were greater than 10 μU/ml. By contrast in gestational diabetes and in insulin-dependent diabetic pregnancy more than 20% and 40% respectively had amniotic fluid insulin concentrations above 10 μU/ml despite good metabolic control with four or more insulin injections a day.

When gestational diabetes is not treated with insulin, or insulin-dependent diabetes is undertreated, elevated amniotic fluid insulin concentrations are associated with fetopathy[8]. In the 1970s gestational diabetic women were treated with diet only, even if the amniotic fluid insulin was elevated. Figure 12.6 shows the amniotic fluid insulin values in these women; the values for healthy born fetuses are lower than those for fetuses born with evidence of diabetic fetopathy.

From these data the third lesson from the fetus can be derived: an elevated amniotic fluid insulin level indicates that metabolic control in insulin-dependent diabetes is not strict enough for the fetal demands, or that the gestational diabetic state is severe enough to damage the fetus.

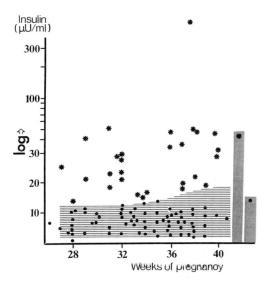

Figure 12.6. Amniotic fluid insulin levels in gestational diabetes under dietary treatment. ✳: 28 amniotic fluid insulin levels in 14 patients with subsequent birth of a child with diabetes-related fetal disease. ●: 75 amniotic fluid insulin values in 61 patients with subsequent delivery of a healthy infant. Hatched zone: normal range*. Bars: mean cord blood insulin (*See legend Figure 12.4)

MATERNAL ORAL GLUCOSE TOLERANCE

Another question is which of the oral glucose tolerance test values (> 95th centile) has the greatest sensitivity and thus the best predictive value for the diagnosis of fetal hyperinsulism. Is it the fasting blood glucose, the 1 h or the 2 h value or a combination of two or more elevated values? Evaluation of 100 oral glucose tolerance tests in gestational diabetic subjects associated with elevated amniotic fluid insulin levels showed that the fasting blood glucose was the least predictive for fetal hyperinsulism (sensitivity of 53%). The sensitivity of the 2 h blood glucose values was 60%, but the 1 h blood glucose had the highest sensitivity and was the most predictive value, being elevated in 99% of gestational diabetic women with a hyperinsulinaemic fetus. While outside pregnancy the 2 h value of an oral glucose tolerance is most important for the diagnosis of present and future diabetes in pregnancy, the 1 h value is of greater physiological importance. Fetal beta cells respond poorly to continuous glucose stimulation, being more responsive to intermittent stimuli[14,15]. Thus, unlike the non-pregnant state, the magnitude of the glucose peak is important, ensuring placental glucose transfer which protects the fetus at lower blood glucose ranges[16]. The greater importance of the 1 h glucose value is further suggested by the finding that while the lowest fasting and 2 h blood glucose values in a women with gestational diabetes and fetal hyperinsulinism were 59 mg/dl (3.3 mmol/l) and 77 mg/dl (4.3 mmol/l) respectively, the lowest 1 h value associated with fetal hyperinsulinism was 160 mg/dl (8.9 mmol/l), corresponding to the 95th percentile for normal pregnancies.

The fourth lesson from the fetus reveals that the 1 h value of an oral glucose tolerance test is the most appropriate to diagnose the potential risk of fetal hyperinsulinism.

ONE-HOUR PEAK MATERNAL ORAL GLUCOSE TOLERANCE TEST LIMITS AND MEAN MATERNAL GLUCOSE VALUES TO PREDICT FETAL HYPERINSULINISM

Figure 12.7 shows the correlation of the glucose peak at 1 h during an oral glucose tolerance test and the rate of fetal hyperinsulinism in 542 gestational diabetic women according to the Graz criteria[16]. One hundred of the 542 gestational diabetic pregnancies were associated with fetal hyperinsulinism. At a maternal 1 h blood glucose peak of 160–169 mg/dl (8.9–9.4 mmol/l) 8% of fetuses were hyperinsulinaemic; at a glucose peak of 215 mg/dl (11.9 mmol/l) 50% of fetuses developed hyperinsulinism, and over a peak of 245 mg/dl (13.9 mmol/l) 75% of fetuses had hyperinsulinism. It is highly likely that at a peak of 280 mg/dl (15.5 mmol/l) every fetus would suffer from hyperinsulinism. Though only 8% of fetuses developed hyperinsulinism at a glucose peak of 165 mg/dl (9.2 mmol/l) the absolute number of children involved is similar to that at higher thresholds, since mild disturbances of carbohydrate metabolism are relatively more common.

The correlation of mean maternal blood glucose, derived from at least six pre- and postprandial blood glucose values, and the rate of fetal hyperinsulinism is shown similarly in Figure 12.8. At a mean maternal

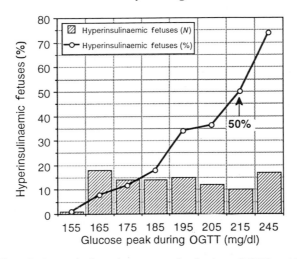

Figure 12.7. Correlation of the glucose peak during OGTT with the rate of subsequent fetal hyperinsulinism in 542 gestational diabetic mothers. Solid line and open circles: rate (%) of hyperinsulinaemic fetuses. Hatched bars: number of hyperinsulinaemic fetuses ($n=100$)

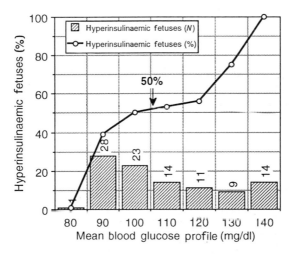

Figure 12.8. Correlation of mean maternal blood glucose profile (six or more pre- and postprandial blood glucose values) prior to amniocentesis with the rate of fetal hyperinsulinism in 542 gestational diabetic mothers. Symbols as in Figure 12.7

blood glucose of 80 mg/dl (4.4 mmol/l) there is practically no fetal hyperinsulinism detectable. At a mean maternal blood glucose of 90 mg/dl (5.0 mmol/l) about 40% of fetuses develop hyperinsulinism. There is a plateau from a mean glucose of 100 to 120 mg/dl (5.5–6.7 mmol/l) associated with about 50% fetal hyperinsulinism. Again, at a mean blood glucose as low as 90 mg/dl (5.0 mmol/l) the absolute number of children involved is the highest, since mild disturbance of carbohydrate metabolism occurs more often.

The fifth lesson from the fetus defines our obstetrically relevant limits. A maternal blood glucose ≥ 160 mg/dl (8.9 mmol/l) for the oral glucose tolerance test at 1 h, or ≥ 90 mg/dl (5.0 mmol/l) for mean pre- and postprandial blood glucose values, indicates a potential fetal risk of fetal hyperinsulinaemia.

THE NEED FOR AMNIOTIC FLUID INSULIN MEASUREMENT

In our experience fetal hyperinsulinism does not develop at a mean maternal blood glucose below 85 mg/dl (4.7 mmol/l) or at a 1 h oral glucose tolerance test value below 160 mg/dl; by contrast a mean maternal blood glucose over 140 mg/dl (7.8 mmol/l) or a 1 h oral glucose tolerance test value over 250 mg/dl (13.9 mmol/l) always predicts hyperinsulinism. When a mean blood glucose is between 80 and 135 mg/dl (4.4–7.5 mmol/l) or a 1 h oral glucose tolerance test value is between 160 and 250 mg/dl (8.8–13.8 mmol/l) as is the case for most gestational diabetic women, fetal hyperinsulinism cannot be accurately predicted or excluded using maternal blood glucose values, although the individual risk increases with increasing maternal glycaemia.

Similar maternal blood glucose levels in different patients do not rule out different fetal insulin production[16]. Figure 12.9 shows the pattern of amniotic fluid insulin in two patients with the same mean blood glucose levels during pregnancy. In the woman with gestational diabetes the amniotic fluid insulin became normal with insulin treatment, but it remained high in the insulin-dependent diabetic woman. The former pregnancy led to a healthy infant with a normal cord blood insulin, while the latter produced a macrosomic hyperinsulinaemic infant. When assessing the metabolic situation of the fetus, it should be remembered that the placenta is interposed between the mother and the fetus. Severe placental damage in diabetes can cause an undersupply as well as an oversupply of glucose to the fetus[16], and the sensitivity of fetuses to glucose stimuli seems to differ. Even in twins, one fetus may be healthy and the other develop fetopathy[11,17].

From these data the sixth lesson from the fetus can be derived. In the middle range of blood glucose values which encompasses most diabetic pregnancies, fetal hyperinsulinism and thus fetal jeopardy may only be proved or excluded by amniotic fluid insulin.

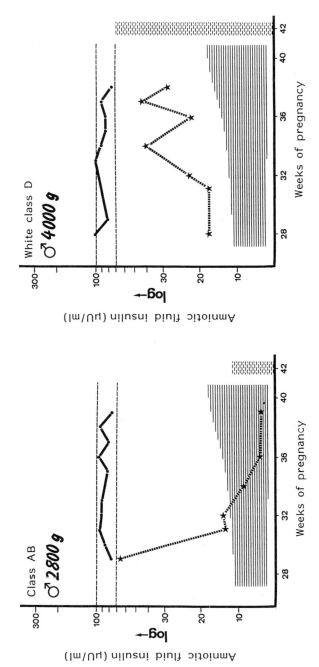

Figure 12.9. Different patterns of amniotic fluid insulin (broken line) in two diabetic mothers with similar mean maternal blood glucose values (solid line), and different fetal outcome (see text). Hatched zone: normal range of amniotic fluid*. Bars: cord blood insulin level (*See legend Figure 12.4)

DIFFERENT GLUCOSE LOADS AND BLOOD SPECIMENS FOR ORAL GLUCOSE TOLERANCE TESTS

There is a lack of consensus on interpreting the oral glucose tolerance test and a lack of agreement on the glucose load to be used. The World Health Organization has suggested the diagnosis of diabetes in pregnancy based on a 75 g oral glucose tolerance test with blood glucose measurement in either capillary blood or venous plasma, while the American Diabetes Association recommends a 100 g glucose load and measurement only in venous plasma. We have recently evaluated a study comparing both methods. We performed a 75 g oral glucose tolerance test in 30 gestational diabetic and 30 control mothers with a 75 g load and capillary blood glucose measurement, and then repeated the test in both groups within three days either with a 75 g or a 100 g load, measuring glucose simultaneously in capillary blood and venous plasma (Figure 12.10).

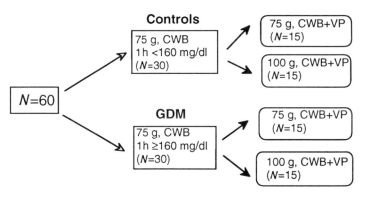

CWB=capillary whole blood, VP=venous plasma

Figure 12.10. Flow sheet of a prospective randomized study on the influence of different glucose loads (75 g vs 100 g) and different blood specimens (capillary blood vs venous plasma) on the OGTT results in gestational diabetes (GDM) and control pregnancies

For the 75 g glucose load in controls there was a significant difference in glucose levels at 1 and 2 h between capillary blood and venous plasma, but there was no difference in the gestational diabetic mothers, most likely due to the elevated peripheral insulin resistance (Figure 12.11a). For the 100 g oral glucose tolerance test there was the same pattern, with a significant difference in glucose between capillary blood and venous plasma glucose in controls but no difference in the gestational diabetic mothers (Figure 12.11b).

Comparing the 75 g and 100 g loads, at 1 h there was no difference in blood glucose in the same patients but the 2 h values differed significantly (Figure 12.12). Thus an upper limit of 160 mg/dl (8.9 mmol/l) at 1 h is valid for a load of 75 g or 100 g, and for capillary blood and venous plasma glucose during an oral glucose tolerance test.

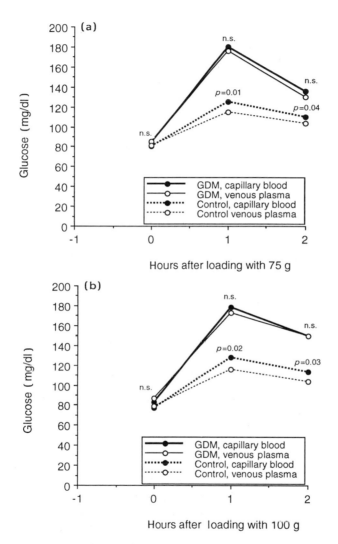

Figure 12.11. Differences of blood glucose between capillary blood and venous plasma during an OGTT with a glucose load of 75 g (a) or 100 g (b). Solid lines: gestational diabetes. Dotted lines: controls. In gestational diabetes (GDM) there is no difference between glucose levels in capillary blood and venous plasma, probably dur to exaggerated peripheral insulin resistance

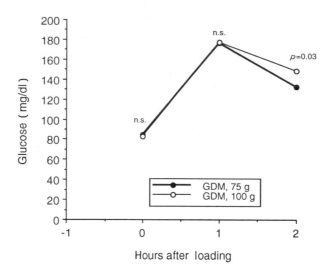

Figure 12.12. Differences between blood glucose levels in gestational diabetes during an OGTT after a glucose load of 75 g or 100 g in the same patients. This applies to capillary blood as well as venous plasma

DIET OR INSULIN TREATMENT?

WHAT IS THE INDICATION FOR TREATMENT—DIET?

The amniotic fluid insulin concentration allows one to predict whether a woman with gestational diabetes can be treated with diet alone. Figure 12.13 shows the fetal outcome in two groups of gestational diabetic mothers with either a normal or an elevated amniotic fluid insulin level during dietary treatment. When the amniotic fluid insulin level was below 10 μU/ml the fetal outcome was similar to that in metabolically healthy patients[2]. However, when the amniotic fluid insulin level was above 20 μU/ml, fetal outcome was poor, despite dietary treatment. In the latter pregnancies diabetes-associated complications, including fetal hyperinsulinaemia, hypoglycaemia, hyperbilirubinaemia, macrosomia, premature birth, respiratory distress syndrome and perinatal mortality, were all more prevalent compared to controls, and to gestational diabetic mothers with normal amniotic fluid insulin levels below 10 μU/ml.

Thus the seventh lesson from the fetus is that in gestational diabetic mothers with a normal amniotic fluid insulin level dietary treatment is appropriate, while in patients with an elevated amniotic fluid insulin level dietary treatment alone is insufficient.

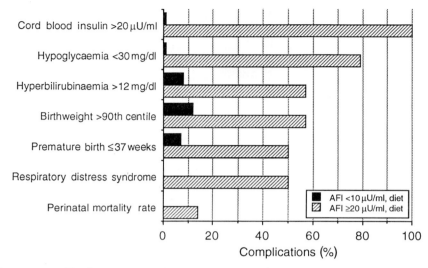

Figure 12.13. Fetal outcome in dietary treatment of gestational diabetes with either normal or elevated amniotic fluid insulin (AFI) level. Dietary treatment in normal amniotic fluid insulin levels is sufficient

INDICATIONS FOR TREATMENT—INSULIN?

Comparison of insulin treatment versus dietary treatment in women with gestational diabetes and elevated amniotic fluid insulin levels shows insulin treatment to be beneficial. Perinatal outcome improved in the insulin-treated group compared with the dietary-treated group (Figure 12.14). Hypoglycaemia, hyperbilirubinaemia, macrosomia and premature birth were all significantly reduced with insulin treatment. Apart from a few cases with a slightly elevated cord blood insulin level, there was no respiratory distress syndrome or perinatal loss in the insulin-treated pregnancies[2].

The eighth lesson from the fetus teaches us that insulin treatment in gestational diabetic pregnancy with elevated amniotic fluid insulin levels may prevent fetopathy.

WHAT IS THE IMPACT OF INSULIN TREATMENT ON THE COURSE OF FETAL INSULIN PRODUCTION?

Figure 12.15 shows the pattern of repeatedly measured amniotic fluid insulin levels in gestational diabetic mothers during strict insulin treatment[12] (left-hand panel). On the right there are amniotic fluid insulin values of those mothers who did not accept insulin treatment. Six insulin-

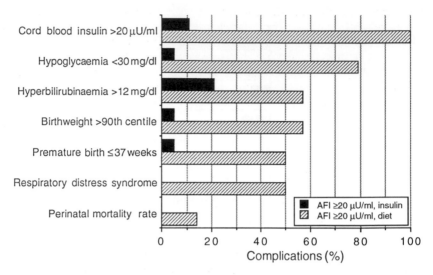

Figure 12.14. Fetal outcome in gestational diabetes with elevated amniotic fluid insulin (AFI) level with either dietary or insulin treatment. Dietary treatment in elevated amniotic fluid insulin levels is insufficient

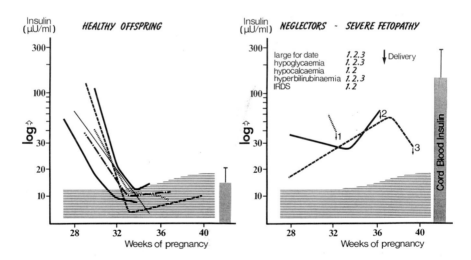

Figure 12.15. Patterns of amniotic fluid insulin levels in strictly treated diabetic women (on the left) and in neglectors (on the right). Hatched zone: normal range of amniotic fluid insulin*. The strictly treated diabetic women gave birth to healthy offspring while the offspring of neglectors suffered from macrosomia, hypoglycaemia, hyperbilirubinaemia, respiratory distress syndrome and hypocalcaemia. Bars: mean cord blood insulin levels (+SD) (*see legend Figure 12.4)

treated gestational diabetic patients who had repeated amniotic fluid measurements throughout pregnancy showed a sharp decrease in amniotic fluid insulin level during pregnancy, and all gave birth to healthy infants with a normal mean cord blood insulin level. In the three women who refused insulin, the amniotic fluid insulin levels remained elevated and all offspring showed severe diabetic fetopathy, and their mean cord blood insulin level was elevated.

The ninth lesson from the fetus is that strict insulin treatment in diabetes with elevated amniotic fluid insulin level may normalize insulin levels within one week and keep them in a normal range during the further course of pregnancy.

The nine lessons from the fetus are thus:

1. Hyperinsulinism has adverse fetal consequences.
2. Amniotic fluid insulin reflects the fetal metabolic situation in the second half of pregnancy.
3. Elevated amniotic fluid insulin indicates too high maternal blood glucose, even if this seems to be normal according to established criteria.
4. A single 1 h value is appropriate for the diagnosis of gestational diabetes.
5. At a 1 h oral glucose tolerance test value ≥ 160 mg/dl (8.9 mmol/l), or a mean blood glucose ≥ 90 mg/dl (5.0 mmol/l) fetal hyperinsulinism becomes increasingly likely.
6. In a middle range of maternal glycaemia, fetal hyperinsulinism is poorly predicted by maternal glycaemia in individual cases.
7. In gestational diabetes mellitus with normal amniotic fluid insulin dietary treatment is sufficient.
8. In gestational diabetes with elevated amniotic fluid insulin, insulin treatment prevents fetopathy.
9. Adequate insulin therapy normalizes fetal insulin homeostasis within one week.

CONCLUSIONS

There are a great number of different screening procedures, glucose loads, blood specimens and blood glucose limits. Many of them are set arbitrarily, derived from experience outside pregnancy, and with maternal endpoints in mind. But gestational diabetes is an obstetric problem, and the obstetrician is caring for the fetus. Thus we used the fetus to determine obstetrically relevant limits, to create guidelines from a fetal point of view. Gestational diabetes should be recognized as a metabolic disturbance severe enough that it can just be recognized by the fetus as abnormal. Treatment in insulin-dependent and gestational diabetes should be aimed to produce a metabolic state so that the fetus does not any longer recognize its mother as diabetic.

THE GRAZ PROTOCOL

We perform an oral glucose tolerance test in the 24th to 28th week of pregnancy with a glucose load of 75 g and capillary blood measurement. If the maternal blood glucose peaks to 160 mg/dl (8.9 mmol/l) or over, the test is positive and we begin dietary treatment and weekly measurement of maternal blood glucose. Between the 28th and 32nd week of gestation we measure the amniotic fluid insulin. If this is elevated we add insulin treatment to the diet. A small number of mothers develop overt diabetes prior to the amniotic fluid insulin measurement and therefore require early insulin treatment. In 84% of gestational diabetic women dietary therapy is appropriate, 11% of gestational diabetic women require insulin therapy due to an elevated amniotic fluid insulin and 5% develop overt diabetes (Figure 12.16).

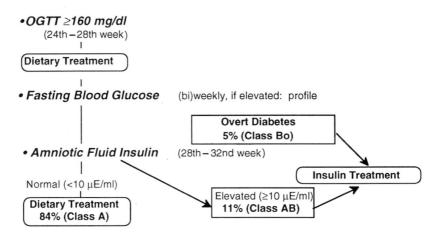

Figure 12.16. The Graz approach to diagnosis and therapy of gestational diabetes

In insulin-dependent diabetic subjects our insulin therapy is aimed at a mean maternal blood glucose of ≤100 mg/dl (5.5 mmol/l)[12]. At about the 32nd week of pregnancy we measure amniotic fluid insulin to adjust the maternal blood glucose to individual fetal requirements (Figure 12.17). In about 30% of cases the insulin level is elevated and we reduce the maternal blood glucose by about 10 mg/dl (0.55 mmol/l). In about 8% of cases the insulin levels are very low, and especially if there is intrauterine growth retardation we now aim to elevate the mean maternal blood glucose by about 20 mg/dl (1.1 mmol/l) in these pregnancies.

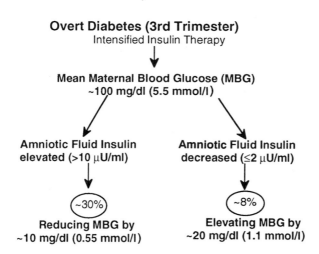

Figure 12.17. The Graz approach to modification of insulin therapy in insulin-dependent diabetic pregnancy

REFERENCES

1 Pedersen J. *The Pregnant Diabetic and Her Newborn: Problems and Management*, 2nd edn. Williams & Wilkins, Baltimore, 1977; 211–20.

2 Weiss PAM, Hofmann HMH, Kainer F, Haas JG. Fetal outcome in gestational diabetes with elevated amniotic fluid insulin levels: dietary versus insulin treatment. *Diabetes Res Clin Pract* 1988; **5**: 1–7.

3 Freinkel N, Metzger BE, Phelps RL *et al*. Heterogeneity of maternal age, weight, insulin secretion, HLA antigens, and islet cell antibodies and the impact of maternal metabolism on pancreatic beta-cell and somatic development in the offspring. Diabetes 1985; **34** (Suppl. 2): 1–7.

4 Metzger BE, Silverman BL, Freinkel N *et al*. Amniotic fluid insulin as a predictor of obesity. *Arch Dis Child* 1990; 65 (Suppl. 10): 1050–2.

5 Landon MB, Gabbe SG, Sachs L. Management of diabetes mellitus and pregnancy: a survey of obstetricians and maternal–fetal specialists. *Obstet Gynecol* 1990; **75**: 635–40.

5a Fraser R. Diabetic control in pregnancy and intrauterine growth of the fetus. *Br J Obstet Gynaecol* 1995; **102**: 275–7.

6 Crandall BF, Howard J, Lebherz TB *et al*. Follow-up of 2000 second-trimester amniocentesis. *Obstet Gynecol* 1980; **56**: 625–8.

7 Baird PA, Yee IML, Sadovnick AD. Population based study of long-term outcomes after amniocentesis. *Lancet* 1994; **344**: 1134–6.

8 Weiss PAM, Hofmann H, Winter R, Purstner P. Gestational diabetes and screening during pregnancy. *Obstet Gynecol* 1984; **63**: 776–80.

9 Weiss PAM, Winter R, Purstner P. Insulin levels in amniotic fluid: management of pregnancy in diabetes. *Obstet Gynecol* 1978; **51**: 393–8.

10 Weiss PAM. Die Überwachung des Ungeborenen bei Diabetes mellitus und Hand von Fruchtwasserinsulinwerten. *Wien Klin Wochenschr* 1979; **91**: 293–304.

11 Weiss PAM. Gestational diabetes: a survey and the Graz approach to diagnosis and therapy. In: Weiss PAM, Coustan DR (eds), *Gestational Diabetes*. Springer, New York, 1988; 1–55.

12 Weiss PAM, Hofmann H. Intensified conventional insulin therapy for the pregnant diabetic patient. *Obstet Gynecol* 1984; **64**: 629–37.
13 Nolan CJ, Proietto J. The feto-placental glucose steal phenomenon is a major cause of maternal metabolic adaptation during late pregnancy. *Diabetologia* 1994; **37**: 976–84.
14 Grasso S, Distefano G, Messina A *et al.* Effect of glucose priming on insulin response in the premature infant. *Diabetes* 1975; **24**: 291–4.
15 Sodoyez-Goffaux F, Sodoyez JC. Effects of intermittent hyperglycemia in pregnant rats on the functional development of the pancreatic beta cells of their offspring. *Diabetologia* 1976; **12**: 73–6.
16 Weiss PAM, Hofmann H. Monitoring pregnancy in diabetes: amniotic fluid. *Diabetes Nutr Metab* 1990; **3** (Suppl. 2): 31–5.
17 Burke BJ, Sheriff RJ, Savage PE, Dixon HG. Diabetic twin pregnancy: an unequal result. *Lancet* 1979; **i**: 1372–3.

13

Monitoring Fetal Well-being in Diabetic Pregnancy

JOANNA C. GIRLING

Hammersmith Hospital, London, UK

Monitoring fetal well-being in diabetic pregnancy incorporates serial assessment of fetal growth and liquor volume, and determining the optimum time for delivery, ensuring minimum risks from prematurity and maximum chance of healthy survival. In many cases, of course, these decisions will be intimately entwined with the assessment of maternal well-being, and decisions regarding delivery may reflect a compromise, giving the best chance for both mother and baby. There has always been concern over fetal well-being in diabetic pregnancy, especially in the third trimester when unexpected intrauterine death can occur.

AVOIDING STILLBIRTH

There still remains a small increased risk of intrauterine death late in diabetic pregnancy, despite excellent glycaemic control. This is perhaps as much as four times greater than the normal population, even after the exclusion of congenital anomaly. Following the observation that the neonatal death rate was lower than the stillbirth rate beyond 36 weeks gestation Peel and Oakley, in 1949[1], recommended delivery at this gestation. By 1980 this policy had been shown not to improve perinatal mortality, largely due to problems of prematurity[2], and there has been a gradual trend again towards later delivery. Some authors advocate delivery at 38 weeks gestation[3], but others[4] allow women with uncomplicated diabetes to go into spontaneous labour irrespective of the gestational age. In

Diabetes and Pregnancy: An International Approach to Diagnosis and Management.
Edited by A. Dornhorst and D. R. Hadden.
© 1996 John Wiley & Sons Ltd.

Murphy's retrospective review[4], 64% of a group of 45 women went into spontaneous labour after 37 weeks gestation, with a mean gestation of 39 weeks. Although there was a decreased need for neonatal tube or intravenous feeding compared to infants delivered during the preceding five years when early induction was recommended, there was no reduction in respiratory distress syndrome, hypoglycaemia, or caesarean section rate which remained almost 50%. There was, however, one unexpected stillbirth at 39 weeks' gestation in this group of diabetic women allowed to go into spontaneous labour. One of the disadvantages of induction at 38 weeks' gestation is that the cervix may be unfavourable and consequently the induction difficult or unsuccessful, but this must be balanced against the still poorly defined risk of late intrauterine death, which is neither fully understood nor predictable and remains a major cause of medical and maternal concern. It is with this in mind that we must carefully monitor fetal well-being.

Although the exact cause for this increased frequency of unexplained late stillbirths in association with diabetic pregnancies is not known, there is a correlation with poor maternal glycaemic control and fetal macrosomia[5]. Various other theories implicate fetal hypoxia and acidosis[6], hypokalaemia leading to dysrhythmias, and placental dysfunction and competition for essential nutrients[7]. Animal studies on primates and sheep have shown that the fetus of a diabetic pregnancy is more susceptible to acidosis than a fetus from a non-diabetic pregnancy[8,9]. Fetal hyperinsulinaemia in the lamb causes fetal hypoxia due to increased oxygen uptake by non-visceral tissues without a corresponding increase in oxygen supply to the fetus[10]. Fetal blood sampling during cordocentesis in insulin-dependent diabetic women has shown that some fetuses have significant acidosis and hyperlacticaemia in the third trimester[6]. The greater oxygen affinity of glycosylated haemoglobin (HbA_1) than the non-glycosylated molecule may also adversely affect fetal placental oxygenation, especially in late pregnancy when fetal haemoglobin F (HbF) with its high oxygen affinity is being replaced by adult haemoglobin with a lower oxygen affinity (HbA)[11].

Whatever the mechanism of intrauterine death, there are no randomized studies to determine the best method of antenatal assessment in diabetic pregnancy, the gestation at which it should begin or how often it is needed. Daily urinary oestriol measurements were used, later being replaced by circulating placental hormones levels[12]: neither are reliable or remain in clinical use. The subsequent introduction of fetal heart rate monitoring using cardiotocography has not clarified the situation. There is also debate regarding the relative merits of the non-stress test and the contraction stress test, with either intravenous oxytocin or nipple stimulation. In the UK the latter has not been introduced into routine antenatal practice due to its invasive and time-consuming nature and lack of proven clinical efficacy. However, in a review of seven studies using non-stress testing in 426 diabetic pregnancies Barrett[13] found a stillbirth incidence of 1.4% within seven days of a normal reactive test, a figure similar to that for pregnancies complicated by intrauterine growth retardation.

Simple methods such as maternal assessment of fetal movements should not be overlooked, but have a poor predictive value. Therefore, in the 1980s, Manning[14] developed the biophysical profile, an ultrasound-based assessment of fetal well-being derived from fetal movement, fetal tone, fetal breathing movements, liquor volume and a non-stress test. Each parameter has a possible score of 0, 1 or 2, the higher score representing normality in each case. In babies without congenital anomaly, a score greater than 8 out of a possible maximum of 10 had a perinatal mortality of 0.65 per 1000, which rose to 22 for a score of 4, 43 for a score of 2 and 187 for a score of 0[15]. However, while oligohydramnios has a low score, polyhydramnios inappropriately has the same maximum score as normal liquor volume. Also, the assessment of reduced fetal tone, breathing and movement by ultrasound is a time-consuming process requiring a minimum of 30 min. Only one study specifically addresses the use of the biophysical profile in diabetic women[16], but unfortunately this muddles insulin-dependent diabetes ($n=50$) with gestational diabetes ($n=178$). Amongst the 50 women with insulin-dependent diabetes, three had an abnormal biophysical profile score but the gestation and associated morbidity are unclear, as is the morbidity in those with a normal score; there were three neonatal deaths, all due to major congenital anomaly, and it is not clear whether these babies had normal profiles. It is therefore difficult to extrapolate their conclusion that the biophysical profile allows safe expectant management in diabetic women to a group of women with insulin-dependent diabetes.

Recently, umbilical artery flow velocity waveforms have been extensively used in the assessment of high-risk pregnancy, but are only validated for use in pregnancy associated with intrauterine growth retardation. Uncomplicated diabetic pregnancy has similar waveforms to non-diabetic pregnancy[17]. Abnormal umbilical artery resistance index appears to be a significant predictor of fetal compromise in diabetic pregnancy, but undue reliance should not be placed on a normal waveform as fetal compromise may occur in the presence of normal Doppler studies[17].

ABNORMAL FETAL GROWTH

Monitoring fetal well-being includes the assessment of growth. Fetal growth is dependent on maternal–fetal nutrient transfer, which is ultimately dependent on placental size, uterine blood flow and nutrient supply, all factors that can be influenced by maternal diabetes[18]. The infant of the diabetic mother is usually 'growth promoted'[19] due to increased maternal–fetal nutrient transfer[20,21]. In diabetic pregnancies complicated by vascular disease, accelerated fetal growth patterns are statistically less likely[22], and growth retardation more likely, suggesting that decreased maternal–fetal nutrient transfer is a consequence of impaired uterine blood flow.

Maternal glycaemic control during fetal pancreatic development, which begins early in pregnancy, may influence the subsequent growth of the fetus. Human studies have shown an increase in pancreatic beta cell mass and insulin secretion in fetuses of poorly controlled diabetic women by 16 weeks gestation[23], which progresses throughout the second trimester until 26 weeks. This priming of the fetal beta cells in mid-gestation may account for the persistence of fetal hyperinsulinaemia, and the consequent accelerated fetal growth, throughout pregnancy, which occasionally occurs despite good maternal metabolic control[24]. The role of the insulin-like growth factors (IGFs) in human fetal growth also needs to be clarified in this respect. Ovine studies suggest that they facilitate maternal–fetal nutrient transfer in late pregnancy, an effect that may be dependent on fetal insulin[25]. Circulating IGF-I is increased in fetal pigs of diabetic sows, in whom a tissue-specific regulation for IGF-I is suggested by the increase in its tissue expression in muscle, heart, liver and placenta but not in fat[26].

The pathogenesis of 'growth promotion' in diabetic pregnancies involves fetal hyperinsulinaemia[27], and it is this rather than glucose itself which is felt to be responsible for the typical pattern of growth. This was demonstrated by animal work, in which fetal hyperinsulinaemia was induced experimentally by insulin infusion, in healthy pregnant euglycaemic Rhesus monkeys, producing similar accelerated fetal growth patterns to those encountered in human diabetic pregnancies[28,29]. These growth abnormalities include excessive abdominal fat disposition, organomegaly (notably liver, spleen and heart), and accelerated skeletal maturation. By contrast fetal lambs rendered hypoinsulinaemic after *in utero* beta cell destruction with streptozocin have decreased somatic and skeletal growth[30]. In humans, as no maternal insulin crosses the placenta (or only negligible amounts), all circulating insulin in the fetus can be presumed to be of fetal origin[31]. In addition, there is a strong correlation between fetal beta cell secretion assessed by amniotic and umbilical cord insulin, C peptide and proinsulin and birth weight[32-38]. The availability to the fetus of glucose, amino acids and lactate is increased in diabetic pregnancy[39], as a result of increased concentrations of these substances in the maternal circulation. Glucose and some amino acids, including arginine and leucine, are fetal beta cell secretagogues and contribute to the fetal hyperinsulinaemia[21,22,27].

The terminology relating to and the definition of 'large for gestational age' babies in diabetic pregnancy is debatable, but often this refers to the largest 10% of all babies. It is therefore of course important to define the percentile weight of an individual baby by comparison with an appropriate population. In humans, birth weight is related to gestational age and fetal gender[40], and is also highly dependent on maternal phenotype, height, weight and ethnicity. Recent work has also suggested that there may be ethnic differences in the influence of maternal hyperglycaemia on infant birth weight, with maternal postprandial plasma glucose concentrations having a significantly greater influence on Asian than white/European infant birth weights[41]. As the frequency of large-for-gestational age infants in diabetic mothers is often used as a surrogate marker of maternal glycaemic control it is essential when defining large-for-gestational age to ensure birth weight percentiles for the correct ethnic group are used, as birth weight differs enormously between ethnic groups[41].

The frequency of large-for-gestational age infants in diabetes is approximately two-fold higher than for non-diabetic pregnancies, atlhough part of this increase, especially in non-insulin-dependent and gestational diabetic pregnancies, is attributable to coexisting maternal obesity[42,43]. However, babies who are large for gestational age may be in an advantageous situation due to possible protection against future adult disease[44-47]. Nonetheless, they remain at increased risk of emergency caesarean section, birth trauma and birth asphyxia[48,49].

The term 'macrosomia' is also best avoided since it is both imprecise and misleading. Definitions vary from birth weights of 4 kg to greater than 5 kg, but rarely take account of gestational age, genetically intended weight, sex or ethnic origin. The term is usually intended to imply that the fetus has exceeded its expected growth, and has an abdominal circumference which is relatively larger than its head circumference. This should be a different concept from that of simply being large, which may occur by chance in 10% of cases (see above). A baby weighing 3 kg at 32 weeks' gestation would be considered large for dates, but one weighing 4.2 kg at 42 weeks' in a Caucasian women might not; a fetus whose abdominal circumference increases from the 3rd to the 50th centile might be considered 'macrosomic' whereas one starting on and remaining at the 70th centile might not. However, size or macrosomia *per se* is not the problem: it is the associated fetal and maternal trauma that may result which influences obstetric practice.

Management is therefore aimed at prevention of excessive fetal growth, by ensuring optimum diabetic control. There is a positive correlation between postprandial maternal glucose concentration and human birth weight[22,50,51], suggesting that the protective, transplacental facilitated diffusion process for glucose which occurs in normal pregnancy may allow higher peaks of fetal insulin to occur when there is maternal hyperglycaemia[52]. In general, therefore, home monitoring of blood glucose should incorporate postprandial testing. Nonetheless, maternal glycaemic control accounts for only part of the fetal hyperinsulinaemia and accelerated growth which can still occur in well-controlled diabetic pregnancies[24] (see above).

Clinically, abdominal palpation is a helpful but imprecise guide to fetal size, particularly in the obese woman. Ultrasound scans should be performed frequently, probably two-weekly beyond 26 weeks' gestation, for assessment of fetal growth and liquor volume. In diabetes, excessive fetal growth presents as an increase in abdominal circumference in relation to the head circumference or biparietal diameter, and usually crossing of the centile lines by the former but not the latter. It is assumed to be due to increased hepatic glycogen storage and subcutaneous fat deposition secondary to poor maternal control of glycaemia and resulting fetal hyperinsulinaemia.

Ultrasound scans have been used to estimate fetal size and to predict which fetuses are at risk from trauma at delivery, in particular shoulder dystocia, fractured clavicle and Erb's palsy. In America, approximately 80% of 471 perinatologists and obstetricians base their decision to deliver by caesarean section on ultrasound-predicted fetal weight[53]. However, in an Australian survey the risk of shoulder dystocia was 2.8–3.4% for an actual birth weight between 4 and 4.5 kg, rising to 10–14% for a weight over 4.5 kg[54], suggesting that a large number of caesarean sections performed in the USA to avoid shoulder dystocia are unnecessary. Therefore, it is not surprising that attempts using ultrasound to predict fetuses at risk of birth trauma are inaccurate, especially as scanning provides only an approximate fetal weight and the degree to which the maternal pelvis will expand in labour is unpredictable. Further only 13% of babies weighing over 4 kg in whom shoulder dystocia occurs actually suffer birth trauma[55]. Computed tomographic measurements of the transverse shoulder diameter provide a reasonable correlation with actual shoulder diameter and birth weight[56] but do not give any additional predictive value when planning delivery. Likewise, complicated formulae based on multiple ultrasound parameters have no more accuracy in predicting birth weight over 4 kg than the use of abdominal circumference and femur length alone[57].

Planning delivery of an apparently large baby must include consideration of maternal factors, including past obstetric history, presence of diabetic or obstetric complications, maternal stature and maternal preference. As 'disproportion' is likely to become apparent after delivery of the head rather than because of 'failure to progress' in the first stage of labour, obstetric decisions regarding planned mode of delivery should be made by senior personnel.

Asymmetrical growth retardation (poor growth of fetal abdominal circumference both in comparison to the centile growth charts and the head circumference) is a feature of pregnancies complicated by diabetic vascular disease, particularly nephropathy and retinopathy, or pre-eclampsia. It results from uteroplacental insufficiency which preferentially spares brain growth at the expense of reduced liver glycogen stores and subcutaneous fat deposition. Asymmetrical growth retardation is rarely detected prior to 24 weeks' gestation. It is associated with increased risk of intrauterine death, intrapartum hypoxia and neonatal complications, including necrotizing enterocolitis. Its detection requires surveillance by clinical palpation, maternal monitoring of fetal movements, serial ultrasound scanning, umbilical Doppler waveform assessment and cardiotocograph recordings. Management decisions are particularly difficult when this occurs at an early gestation, when fetal survival is likely to be poor. Once these biophysical tests become abnormal, delivery is likely to be necessary.

MONITORING LIQUOR VOLUME

Fetal well-being is in part reflected by liquor volume, the main concern in diabetic pregnancy being whether polyhydramnios has developed. In some cases, this can be obvious clinically, with discomfort, distension and increased heartburn. On abdominal palpation, the uterus may be larger than expected, and tense, such that it is not possible to distinguish the fetal parts. However, as lesser degrees are difficult to diagnose clinically, and there are potentially serious implications and repercussions of this diagnosis, it should be sought actively, by serial ultrasonography. Although it is most likely to be due to fetal polyuria, secondary to fetal hyperglycaemia[58], congenital anomaly of the gastrointestinal tract, which has an incidence of 2.4 per 1000 diabetic pregnancies[59,60], must always be excluded by careful ultrasonography.

Polyhydramnios may be defined as a four-quadrant liquor volume greater than the 90th percentile for gestational age, or a single liquor pool greater than normal. Its incidence in diabetes varies from 16[61] to 29%[62], depending at least in part on definitions used. Other than causing considerable maternal discomfort, it may be associated with preterm labour, pre-labour rupture of membranes, unstable lie and cord prolapse. Polyhydramnios has also been associated with an increase risk of stillbirth in diabetic women at term[63]. Non-steroidal anti-inflammatory drugs such as indomethacin have been used to reduce fetal urine production and consequently the liquor volume. However, maximum control of the diabetes should be the goal, as this has been helpful in some cases.

Oligohydramnios is less frequent in diabetic pregnancy. Assuming that the fetal renal tract is normal (which is not the case in over four per 1000 diabetic pregnancies[59,60]) it reflects either ruptured membranes or most importantly in this context poor fetoplacental perfusion. The latter may be due to development of pre-eclampsia or as a consequence of microvascular complications of diabetes, and is usually associated with a slowing in the rate of fetal growth.

ASSESSMENT OF FETAL MATURITY – Qu 4.

Assessment of fetal well-being may involve consideration of lung maturity. The respiratory distress syndrome historically was a major cause of neonatal morbidity and mortality in diabetic pregnancies, with a six-fold higher incidence for any given gestational age, compared to non-diabetic pregnancies[64]. Its incidence has fallen dramatically in the last four decades, from 27% in the 1960s[171] to 2.4% in the 1980s[65], corresponding to the fall in elective premature delivery and in elective caesarean section rates, and the overall improvements in diabetic control.

The pathogenesis has been postulated to be due to poor diabetic control[66], or more specifically to fetal hyperinsulinaemia inhibiting the synthesis of the phospholipid component of surfactant[67], but this theory is not universally accepted[68]. When diabetes is well controlled, surfactant production is similar to that of non-diabetic pregnancies[69]. The reason for this high incidence is therefore unclear. It may in part be due to the high caesarean section rate which is associated with an increased incidence of the more benign component of the respiratory distress syndrome, transient tachypnoea of the newborn or 'wet lung' syndrome, rather than life-threatening hyaline membrane disease.

Previously amniocentesis was widely used to assess pulmonary maturity even though concerns existed that the lecithin : sphingomyelin ratio was less reliable in diabetes[70]. Today any indications for preterm delivery are usually sufficiently urgent to override concerns about lung immaturity and the assessment of test results. The use of dexamethasone to improve fetal lung maturity is debatable in diabetic pregnancy, as it usually has such a profoundly adverse influence on glycaemic control, for at least 48 h after the 12 h course. Careful consideration should be given before embarking on this course of treatment.

SUMMARY

Relatively little is known about the best way in which to monitor the well-being of the fetus in a diabetic pregnancy. The main concerns relate to late intrauterine death and either excessive or insufficient fetal growth or liquor. Regular, probably two-weekly ultrasound scans for fetal growth and liquor volume are useful additions to clinical assessment. There is no evidence that assessments of Doppler waveforms in the umbilical artery are valid, although they are frequently used. Cardiotocography does not seem to be predictive and fetal movements are too imprecise. Certainly glycaemic control should be optimal, and in cases where this has not been achieved and the consequent risk of intrauterine death is higher, careful consideration should be given to delivery, by the safest route, bearing in mind the possible risk of prematurity.

REFERENCES

1 Peel J, Oakley W. The management of pregnancy in diabetics. In: *Transactions of the 12th British Congress of Obstetrics and Gynaecology*. Royal College of Obstetricians and Gynaecologists, London, 1949; 161.
2 Beard RW, Lowy C. The British survey of diabetic pregnancies. *Br J Obstet Gynaecol* 1982; **89**: 783–6.

3 Barss VA. Obstetrical management. In: Hare JW (ed.), *Diabetes Complicating Pregnancy: The Joslin Clinic Method*. Liss, New York, 1989; 112.

4 Murphy J, Peters J, Morris P *et al.* Conservative management of pregnancy in diabetic women. *Br J Med* 1984; **288**: 1203–5.

5 Karlsson K, Kjellmer I. The outcome of diabetic pregnancies in relationship to the mothers' blood sugar level. *Am J Obstet Gynecol* 1972; **112**: 213–20.

6 Bradley RJ, Brudenell JM, Nicolaides KH. Fetal acidosis and hyperlacticaemia diagnosed by cordocentesis in pregnancies complicated by maternal diabetes mellitus. *Diabetic Med* 1991; **8**: 464–8.

7 Salafia CM. The fetal, placental, and neonatal pathology associated with maternal diabetes. In: Reece EA, Coustan DR (eds), *Diabetes Mellitus in Pregnancy: Principles and Practice*. Churchill Livingstone, Edinburgh, 1988; 143–204.

8 Myers RE. Brain damage due to asphyxia: mechanism of causation. *J Perinat Med* 1981; **9**: 78–86.

9 Philips AF, Dublin JW, Matty PJ, Raye JR. Arterial hypoxemia and hyperinsulinemia in the chronically hyperglycemic fetal lamb. *Pediatr Res* 1982; **16**: 653–8.

10 Milley JR, Papacostas JS. Effect of insulin on metabolism of fetal sheep hindquarters. *Diabetes* 1989; **38**: 597–603.

11 Fadel HE, Hammond SD, Huff TA, Harp RJ. Glycosylated hemoglobins in normal pregnancies and gestational diabetes mellitus. *Obstet Gynecol* 1979; **54**: 322–6.

12 Gillmer MDG, Beard RW. Fetal and placental function tests in diabetic pregnancy. In: Sutherland HW, Stowers JM (eds), *Carbohydrate Metabolism in Pregnancy and the Newborn*. Livingstone, Edinburgh, 1975; 168–94.

13 Barrett JM, Salyer SL, Boehm FH. The nonstress test: an evaluation of 1000 patients. *Am J Obstet Gynecol* 1981; **141**: 153–7.

14 Manning FA, Baskett TF, Morrison I, Lange IR. Fetal biophysical profile scoring: a prospective study in 1,184 high risk patients. *Am J Obstet Gynecol* 1981; **140**: 289–94.

15 Manning FA, Morrison I, Lange IR *et al.* Fetal assessment based on fetal biophysical profile scoring: experience in 12,620 referred high-risk pregnancies. *Am J Obstet Gynecol* 1985; **151**: 343–50.

16 Johnson JM, Lange IR, Harman CR *et al.* Biophysical profile scoring in the management of diabetic pregnancy. *Obstet Gynecol* 1988; **72**: 841–6.

17 Johnstone FD, Steel JM, Haddad NG *et al.* Doppler umbilical artery flow waveforms in diabetic pregnancy. *Br J Obstet Gynaecol* 1992; **99**: 135–40.

18 Hay WWJ. The role of placental–fetal interaction in fetal nutrition. *Semin Perinatol* 1991; **15**: 424–33.

19 Bradley RJ, Nicolaides KH, Brudenell JM. Are all infants of diabetic mothers 'macrosomic'? *Br Med J* 1988; **297**: 1583–5.

20 Cano A, Barcelo F, Fuente T *et al.* Relationship of maternal glycosylated hemoglobin and fetal beta-cell activity with birth weight. *Gynecol Obstet Invest* 1986; **22**: 91–6.

21 Metzger BE. Biphasic effect of maternal metabolism on fetal growth: quintessential expression of fuel-mediated teratogenesis. *Diabetes* 1991; **40** (Suppl. 2): 99–105.

22 Jovanovic-Peterson L, Peterson CM, Reed CF *et al.* Maternal postprandial glucose levels and infant birth weight: the Diabetes in early Pregnancy Study Group. *Am J Obstet Gynaecol* 1991; **164**: 103–11.

23 Reiher H, Fuhrmann K, Noack S *et al.* Age-dependent insulin secretion of the endocrine pancreas in vitro from fetuses of diabetic and non-diabetic patients. *Diabetes Care* 1983; **6**: 446–51.

24 Schwartz R, Gruppuso PA, Petzold K *et al.* Hyperinsulinemia and macrosomia in the fetus of the diabetic mother. *Diabetes Care* 1994; **17**: 640–8.

25 Gluckman PD. The endocrine role of fetal growth in late gestation: the role of insulin-like growth factors. *J Clin Endocrinol Metab* 1995; **80**: 1047–50.

26 Ramsay TG, Wolverton CK, Steele NC. Alteration in IGF-1 mRNA content of fetal swine tissues in response to maternal diabetes. *Am J Physiol* 1994; **267**: R1391–6.

27 Pederson D. *Hyperglycaemia–Hyperinsulinism Theory and Birthweight*. Williams & Wilkins, Baltimore, 1977; 211–20.

28 Schwartz R, Susa J. Fetal macrosomia: animal models. *Diabetes Care* 1980; **3**: 430–2.

29 Schwartz R. Hyperinsulinemia and macrosomia. *N Engl J Med* 1990; **323**: 340–2.

30 Philips AF, Rosenkrantz TS, Clark RM *et al.* Effects of fetal insulin deficiency on growth in fetal lambs. *Diabetes* 1991; **40**: 20–7.

31 Katz AI, Lindheimer MD, Mako ME, Rubenstein AH. Peripheral metabolism of insulin, proinsulin, and C-peptide in the pregnant rat. *J Clin Invest* 1975; **56**: 1608–14.

32 Sosenko IR, Kitzmiller JL, Loo SW *et al.* The infant of the diabetic mother: correlation of increased cord blood C-peptide levels with macrosomia and hypoglycemia. *N Engl J Med* 1979; **301**: 859–62.

33 Ogata ES, Freinkel N, Metzger BE *et al.* Perinatal islet function in gestational diabetes: assessment by cord plasma C-peptide and amniotic fluid insulin. *Diabetes Care* 1980; **3**: 425–9.

34 Persson B, Heding LG, Lunell NO *et al.* Fetal beta cell function in diabetic pregnancy: amniotic fluid concentrations of proinsulin, insulin, and C-peptide during the last trimester of pregnancy. *Am J Obstet Gynecol* 1982; **144**: 455–9.

35 Sosenko JM, Kitzmiller JL, Fluckiger R *et al.* Umbilical cord glycosylated hemoglobin in infants of diabetic mothers: relationships to neonatal hypoglycemia, macrosomia, serum C-peptide. *Diabetes Care* 1982; **5**: 566–70.

36 Lin C-C, Moawad MD, River P *et al.* Amniotic fluid C-peptide as an index for intrauterine fetal growth. *Am J Obstet Gynecol* 1981; **139**: 390–6.

37 Lin CC, River P, Blix PM *et al.* Prenatal assessment of fetal outcome by amniotic fluid C-peptide levels in pregnant women. *Am J Obstet Gynecol* 1981; **141**: 671–7.

38 Dornhorst A, Nicholls JSD, Ali K *et al.* Fetal proinsulin and birth weight. *Diabetic Med* 1993; **11**: 171–81.

39 Challier JC, Schneider H, Dancic J. In vitro perfusion of human placenta. V. Oxygen consumption. *Am J Obstet Gynecol* 1976; **126**: 261–5.

40 Altman DG, Coles EC. Nomograms for precise determination of birth weight for date. *Br J Obstet Gynaecol* 1980; **87** (New Series): 81–6.

41 Dornhorst A, Nicholls JSD, Welch A *et al.* Correcting for ethnicity when defining large-for-gestational-age infants in diabetic pregnancies. *Diabetic Med* 1996; **13**: 226–31.

42 Maresh M, Beard RW, Bray CS *et al.* Factors predisposing to and outcome of gestational diabetes. *Obstet Gynecol* 1989; **74**: 342–6.

43 Green JR, Schumacher LB, Pawson IG *et al.* Influence of maternal body habitus and glucose tolerance on birth weight of their infants. *Obstet Gynecol* 1991; **78**: 235–40.

44 Barker DJP, Winter PD, Osmond C *et al.* Weight in infancy and death from ischaemic heart disease. *Lancet* 1989; **ii**: 577–80.

45 Barker DJP. Fetal origins of coronary heart disease. *Br Heart J* 1993; **69**: 195–6.

46 Barker DJP, Hales CN, Fall CHD *et al.* Type 2 (non-insulin-dependent) diabetes mellitus, hypertension and hyperlipidaemia (syndrome X) In relation to reduced fetal growth. *Diabetologia* 1993; **36**: 62–7.

47 Barker DJP. Fetal origins of coronary heart disease. *Br Med J* 1995; **311**: 171–4.

48 Boyd ME, Usher RH, McLean FH. Fetal macrosomia: prediction, risk, proposed management. *Obstet Gynecol* 1983; **61**: 715–22.

49 Spellacy WN, Miller S, Winegar MPH, Peterson PQ. Macrosomia: maternal characteristics and infant complications. *Obstet Gynecol* 1985; **66**: 158–61.

50 Combs CA, Gunderson E, Kitzmiller JL *et al.* The relationship of fetal macrosomia to maternal postprandial glucose control during pregnancy. *Diabetes Care* 1992; **15**: 1251–7.

51 De Veciana M, Major CA, Morgan MA *et al.* Postprandial versus preprandial blood glucose monitoring in women with gestational diabetes mellitus requiring insulin therapy. *New Eng J Med* 1995; **533**: 1237–41.

52 deSwiet M. Medical disorders in pregnancy: diabetes, thyroid diseases and epilepsy. In: Chamberlain G (ed.), *Turnbull's Obstetrics*, 2nd edition. Churchill Livingstone, Edinburgh, 1995; 383–405.

53 Landon MB, Gabbe SG, Sachs L. Management of diabetes mellitus and pregnancy: a survey of obstetricians and maternal–fetal specialists. *Obstet Gynecol* 1990; **75**: 635–40.

54 Oats JN. Obstetrical management of patients with diabetes in pregnancy. *Baillieres Clin Obstet Gynaecol* 1991; **5**: 395–411.

55 Acker DB, Sachs BP, Friedman EA. Risk factors for shoulder dystocia. *Obstet Gynecol* 1985;

66: 762–8.

56 Kitzmiller JL, Mall JC, Gin GD *et al.* Measurement of fetal shoulder width with computed tomography in diabetic women. *Obstet Gynecol* 1987; **70**: 941–5.

57 McLaren RA, Puckett JL, Chauhan SP. Estimators of birth weight in pregnant women requiring insulin: a comparison of seven sonographic models. *Obstet Gynecol* 1995; **85**: 565–9.

58 Yasuhi I, Ishimaru T, Hirai M, Yamabe T. Hourly fetal urine production rate in the fasting and the postprandial state of normal and diabetic pregnant women. *Obstet Gynecol* 1994; **84**: 64–8.

59 Kucera J. Rate and type of congenital anomalies among offspring of diabetic women. *J Reprod Med* 1971; **7**: 61–70.

60 Mills JP, Simpson JL, Driscoll SG *et al.* Incidence of spontaneous abortion among normal women and IDDM women whose pregnancies were identified within 21 days of conception. *N Engl J Med* 1988; **319**: 1617–23.

61 Cousins L. Pregnancy complications among diabetic women: review 1965–1985. *Obstet Gynecol Survey* 1987; **42**: 140–9.

62 Lufkin EG, Nelson RL, Hill LM *et al.* An analysis of diabetic pregnancies at Mayo Clinic. *Diabetes Care* 1984; **7**: 539–47.

63 Rasmussen MJ, Firth R, Foley M, Stronge JM. The timing of delivery in diabetic pregnancy. *Aust NZ J Obstet Gynaecol* 1992; **32**: 313–17.

64 Robert MF, Neff RK, Hubbell JP *et al.* Association between maternal diabetes and respiratory distress syndrome in the newborn. *N Engl J Med* 1976; **294**: 357–60.

65 Hubbell JP, Muirhead DM, Drorbough JE. The newborn infant of the diabetic mother. *Med Clin North Am* 1965; **49**: 1035–52.

66 Drury MI, Stronge JM, Foley ME, MacDonald DW. Pregnancy in the diabetic patient: timing and mode of delivery. *Obstet Gynecol* 1983; **62**: 279–82.

67 Ylinen K. High maternal levels of hemoglobin Alc associated with delayed fetal lung maturation in insulin-dependent diabetic pregnancies. *Acta Obstet Gynecol Scand* 1987; **66**: 263–6.

68 Bourbon JR, Farrell PM. Fetal lung development in the diabetic pregnancy. *Pediatr Res* 1985; **19**: 253–67.

69 Fadel HE, Saad SA, Davis H, Nelson GH. Fetal lung maturity in diabetic pregnancies: relation among amniotic fluid insulin, prolactin, and lecithin. *Am J Obstet Gynecol* 1988; **159**: 457–63.

70 Dudley DK, Black DM. Reliability of lecithin/sphingomyelin ratio in diabetic pregnancy. *Obstet Gynecol* 1985; **66**: 521–4.

14

A Protocol for Diabetes in Pregnancy: The Practical Organization of a Regional Combined Obstetric/Diabetic Clinic

PAULINE WATT[1], JENNIFER HUGHES[2], ALYSON MOORE[1], ANTHONY I. TRAUB[1] and DAVID R. HADDEN[2]

[1]The Royal Maternity Hospital, Belfast, UK and
[2] Royal Victoria Hospital, Belfast UK

Readers of this book will be interested in the practicalities of providing special care for the high-risk diabetic pregnancy. This has been addressed in different ways in different places, and it is not possible to make specific guidelines that will be appropriate worldwide. More than 100 years ago, one of the first medical specialties to be recognized was the art of obstetrics, and the ability of the specialist obstetrician and midwife to focus on a particular situation such as diabetes in pregnancy undoubtedly established the initial interest in this subject. The more gradual development of the concept of a diabetes specialist following the discovery of insulin, often an internist or endocrinologist, brought the skills required for better control of blood glucose. More recently the recognition of the crucial roles of a trained diabetes nurse specialist, and of a midwife with special diabetes experience, has allowed their position to be better established. Dietetic advice in pregnancy has always been important, and the particular metabolic aspects of diabetic pregnancy require a nutritional knowledge of many aspects of insulin-dependent and non-insulin-dependent diabetes: an interested

Diabetes and Pregnancy: An International Approach to Diagnosis and Management.
Edited by A. Dornhorst and D. R. Hadden.
© 1996 John Wiley & Sons Ltd.

dietician is an important part of the team. The evolution of the concept of this team approach has taken time, and it is now necessary to establish the role of such a team in current practice protocols.

It is not the aim of this chapter to review the history of joint clinics, but it is appropriate to mention a few seminal names. Dr Jorgen Pedersen (internist) was soon joined by Dr Lars Molsted-Pedersen (obstetrician) in Copenhagen, and their combined experience over 50 years has set a standard for others to follow[1,2]. In Boston the pioneering work of Dr Eliot Joslin (internist) and Dr Priscilla White (paediatrician) at the Joslin Diabetes Clinic and the New England Deaconess Hospital established a core of interest in the USA[3]. At about the same time Dr Wilfred Oakley (physician) and Dr (later Sir) John Peel at King's College Hospital in London continued the pioneering diabetes service first established there by Dr Robin Laurence, himself a diabetic whose life was saved by the discovery of insulin in 1921[4].

The actual concept of a joint clinic to facilitate the better care of the mother without her having to attend separate offices on different days came somewhat gradually, and there are several well-remembered pairs of obstetrician and diabetologist in a number of places: Harley and Montgomery in Belfast[5], Sutherland and Stowers in Aberdeen[6,7], Peterson and Jovanovic in New York and subsequently California[8]. There are also a number of well-known places where the concept of a joint clinic has evolved, but under the aegis of one or other specialist depending on circumstances. Coustan in Rhode Island[9], Gabbe in Ohio, Weiss in Austria[10], Beard at St Mary's Hospital, London, and Gillmer in Oxford are all obstetricians. Drury in Dublin, Freinkel and Metzger in Chicago, Jervell in Oslo, Hollingsworth in California[11] and many others have practised or still practise as diabetes specialists or internists; Persson in Stockholm focuses on the problem from a paediatric viewpoint. There are many other centres that have developed the team concept. Basic scientific work, for example, in Belgium by a number of colleagues over the years (Hoet, Van Assche, Gepts, de Hertogh and others), and in Uppsala, Sweden (Hellerstrom, Eriksson) has served as another point of entry into the team approach. We have referenced only a number of books which will serve as introductions to the published work of these teams.

In Australia, Japan and the Far East, in India, in Middle Eastern and Mediterranean countries, in the West Indies, in Africa, in South America, and under some difficulties in the former USSR, in all these countries there have been groups dedicated to providing better care on a joint basis for diabetic pregnancy. Each and every one of these places will have identified particular ways of providing the joint service—this chapter offers a view of a single situation for purposes of comparison.

A PROTOCOL FOR A COMBINED CLINIC

This scheme represents the present practice at the combined diabetes/endocrine antenatal clinic, and the delivery and postnatal arrangements for diabetic mothers, at one regional centre in the UK National Health Service. This protocol is used for 40–50 diabetic pregnancies annually, representing about half of those in the region. The Royal Maternity Hospital, Belfast, is responsible for about 3000 pregnancies in total out of about 28 000 annually in Northern Ireland, where the overall population has been stable at 1 500 000 persons for several decades. The prevalence of known cases of insulin-dependent diabetes in Northern Ireland is about 8000 and of non-insulin-dependent diabetes about 30 000 by estimate, although there is no regional register. Accurate figures are available for newly diagnosed insulin-dependent diabetes in Northern Ireland for the years 1988–1994 when on average 70 new cases were diagnosed annually in the age group 0–16 years[12]. This places Northern Ireland at the upper end of the frequency distribution of insulin-dependent diabetes incidence in Europe. Screening for unrecognized hyperglycaemia in pregnancy has been carefully carried out over the past 30 years at the Royal Maternity Hospital and the incidence of newly diagnosed impaired glucose tolerance, or diabetes (75 g oral glucose tolerance test—World Health Organization criteria) persistently has been very low in pregnancy. This may represent in part an efficient recognition process by the primary care family doctors prior to pregnancy, but must also recognize the relatively late age of onset of non-insulin-dependent diabetes in Northern Ireland, in general well past the childbearing years. In most developing countries this condition has an earlier onset, and their prevalence of true gestational diabetes is much greater.

The recent changes in health care provision which are worldwide, and often financially driven, have also affected our combined clinical activities. There has not been any significant amount of diabetes-related private practice, either obstetrically or for diabetes care in this hospital for many years, and the clinic has been attended regularly by the senior consultant obstetrician and the senior diabetologist, in conjunction with the junior obstetric and diabetes medical staff. This has led to a close relationship between the pregnant mother and the team, which is often maintained for several pregnancies, and for subsequent long-term diabetes review at the Royal Victoria Hospital Diabetes Clinic.

It is clear that this protocol will not be appropriate in many other countries, but it should be of interest for purposes of comparison[2,13]. The combined antenatal diabetes clinic has been held in the usual maternity hospital antenatal area; initially separate consulting rooms were not available but with new buildings these facilities now exist. The clinic is held at the same time as other specialist clinics, but maintains a momentum of its own, due to the enthusiasm of all members of nursing, midwifery and medical staff, and especially that of the mothers. In an increasingly cost-conscious economy it will be necessary to prove the efficiency of such joint clinics, as they tend to run across the established contracting processes for a purchaser/provider-driven market. We have established the benefit of such a combined clinic in our regional environment[14], and we have no doubt that such a service will continue[15]. There is considerable opportunity for individual local management schemes, such as early-morning or late-evening clinics to facilitate the working mother, and special arrangements for fathers and for care for other children. The growing concept of shared care between family doctor and maternity hospital will need a carefully agreed protocol for successful partnership amongst all the health care professionals involved; in general as diabetic pregnancy is still a high-risk situation, the responsibility should remain that of the combined hospital clinic. If it is not possible to organize a combined clinic then extra care is necessary by each party to the pregnancy to ensure proper communication before, during and after the event for the ultimate benefit of the mother and baby[16].

SCREENING

Screening for the onset of hyperglycaemia in pregnancy is carried out on all pregnant women attending this hospital (Box 14.1). This is an unusual occurrence in this obstetric environment. When hyperglycaemia is detected for the first time in pregnancy, and confirmed by a 75 g oral glucose tolerance test, the woman will be asked to attend the combined antenatal/diabetic clinic and appropriate management with diet or insulin instituted.

PRE-PREGNANCY COUNSELLING

This important function is usually undertaken by the diabetes team at the routine diabetic clinic. A special leaflet is available and will be discussed with all patients at risk of pregnancy. Further special pre-pregnancy discussion will be necessary with the obstetrician and midwife in certain cases, particularly where there are serious maternal diabetic complications such as advanced kidney or eye disease. The specialist midwife will also be able to counsel diabetic mothers as the pregnancy progresses, and in relation to possible future pregnancies.

THE DIABETIC WOMAN'S FIRST ANTENATAL VISIT TO THE COMBINED CLINIC

The woman and her partner are welcomed by the midwife-in-charge. She will introduce them to her named midwife, who will follow her progress and provide her care throughout the pregnancy, delivery and postnatal period in hospital. Team midwifery is practised in this hospital and the named

BOX 14.1. Screening for hyperglycaemia in pregnancy: protocol at the Royal Maternity Hospital, Belfast

1. *Urine test for glucose* (and protein) at every antenatal visit. If glycosuria present, consider blood glucose at any time.
2. *Random, untimed blood glucose:* at first booking, at any other time if desired and at 28 weeks.
   (a) Capillary—self-monitoring strip or micro-cuvette.
   (b) Venous plasma laboratory glucose.
3. If blood glucose at any time is > 6.6 mmol/l (120 mg/dl), to have *standard breakfast meal test* (fasting)—40 g CHO as normal breakfast (two rounds toast, portion fruit)—laboratory or micro-cuvette, plasma glucose at 0 and 2 h.
4. If fasting plasma glucose at standard breakfast meal test is > 6.6 mmol/l (120 mg/dl) and/or 2 h plasma glucose > 8.0 mmol/l (144 mg/dl) to have *75 g oral glucose tolerance test.* If 2 h plasma glucose > 9.0 mmol/l (160 mg/dl) the diagnosis of hyperglycaemia in pregnancy is made and treatment with insulin considered. (A full oral glucose tolerance test has venous plasma glucose at 0, 30, 60, 90, 120 min: a minimal oral glucose tolerance test has only the fasting and 120 min samples.)
5. Treatment with insulin is usually necessary when random plasma glucose is persistently above 8.0 mmol/l (144 mg/dl), when the breakfast tolerance test shows 2 h venous plasma glucose > 8.0 mmol/l (144 mg/dl), and/or when the 75 g oral glucose tolerance test shows a 2 h plasma glucose > 9.0 mmol/l (160 mg/dl). Prior to starting insulin, assessment by a dietician and advice on sensible eating patterns are necessary. If blood glucose is above 11.0 mmol/l (200 mg/dl) at any time, the diagnosis of diabetes is established and insulin must be seriously considered.
6. Mothers diagnosed as having hyperglycaemia in pregnancy may have subsequent insulin-dependent diabetes or non-insulin-dependent diabetes. Postpartum review is necessary and subsequent measurement of urine glucose and capillary blood glucose at six weeks. Non-pregnant criteria for diagnosis of diabetes mellitus would then apply.

midwife is part of the team. If the named midwife is not on duty when the woman is at hospital, then her team colleague will carry on her care.

Many insulin-dependent diabetic women attend as early as five to six weeks amenorrhoea, when a vaginal ultrasonic scan is carried out to ensure the presence of an ongoing intrauterine pregnancy. A repeat ultrasound scan may be necessary a week later. Such an early visit to the antenatal clinic is very beneficial, as it provides an opportunity for the woman to be seen by the diabetic team to discuss blood glucose control and monitoring.

ANTENATAL BOOKING PROCEDURE

Once an ongoing pregnancy has been confirmed, the woman's named midwife explains the clinical procedures, her role and the role of each member of the team. The midwife interviews the woman in the booking room where her relevant medical, obstetric, family history and present pregnancy details are recorded. The history printout from the computer is filed in her antenatal chart.

The midwife also documents the woman's weight, height, blood pressure and urinalysis. A mid-stream specimen of urine is sent for culture and a sample of blood obtained for routine antenatal investigations, including haemoglobin A_{1c} (HbA$_{1c}$). The obstetrician will then review the woman's booking history and carry out a general physical examination. An outline of the plan for her antenatal care is discussed (Box 14.2). As this is a regional clinic, consideration is taken of the distance the woman lives from the hospital and whether or not she has ready access to transport.

BOX 14.2. Patient handout: protocol for diabetic mothers attending the joint antenatal clinic

'This is a joint clinic so that you can be seen by both the diabetic team and the obstetrician on the same afternoon.

On the booking day you will be seen in detail by the midwife who will complete all the computer details and take blood tests as needed. After this is completed and the metabolic blood tests are measured you will be seen by the metabolic nurse who will give the diabetic mothers the blood test recording book and discuss the clinic arrangements.

On a usual day you should check in with both the obstetric receptionist and the diabetes receptionist. The diabetes staff nurse will then see you and take your blood tests (blood glucose and HbA$_{1c}$). It is necessary to wait about 20–30 minutes for the results of these tests to be telephoned back from the laboratory. You will use this time to see the dietician, and to learn any new developments regarding your diabetes. When the blood result is returned, you will see the metabolic doctor. You may or may not need another test after this.

You will then be seen by the obstetric doctor. Following this you should book you next appointment with the obstetrical receptionist.

During *admission* and *delivery* you will be seen daily by the diabetes doctor on call who will keep in close touch with your treatment. You should also be referred to the dietician.

At the six-week postnatal visit you will have the usual blood tests and be seen by the diabetes doctor before you see the obstetrician. Following the postnatal appointment, arrangements are made for a review appointment at your usual diabetic clinic.'

She will then see the diabetes specialist nurse, who ensures the woman has a suitable blood glucose meter and knows how to use it correctly. If the woman does not have one then she will be lent one for the duration of the pregnancy and puerperium (Figure 14.1).

The woman then meets the diabetic specialist who will discuss her blood glucose control and management. If blood glucose control is good, then the woman will not need admission to hospital for stabilization. She will be

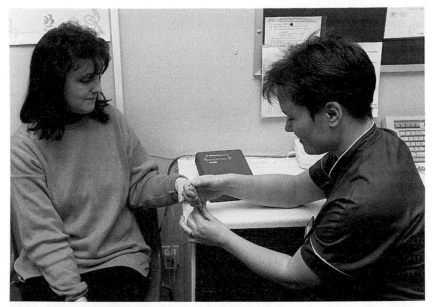

Figure 14.1. The diabetes nurse specialist instructing the mother in blood glucose monitoring

given the Royal Maternity Hospital Diabetes Pregnancy Booklet to take home with her to record her capillary blood glucose readings before and after each meal, and the physician will write the usual dose of insulin that the woman requires at the top of the page.

The dietician will also see the woman to discuss and promote healthy eating and good diet control, and to sort out any worries about her diet. An eating plan is given to the woman to take home.

Before leaving the clinic, the woman is given the opportunity to meet the parentcraft midwife, who will give her information books and leaflets on various aspects of pregnancy, inform her of the hospital parentcraft classes, and the concept of a birth plan is also raised. The date of the next clinic appointment is confirmed. In general, she will be seen by the obstetrician and the diabetes specialist at each visit, although in cases where there is difficulty with control of blood glucose a visit to the diabetes specialist alone may need to be more frequent.

SUBSEQUENT ANTENATAL VISITS

At each antenatal review visit the woman first sees the diabetic specialist nurse who will take a venous blood sample for HbA$_{1c}$ and blood sugar estimation. At this clinic both these results are available within 20 min. She is then seen by the midwife or obstetrician for routine antenatal examination, including urinalysis and blood pressure measurement.

At each visit an ultrasound scan is performed by the obstetric team with a view to assessing fetal well-being and to allow early detection of polyhydramnios (Figure 14.2). The visit to the diabetes specialist follows and she may also see the dietician at any visit, or on request throughout the pregnancy.

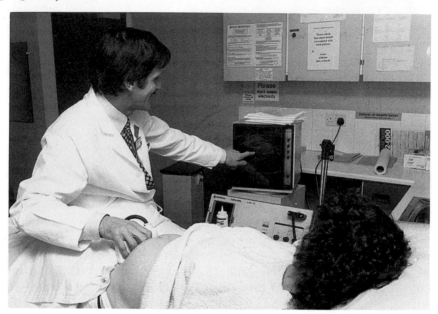

Figure 14.2. The obstetrician explaining the ultrasound examination

All women have an ultrasound scan at approximately 18–20 weeks gestation carried out by a radiographer. This is aimed at studying the fetus to confirm the dates and exclude as far as possible any obvious structural anomalies. The midwife-in-charge of the fetal assessment clinic is available at the time of the antenatal clinic to perform any extensive fetal assessment tests that may be necessary, such as cardiotocography or ultrasound scan of the fetal artery umbilical blood flow. The findings would then be discussed with the obstetrician and further management decided.

The parentcraft midwife will meet the couple again at the 26-week visit to arrange the parentcraft classes, if this is the woman's wish. She is also available at each visit for any questions the woman may want to discuss.

DELIVERY

The woman's delivery is normally planned for term but this is dependent on the blood glucose control and fetal and maternal well-being. The decision regarding the mode of delivery is made following a full assessment by the obstetrician at the antenatal clinic. Induction of labour is either by use of prostaglandin gel or Syntocinon infusion. If there are any perceived obstetric problems, the decision may be for an elective caesarean section.

The woman will be admitted to hospital the day before delivery. When admitted, the woman will be cared for by her 'named midwife'. If she is not on duty then another midwife in her team will continue her care. The woman will be visited in the ward by the metabolic registrar and diabetic management organized and an individual dose of insulin ordered.

Regardless of the mode of delivery the woman will be requested not to eat from 10.00 p.m., prior to which she will be given a light supper. If the blood glucose levels have been unstable, the midwife may wake the woman around 2.00 a.m. to check a capillary blood glucose to ascertain if she is becoming hypoglycaemic. If this is diagnosed, intravenous fluids with insulin will be erected. At approximately 7.00 a.m. a capillary blood glucose reading will be taken and a fasting blood glucose sample sent to the laboratory for confirmation (Box 14.3: see also pages 130 and 300).

When the woman is transferred to the delivery suite or theatre, if not previously erected, an intravenous infusion will be connected with 5% dextrose and insulin. If a Syntocinon infusion is required, the drug is added to normal saline solution and given through a second intravenous infusion. All intravenous infusions are monitored by use of infusion pumps. When an amniotomy is performed, the woman is given tea and toast with short-acting insulin given subcutaneously. Throughout labour, blood glucose readings are monitored hourly and closely observed by midwifery and obstetric staff. The diabetic team may be contacted at any time.

The diabetic woman, as is the case for any woman admitted for induction of labour, will have fetal monitoring throughout labour to observe the fetal heart and uterine activity. She may, in early labour, sit in an obstetric chair, whilst being continuously monitored. Regular maternal and fetal observations are recorded on the partograph. Vaginal examination is carried out four-hourly.

Antenatally the woman may have written a birth plan. The midwife will respect the woman's wishes regarding her care and should her condition change due to maternal or fetal complications, then the woman is kept fully informed. Methods of analgesia are discussed and she will be given a choice. An epidural anaesthetic is available for any woman who wishes it. The midwife will remain with the woman throughout labour on a one-to-one basis, and if the labour continues uncomplicated she will also deliver the woman. If any complication of labour does occur then the obstetrician will carry out the delivery.

A paediatrician will be present for the delivery. A sample of cord blood is sent to the laboratory to obtain the infant's blood glucose level. Heel prick capillary blood glucose (glucose oxidase strip or preferably the Haemocue technique, which is more accurate at low glucose levels) readings are taken

BOX 14.3. Management of diabetes in labour: a labour ward guide

Blood glucose should be 3–6 mmol/l before and during delivery. Ensure that self-monitoring meters are accurately calibrated, and if in doubt get a laboratory check.

Spontaneous labour

It is not necessary for the mother to take her full regular diet and insulin dose while in labour. Light food and fluids are prescribed: maintain capillary blood glucose 3–6 mmol/l, hourly measurement. Usually a 5% dextrose infusion is erected in the labour ward and the insulin dose adjusted as below: this is kept running until the mother is able to eat light meals and return to her pre-pregnancy insulin regimen.

Induction of labour

Either by oxytocin infusion or prostaglandin pessary in early morning. Give usual doses of insulin the day before but omit the late evening long-acting insulin for those on four daily injections. No morning breakfast or insulin in antenatal ward. Measure capillary blood glucose hourly from 6.00 a.m.

In labour ward 5% dextrose infusion with insulin as below. A light breakfast meal may be given as well if trial of labour is unsuccessful.

Elective caesarean section

Give usual doses of insulin the day before, but omit any late evening long-acting insulin. No morning breakfast or insulin in antenatal ward. Measure capillary blood glucose hourly from 6.00 a.m.

In labour ward 5% dextrose infusion with insulin throughout procedure.

5% dextrose and insulin guidelines in labour ward

Capillary blood glucose (mmol/l)	Infusion 5% dextrose	Insulin (short-acting) added to each 500 ml	Time for 500 ml infusion	Drops per minute	Supplementary subcutaneous short-acting insulin every 6 h
<2.0	500 ml	0	2 h	84	0
2.0–3.9	500 ml	0	6 h	28	0
4.0–7.9	500 ml	6 U	6 h	28	0
8.0–11.9	500 ml	6 U	6 h	28	6 U
12.0–15.9	500 ml	6 U	6 h	28	10 U
16.0 plus	Contact diabetes staff				

Post partum

On first day give approximately half of normal pre-pregnancy dose and light meals. Mother's blood glucose in range 6–8 mmol/l before meals.

Breastfeeding

Dietician to arrange to increase mother's diet. Insulin dose not to be increased and may need to be decreased. Mother's food always before breastfeeding to avoid risk of maternal hypoglycaemia if baby is slow to feed.

from the infant at 30 min intervals for 2 h, and thereafter three-hourly for 24 h. The infant is breast or bottle fed within 1 h of birth and if the capillary glucose level is above 1.5 mmol/l (27 mg/dl), every 2–3 h subsequently. If the capillary blood glucose is 1.5 mmol/l (27 mg/dl) or lower an extra feed is given immediately and a repeat measurement taken 30–60 min later. If the capillary blood glucose is 1.1 mmol/l (20 mg/dl) or less and/or the baby has symptomatic hypoglycaemia, then the paediatrician is informed and the baby fed immediately. A capillary blood glucose sample is sent to the laboratory. Occasionally the infant may need to be transferred to the 'special care baby unit' for intravenous dextrose and stabilization. The low-risk infant of a diabetic mother remains with her and if all is well both are transferred back to the maternity ward 2 h after birth.

POSTNATAL CARE

The woman's capillary blood glucose readings continue to be observed and, depending on the method of delivery, intravenous fluids are continued until normal eating has resumed. At this stage capillary blood glucose is checked before and after each meal, and insulin requirements adjusted by the diabetic team. The named midwife plans the postnatal care with the woman, who is assisted with the care of her baby. Parentcraft education continues each day to enable the woman to become confident with feeding and caring for her baby. The physiotherapist calls to the ward daily and encourages her to practise postnatal exercises. Her time spent in hospital depends on her own and the baby's health, and her diabetic restabilization. Nowadays the woman is usually home as quickly as any other non-diabetic woman. The diabetic woman can also successfully breastfeed her baby and the dietician will increase her dietary intake to compensate for this.

Prior to discharge the paediatrician will examine the baby. The midwife evaluates her care with the woman and contraceptive advice is offered. The midwife completes a discharge form on computer that provides the community midwife and health visitor with information on the woman's delivery, medical condition and both her and the baby's care. The woman is given this information to give to the community midwife who visits her at home the next day. She is also given a six-week postnatal review appointment for the hospital clinic, where she is seen by the obstetrician, diabetic physician and dietician, to ensure her diabetes and physical condition have returned to pre-pregnancy levels, and this also enables her to discuss any questions she may have.

REFERENCES

1 Pedersen J *The Pregnant Diabetic and her Newborn: Problems and Management*, 2nd edn. Munksgaard, Copenhagen, 1977; 280.
2 Molsted-Pedersen L, Damm P. How to organise care for pregnant diabetic patients. In:

Mogensen CE, Strandl E (eds), *Concepts for the Ideal Diabetes Clinic*. de Gruyter, Berlin, 1993; 199–214.

3 Hare JW (ed.). *Diabetes Complicating Pregnancy: The Joslin Clinic Method*. Liss, New York, 1989; 194.

4 Brudenell M, Doddridge MC. *Diabetic Pregnancy*. Churchill Livingstone, Edinburgh, 1989; 152.

5 Harley JMG, Montgomery DAD. Management of pregnancy complicated by diabetes. *Br Med J* 1965; i: 14–16.

6 Sutherland HW, Stowers JM (eds). *Carbohydrate Metabolism in Pregnancy and the Newborn*. Churchill Livingstone, Edinburgh, 1975; 252.

7 Sutherland HW, Stowers JM, Pearson DWM (eds). *Carbohydrate Metabolism in Pregnancy and the Newborn*, Vol. IV. Springer-Verlag, London, 1989; 377.

8 Jovanovic L (ed.). *Controversies in Diabetes and Pregnancy*. Springer-Verlag, New York, 1988; 205.

9 Reece EA, Coustan DR (eds). *Diabetes Mellitus in Pregnancy: Principles and Practice*. Churchill Livingstone, Edinburgh, 1988; 545.

10 Weiss PAM, Coustan DR (eds). *Gestational Diabetes*. Springer-Verlag, Vienna, 1988; 240.

11 Hollingsworth DR. *Pregnancy, Diabetes and Birth: A Management Guide*, 2nd edn. Williams & Wilkins, Baltimore, 1992; 288.

12 Green A, Gale EAM, Patterson CC. Incidence of childhood onset insulin dependent diabetes mellitus: the Eurodiab ACE study. *Lancet* 1992; **339**: 905–9.

13 Tattersall RB, Gale EAM. Pregnancy and genetic counselling. In: Tattersall RB, Gale EAM (eds), *Diabetes: Clinical Management*. Churchill Livingstone, Edinburgh, 1990; 156–69.

14 Traub AI, Harley JMG, Cooper TK *et al*. Is centralized hospital care necessary for all insulin dependent pregnant diabetics? *Br J Obstet Gynaecol* 1987; **94**: 957–62.

15 Hadden DR. Medical management of diabetes in pregnancy. *Ballieres Clin Obstet Gynaecol* 1991; **5**: 369–94.

16 Hadden DR. The medical management of diabetes in pregnancy. *Postgrad Med J* 1996 (in press).

15

Addressing the Needs of the Inner City Clinics

JENNY WOOTTON[1] and JOANNA C. GIRLING[2]
[1]Central Middlesex Hospital, London, UK and
[2]Hammersmith Hospital, London, UK

SOCIAL AND CULTURAL ASPECTS OF DIABETIC PREGNANCY

The incidence of diabetes in pregnancy and its impact on a woman are dependent on a wide range of sociological factors, some of which will be discussed in this chapter. However, generalizations relating to any individual factor may be misleading or inappropriate. It is simplistic to assume that all women of one ethnic origin or social situation have the same problems or require the same support. Thus the influence of ethnicity, for example, is affected by family support, place of birth, degree of adoption of Western lifestyle and fluency in English. The extended family may be responsible for shopping and cooking such that it is difficult to adhere to the diabetic diet; religious beliefs may render screening for lethal congenital abnormalities less important if termination of pregnancy is not an option; language difference may make communication difficult, and this may be only partially overcome by the use of a translator.

Women who develop gestational diabetes tend to be older, more obese and of higher parity and these factors may interact with social and cultural factors, and thereby influence both obstetric and diabetic risk factors and management.

Diabetes and Pregnancy: An International Approach to Diagnosis and Management.
Edited by A. Dornhorst and D. R. Hadden.
© 1996 John Wiley & Sons Ltd.

ETHNICITY AND DEPRIVATION IN THE UK

Britain has had an ethnic minority population for many years. In the 1950s, there was considerable immigration from the West Indies in response to post-war labour shortages. This was followed in the 1960s and 1970s by immigrants from India, Pakistan and Balgladesh, and in the 1970s many Asian people came from East Africa. Recent arrivals include refugees and asylum seekers from Vietnam, Sri Lanka, Somalia, Turkey, the Middle East and the former Yugoslavia.

The 1991 census[1] was the first to record the ethnic origin of all residents in the UK, and included place of birth and place of residence. This showed (Table 15.1) that half of all non-Caucasian people living in England were born here, being second- and third-generation descendants of families who themselves had immigrated since the 1950s. The majority of people of ethnic minority origin (97%) live in England, and many of these (45%) live in the Greater London area. Two per cent live in Scotland, mainly in Edinburgh, Glasgow and Aberdeen, and 1.4% live in Wales, principally in Cardiff and Newport. In some parts of Britain, people of so-called ethnic minority origin in fact form a major part of the population (Table 15.2). However, in such areas it is likely that the population will comprise individuals of many different cultural backgrounds, requiring the health care teams to have a broad understanding of varying needs. Each ethnic group has its own language, traditions, religious customs, dietary habits and associated tendency to diabetes and other health problems.

Table 15.1. Ethnic minority population in Britain (1991 census)

	Population	% of total population	% born in the UK
	54 888 844	100.0	93.0
White	51 874 000	94.5	95.9
All ethnic minorities	3 015 050	5.5	47.0

Table 15.2. Ethnic minorities as percentage of total population in 15 local authorities in England

Brent	44.9	Slough	27.7
Newham	42.4	Harrow	26.3
Tower Hamlets	35.4	Waltham Forest	25.6
Hackney	33.7	Southwark	24.4
Ealing	32.4	Hounslow	24.3
Lambeth	30.1	Lewisham	22.0
Haringey	29.0	Birmingham	21.5
Leicester	28.5		

Studies have shown that women from ethnic minority groups have a significantly increased risk of gestational diabetes compared to white women[2,3]. Dornhorst[2] demonstrated, following adjustment for age, obesity and parity, that this risk of gestational diabetes ranged from a three-fold increase in black women to an 11-fold increase in Asian women compared to Caucasian women. She found that this influence of ethnic origin was independent of and much greater than the effects of increasing age or body mass index. In addition, a woman's cultural, religious, personal and social background may influence how she manages the restrictions imposed by a diabetic pregnancy.

The problems associated with living in an 'inner city' area are similar throughout the country, and include poor housing, perhaps in high-rise flats, unsupported mothers often only just beyond childhood themselves, unemployment and low educational achievements. This may be compounded by either insufficient health care provisions or inability to access them properly. These factors alone may be sufficient to influence a woman's ability to cope with the restrictions of a diabetic pregnancy. For economic and social reasons, inner city populations often have a high proportion of people from the so-called ethnic minorities, who migrate towards areas where housing and employment opportunities are perceived to be more densely concentrated. Individuals from ethnic minority groups living in the inner city may be even less able to adapt to the demands of a diabetic pregnancy, due to the stress this places on their cultural beliefs.

Personal and financial circumstances, as well as cultural factors, can influence a woman's acceptance, understanding or compliance with the restrictions imposed by a diabetic pregnancy. It is in appreciating the customs and needs of women belonging to a social class or ethnic group different from that of the health care worker that there is the greatest need for sensitivity.

Our experience is in the London Borough of Brent, which has the largest ethnic population in the UK. In total 45% of the population is non-white. These people come from a wide range of ethnic groups, speaking a large number of different languages and following many different religions. Brent has the eighth largest population of all the London boroughs with the highest residential density in outer London.

The antenatal clinic at the Central Middlesex Hospital serves a large part of the Borough of Brent. The population attending it reflects the ethnic mix of the area. In 1992, 2150 women were delivered at the hospital, of whom 38% were European, 26% were Asian (Indian subcontinent) and 13% Afro-Caribbean. The prevalence of gestational diabetes was 3%, 8% and 5% respectively in these ethnic groups. These categorizations by ethnic group are obviously a gross simplification, and the needs of each woman should be determined on an individual basis. It is important for all staff to understand the implications of a woman's beliefs for her understanding and acceptance of medical and obstetric advice. This applies particularly to language, diet and religious beliefs, which are discussed later.

Deprivation is used as an indicator of the lack of basic requirements for daily living, such as employment, adequate income and decent housing. Following the 1991 census, a number of statistical studies have been carried out to measure the extent of deprivation in Brent, including the Jarman score[4]. This is widely recognized as a way of measuring the extent of deprivation in an area, and is used to determine environmental, social and economic factors, and health care needs. The 1991 census data used in the score include population density, lone pensioners, children under five years, lone parent households, unskilled workers, overcrowding, ethnicity, population migration and unemployment rate.

Jarman scores for Brent show that about a third of the borough's wards are underprivileged areas with high health care needs. These are all situated in the south of the borough. Since the 1981 census the Jarman score has increased, reflecting a sharp rise in deprivation compared to other local authorities. Further, a distinct pattern of ethnicity appears, with the southern wards having the highest proportion of black residents and the north of the Borough having a high proportion of the Asian households.

Low income is an obvious cause of poverty. The London Area Transport Survey[5] showed that around a third of Brent households have a gross income less than £200 a week, which is below the average for Greater London. Social security benefits are paid to people whose income is deemed insufficient to meet their needs and entitlement to these benefits is a reliable indicator of the poverty levels within an area. Nearly one in six (16%) of the total adult population of Brent claim income support, and 20% of these are single parents. Over the past 10 years there has been a large increase, from 2840 in 1981 to 5460 in 1991, in the number of households in Brent in which children are looked after by a single parent. This also varies according to cultural beliefs (Table 15.3) and may influence a woman's attitude towards diabetes in pregnancy.

Table 15.3. Household composition of lone parents (%)

Total	White	Black Caribbean	Black African	Black other	Indian	Pakistani	Bangladeshi	Chinese	Other Asian	Other
6.5	4.2	18.2	17.0	28.4	2.4	4.0	3.4	4.0	3.9	9.7

LANGUAGE

The majority of young Asian and Afro-Caribbean women are second or third generation and have no language problems. However, many of the older women and new immigrants need the assistance of an interpreter. Some women, particularly from the Asian subcontinent, may be too shy to express their beliefs, or openly to decline advice which they find unacceptable, even if they have sufficient English to do so, but also if they are dependent on a translator. Effective care cannot be achieved unless there is good communication, with mutual understanding of language.

A family member or friend is often asked to translate. Despite some advantages, this may result in embarrassment on the behalf of the translator or the patient, and therefore answers may be of dubious reliability. The attitudes of the interpreter may influence the translation, and frequently only 'selected highlights' are conveyed to the woman; they may be too self-conscious to tell the health worker that the advice is inappropriate. The use of an impartial, trained interpreter eliminates this problem, but still is not easy. It is important that the interpreter is familiar with the appropriate culture and that there is good feedback to ensure that the information is understood. Consultation through an interpreter may take two to three times as long as 'direct' interviews. In the Borough of Brent there is a large interpreting service which covers over 30 languages. When possible the same interpreter attends each outpatient appointment with an individual woman with diabetes in pregnancy, thus enabling good rapport.

In other areas of London where there are many women speaking a single non-English language, trained 'link persons' have been used, such as Tower Hamlets where 22.9% of a population of 161 064 are from Bangladesh. Parsons[6] describes a similar scheme in Hackney where the 'health advocate' both interprets language and provides support throughout the pregnancy, mediating between the professionals and the patient, and providing a degree of continuity. However, these schemes are expensive, and future financial restraints may curtail their availability.

FOOD AND POVERTY

Poorer people pay a larger proportion, although smaller absolute amount, of their income on food, than do wealthier people[7]. Typically an adult on income support can afford about £10–12 a week on food. The cost of 'healthy' food is much higher than that of 'less healthy' food, and therefore poorer people tend to have a diet which is cheap and filling, but unnutritious. It is inclined to have a high sugar and fat content, and to be low in vitamins and fibre. The consumption of fruit and vegetables is also much lower, for the same reason. Food may also be relatively more expensive if access to transport, such as a car, is limited, and local shops are relied upon rather than larger but less expensive supermarkets.

Thus, in Brent, women on a low income have an increased risk of gestational diabetes not only because of their inherent ethnic tendencies towards the condition, but also because of obesity due to their poor diet. Ironically, they are the least likely to be able to afford the dietary adjustments recommended. Special payment of a dietary allowance to meet medically indicated food requirements was abolished in 1988, and since then Social Security payments have not explicitly included a costing for food.

RELIGION, ETHNICITY AND DIET

The relationship between ethnicity, religion and food is complex. Health care workers should be aware of a woman's religion so that advice, both dietary and obstetric, may be given accordingly.

Many religions have food taboos, periods of fasting and other rituals which may have a bearing on the treatment of diabetes. However, there is no evidence that any specific aspects of traditional diets are responsible for the high incidence of diabetes in women from ethnic minority groups. Further, Westernized 'fast food', high-sugar fizzy drinks and lack of traditional ingredients are increasingly influencing the diets of the young from all ethnic groups. It is important that the dietary advice given to pregnant women not only meets the requirements of their glycaemic control, but also that it is acceptable, affordable and available. An understanding of the implications of their religious beliefs in this respect is important.

A knowledge of the six main religions in this part of the world—Christianity, Hinduism, Islam, Sikhism, Buddhism and Judaism—is helpful when providing antenatal care to a multi-ethnic population. It is not possible here to give a detailed and accurate profile of the diet of each of the different ethnic and religious groups, not least because many of the religions are subdivided and the types of foods eaten may depend on this and on the food available in the original homeland. The availability and cost of traditional foods in the local shops will also have an important influence. In extended families, the older women may prepare and cook the food for everyone, making it more difficult to undertake the changes necessary for a diabetic diet. It is therefore helpful if the family member who does the cooking is seen and advised by a dietician. For those who read, explanatory sheets in the appropriate language may be a useful adjunct. Younger women living in smaller family groups are more likely to have moved towards a more Western style diet, at least in part because traditional food often takes longer to prepare, a feature which is not easily compatible with full-time employment.

CHRISTIANITY

The majority of people of Caucasian and Afro-Caribbean origin in the UK are Christian and in most cases their diets are free from religious influences. However, there are many different denominations within the Christian faith, including Church of England, Roman Catholic, Methodist, Baptist, Seventh Day Adventist, Pentecostal, Jehovah's Witness, Church of God and Rastafarian.

Seventh Day Adventists do not eat pork and pork products or fish without scales, and do not drink anything regarded as a stimulant, such as tea, coffee and alcohol. An increasing number of young Afro-Caribbean people are Rastafarians, some of whom may be vegan or vegetarian. They prefer pure foods, and avoid processed or canned products, since they believe that food additives pollute the body.

Food consumption amongst black ethnic groups has not been investigated to the same extent as other groups. Traditional foods remain popular but there is little information about the diet of the younger Afro-Caribbean woman. It is thought that if a young person lives within an extended family they are more likely to eat traditional food.

The Caribbean staple diet is based on rice, maize (corn meal) and wheat. The African staple cereal is cassava, which can be made into bread (bammie) dumplings, or eaten as a porridge (farine). Popular vegetables are yams, sweet potatoes, green bananas and plantains, and these are eaten with meat or fish. Condensed and evaporated milk is frequently used in cooking, and when mixed with carrot juice it is a popular Caribbean drink.

HINDUISM

Most of the Hindus in Britain originated from the Indian states of Gujarat and Punjab, although a number came from East Africa. The majority of Hindus are vegetarian, believing that all living things are sacred. However, the cow is particularly sacred and the eating of beef is strictly forbidden. Many devout Hindus do not eat eggs, or foods which contain eggs.

Some Hindu women may 'fast' one or two days a week, a process which involves restricted food intake or eating only certain food types such as fruits and nuts. Fasting is considered to be beneficial both physically and spiritually, and may be specifically to 'ensure' a successful pregnancy. Way[8] found that some Hindu women will fast during the last month of pregnancy in the belief that this will limit the baby's growth and make delivery less difficult. This should be considered if there is maternal weight loss at the end of pregnancy.

The traditional staple foods amongst Hindus are chapattis, puris and parathas—types of bread made from wheat flour. These reduce intestinal absorption of supplemental iron, which should therefore be taken separately. Ghee (clarified butter) or oil is used for cooking and a variety of pulses and lentils (known as dhals) and other vegetables are eaten once or twice a day.

Hindu women[9] may follow the *Ayurvedic* philosophy which encompasses both food and health concepts. This considers the healthy body to be in a state of harmony and balance, which the individual achieves by maintaining an equilibrium between 'hot' and 'cold' states. Food within this system is also classified as being either 'hot' or 'cold', the terms referring not to the temperature of the food but to the cooling or heating effect on the body. Pregnancy is considered to be a 'hot' state and therefore 'hot' foods should be avoided.

'Hot' foods include animal products, especially those high in protein (often associated with their blood content), chillies, radishes, ginger, fizzy drinks and many of the spices.

'Cold' foods include milk products, cream, yoghurt, lassi, butter, most vegetables, most sweeteners and foods with a sour or astringent flavour such as lemons. Some other foods may be classified according to the manner of preparation and how they are mixed with other foods. The classification of some foods may also vary according to local culture and traditions.

ISLAM

Muslims in Britain originate from the Indian subcontinent, Africa and the Middle East. Their dietary restrictions, food preparation and eating are laid down in their holy book, the Koran. These are regarded as a direct command of God and are part of a set of rules designed to create a disciplined life.

Muslims may not eat pork or pork products. The only meat permitted is that from cloven-hoofed animals that chew the cud and it must be halal, i.e. ritually slaughtered. Only fish with fins and scales may be eaten and dairy products and cheese should be vegetarian, made without animal rennet. The staple food varies according to the country of origin, e.g. for Pakistani Muslims the chapatti is made from wheat, whilst rice plays an important part in the Muslim diet from other regions.

Ramadan is the month of fasting, its date varying each year. Fasting takes place between sunrise and sunset, with a meal being eaten after sunset and again before dawn. Pregnant women are excused from fasting provided they 'make up' the days on another occasion. However, many Muslim women either prefer to fast with the rest of the family or feel pressurized to do so. They may find it difficult to maintain the diabetic diet during this time and, particularly if insulin is required, control may be poor.

SIKHISM

The Sikh community primarily originates from the Punjabi region of India. Their religion developed as an offshoot of Hinduism. Although meat is not specifically prohibited, many devout Sikhs are vegetarians. Amongst those who do eat meat, many will not eat beef, and others will not eat pork. Eating meat killed according to the halal method is strictly forbidden. The staple foods are similar to the Hindus, with chapattis and parathas being important. Ghee is used for cooking, and dairy products are an important part of the diet. Some Sikhs eat only certain foods, such as fruits, on a personal special religious day.

BUDDHISM

Buddhism is more of a philosophy and a system of ethics than a religion with a set of social rules, and as such has quite a wide range of practices. Some strict Buddhists are vegetarian, some will not eat beef and some have no dietary regulations. Some Buddhists fast on the first and 15th days of each lunar month, but fasting may merely be abstinence from meat. Festivals provide an opportunity to indulge in special foods including sweets, special meats, fruits and vegetables.

In the UK most Buddhists originate from the Far East, China, Hong Kong, Taiwan, Malaysia and Vietnam. The largest group of these (70%) are from Hong Kong. According to Chinese and Vietnamese tradition[10], diet plays an essential part in health during pregnancy. The diet is based on the principles of *yin* and *yang*. This is similar to the 'hot' and 'cold' beliefs of the *Ayurvedic* philosophy and, like those, it is independent of the actual temperature. Pregnancy is regarded as *yang*, so if a woman feels her health is not good she is likely to cut down on *yang* foods. These include meats, herbs, ginger, spices, oils and fats. *Yin/yang* foods, which are regarded as balanced, include fish, rice and some vegetables. *Yin* foods include some fruits and vegetables. Rice is the staple food and is regarded as an essential source of energy and nourishment.

JUDAISM

Most of the Jewish population originally migrated from the central European countries and very few do not speak English. Their religious practices vary according to how orthodox their beliefs are, but most observe some of the traditional dietary regulations. Pork and shellfish are strictly prohibited. Whilst orthodox Jews will only eat kosher foods and do not mix milk and meat, there are no Jewish traditional dietary regulations that will affect the diet of a diabetic woman in pregnancy.

THE INFLUENCE OF RELIGIOUS AND CULTURAL VIEWS ON OBSTETRIC CARE

Many of the aspects of pregnancy care are determined by individual choice, particularly concerning the pattern of antenatal care and delivery, the choice of analgesia in labour and the amount of postnatal care which is received in hospital. For women without medical complications, there is a wide range of options available. These, however, will automatically be restricted by the diagnosis of diabetes, whether gestational or established.

For some women, this restriction may cause difficulties or frustrations, particularly if language barriers limit free communication.

PLACE OF ANTENATAL CARE

The place of antenatal care for women with diabetes should be at a joint endocrine and antenatal clinic in the hospital. Appointments may be more frequent than for women without diabetes, particularly at times when rapid adjustment of therapy is required. This may entail additional travelling expenses, stretching an already tight budget; it will reduce contact with the general practitioner, who may have been selected because of a common ethnic or cultural approach; it may be more difficult for relatives who are in employment to attend a clinic during working hours to assist with translation. Although these factors may cause problems for the individual woman, it is anticipated that the increased quality of care will be beneficial to her and to her baby.

ANTENATAL SCREENING FOR AND DIAGNOSIS OF CONGENITAL ANOMALIES

As women with diabetes have an increased risk of having a child with a congenital anomaly, most centres offer detailed ultrasound scanning, with a particular focus on the spine, heart and kidneys. The implication of these scans, often unspoken, is that the woman is able to terminate the pregnancy if a serious abnormality is detected. However, for some women and in particular those of certain religious beliefs, termination of pregnancy may not be a course of action which is acceptable to them. Doctors should be aware of this, and should discuss the potential repercussions of anomaly scanning with a woman and allow her to decide whether to have this performed.

Many obstetric units offer universal serum screening for chromosomal abnormality in the early second trimester. The result is based on the woman's age, the gestational age of the pregnancy and the concentrations of maternal α-fetoprotein, β-subunit of human chorionic gonadotrophin and in some centres oestriol. This allows an individual risk assessment to be made regarding the chance of a chromosomal anomaly, predominantly Down's syndrome, enabling a woman to choose whether to have a diagnostic but invasive and therefore potentially dangerous procedure, such as an amniocentesis, performed. This raises the issue discussed above concerning the acceptability of aborting an abnormal fetus. However, of even greater importance is the fact that women with insulin-dependent diabetes mellitus have lower serum concentrations of α-fetoprotein than their non-diabetic counterparts. This is one of the features which gives a high risk of Down's syndrome, and therefore may be falsely applied to the diabetic woman; calculation of the risk assessment must be adjusted to allow for the influence of her diabetes on the α-fetoprotein concentration.

HIGH PARITY

Women of high parity pose obstetric risks of their own. If they also have diabetes (which when gestational is associated with high parity) and belong to certain religious sects (some of which may be associated with large family size such as orthodox Judaism), the team caring for them should be aware of these possible compounding issues. Thus postpartum haemorrhage is associated with large babies, rapid labour and grand multiparity, each of which is associated with diabetes. Therefore the third stage of labour should be managed actively, with intravenous access and the facility for rapid cross-matching of blood if required. For women who are Seventh Day Adventists or Jehovah's Witnesses, use of blood products is not usually acceptable, even in a life-threatening situation. Their wishes should be discussed and clearly documented prior to the onset of labour.

CONTRACEPTION

Although there is little evidence that repeated pregnancy hastens the onset of complications in established diabetes, there is no doubt that each pregnancy is a time of considerable emotional and physical commitment for a diabetic woman, and one which should not be undertaken lightly. Ideally, each pregnancy should be planned, so that diabetic control is optimized prior to conception. Some diabetic women will choose to restrict the size of their family because of worries about their own health or their ability to look after children in the future if their diabetes deteriorates.

However, women from some religious groups may not feel able to use contraception, even though there is usually a 'clause' allowing this if the woman's health is at risk as is the case in orthodox Judaism. These issues should be discussed sensitively with the couple.

Pregnancy is an important time for all families. If it is complicated by diabetes, there are additional ramifications which may need careful and sympathetic explanation, with allowance being made for the social, religious, cultural and ethnic beliefs of the individual woman. This chapter gives general guidelines regarding some of these factors. However, in local areas, the requirements may be different from those emphasized here. In addition, there are other ethnic groups which we have not discussed here, including many European, Southeast Asian and African people.

REFERENCES

1 Balarajan R, Raleigh VS. The ethnic population of England and Wales: the 1991 Census. *Health Trends* 1992; **24**: 113–16.
2 Dornhorst A, Paterson C, Nicholls JSD *et al*. High prevalence of gestational diabetes in women from ethnic minority groups. *Diabetic Med* 1992; **9**: 820–5.
3 Berkowitz GS, Lapinski R, Wein R, Lee D. Race/ethnicity and other risk factors for gestational diabetes. *Am J Epidemiol* 1992; 135: 965–73.
4 Jarman B. Identification of underprivileged Areas. *Br Med J Clin Res Ed* 1983; **286**: 1705–9.
5 The London Area Transport Survey. London Research Centre, London, 1991.
6 Parsons L, Day S. Improving obstetric outcomes in minorities: an evaluation of health advocacy in Hackney. *J Publ Health Med* 1992; **14**: 183–91.
7 *Food and Low Income: A Conference Report*. Drafted by Peta Cottee for the National Food Alliance Working Party on Low Income. National Food Alliance, London, 1995.
8 Way S. Food for Asian mothers-to-be. *Nursing Times* 1991; **87**: 50–2.
9 Shircore R, Biachoo S. Understanding Asian diets. *Community Outlook* 1985; 16–17.
10 Hill S. *More Than Rice and Peas: Guidelines to Improve Food Provision for Black and Ethnic Minorities in Britain*. Food Commission, London, 1990.

16

Gestational Diabetes in Developing Countries

R. MADAN[1] and J. S. BAJAJ[2]

[1]Government Medical College, Jammu, India and
[2]All-India Institute of Medical Sciences, New Delhi, India

Epidemiological surveys conducted in several developing countries show that prevalence rates of diabetes mellitus vary from 2% to 4% in different population groups. The world population has crossed the 5.5 billion mark, and population projections indicate that by the turn of the century the total world population will be 6.26 billion. Of these, 4.97 billion people will be inhabitants of developing countries. With rapid increases in the population and changes in the demographic profile leading to a marked increase in the middle-aged population in these countries, the number of people with diabetes in the Third World is likely to show a steep increase[1]. Socioeconomic changes, resulting in alterations in lifestyles, may act as additional contributory factors. Thus the present estimate of 45 million individuals with diabetes in developing countries by the end of the 1990s may be realistically revised to 65 million[2], amongst whom will be 15 million women in the reproductive age group. There is, therefore, a colossal problem that needs urgent attention not only with respect to diabetes, but equally in view of its impact on reproductive health.

The prevalence of insulin-dependent diabetes mellitus is extremely low in Asian and some of the other developing countries. Tandhanand and Vannasaeng[3] provide a critical review of the data from a large number of Asian countries and reinforce the earlier observation that insulin-dependent diabetes is unknown or rare in certain ethnic groups, including Japanese, Indians, Filipinos and Sri Lankans. In contrast, malnutrition-related diabetes mellitus may constitute 30–70% of all cases of youth-onset diabetes

Diabetes and Pregnancy: An International Approach to Diagnosis and Management.
Edited by A. Dornhorst and D. R. Hadden.
© 1996 John Wiley & Sons Ltd.

in several developing countries. Finally, traditional modes of life and behavioural patterns have undergone alterations, mainly in response to urbanization, industrialization and changes in socioeconomic profile. All this has resulted in an increased prevalence of non-insulin-dependent diabetes, which is also reflected in the geographic epidemiology of other non-communicable diseases, bringing in its wake a shift in public health priorities and strategies. This may be further amplified for gestational diabetes in developing countries, in view of the role of ethnicity as highlighted by Hadden[4]. Compared with white/European women, Dornhorst[5] reported a higher prevalence rate of gestational diabetes in London of approximately 11-fold in women from the Indian subcontinent, eight-fold in Southeast Asian women and six- and three-fold in Arab/Mediterranean and black/Afro-Caribbean women respectively.

MATERNAL HEALTH IN DEVELOPING COUNTRIES

Maternal death rate for the 10 most populous nations of the developing world is summarized in Table 16.1.

Table 16.1. Maternal mortality in developing nations with high population growth rate[6]

	Maternal mortality (per 100 000 live births)	Lifetime chance of dying in pregnancy or childbirth
China	95	1 in 400
Philippines	100	1 in 400
Mexico	110	1 in 240
Vietnam	120	1 in 180
Brazil	200	1 in 150
Indonesia	450	1 in 60
India	460	1 in 45
Pakistan	500	1 in 30
Bangladesh	600	1 in 30
Nigeria	800	1 in 16

Several developing nations, which are not amongst the most populous and therefore are outside the purview of Table 16.1, have an estimated maternal mortality rate of 800 or more. The highest maternal mortality rate of 2000, reported from Mali, is more than 300 times that for Western Europe, which is six per 100 000 live births (Table 16.2).

A major public health approach for reducing maternal mortality is to focus sharply on the determinants of high-risk pregnancy and to build appropriate intervention programmes.

Table 16.2. Maternal mortality in other developing countries[6]

	Maternal mortality (per 100 000 live births)	Lifetime chance of dying in pregnancy or childbirth
Guinea	800	1 in 15
Zaire	800	1 in 16
Burkina Faso	810	1 in 16
Nepal	830	1 in 18
Congo	900	1 in 15
Papua New Guinea	900	1 in 19
Chad	960	1 in 15
Ghana	1000	1 in 14
Somalia	1100	1 in 11
Bhutan	1310	1 in 11
Mali	2000	1 in 6

DETERMINANTS OF HIGH-RISK PREGNANCY

Several social, nutritional and obstetrical factors like teenage pregnancy, anaemia, maternal anthropometric status and poor quality and outreach of antenatal care contribute to the problem of high maternal mortality and low birth weight babies (Table 16.3). Low birth weight is not only an indicator of poor maternal nutritional status but also a determinant of high perinatal mortality and of poor future growth and development of the baby.

Table 16.3. Prevalence of risk factors in women who delivered infants < 2500 g[7]

Maternal risk factor	Urban	Rural
Teenage pregnancy	16.9	38.4
Primiparity	37.8	40.6
Height below 140 cm	2.9	2.6
Weight below 40 kg	28.8	38.6
Haemoglobin < 8 g	22.5	16.2
Previous bad obstetric history	18.2	8.9
Single risk factor	23.1%	21.6%
One or more risk factors	76.9%	78.4%
Number of women studied	823.0	514.0

ANAEMIA

Iron deficiency anaemia is recognized as a major cause of maternal mortality in developing countries. Recent data, based on World Health Organization (WHO) surveys in developing countries with over three million births a year, are summarized in Table 16.4.

Table 16.4. Anaemia in pregnancy (developing countries) (based on WHO surveys 1985–1990, unpublished data[6])

Country	Pregnancy anaemia rate (%)
India	83
Indonesia	74
Pakistan	65
Bangladesh	62
Nigeria	60
Brazil	42
China	37

Detailed observations from Indian studies show that a great majority, nearly two-thirds or more, of young adolescent girls of 6–14 years of age as well as women in the reproductive age group are anaemic (Table 16.5), and in a considerable proportion the anaemia is of moderate or severe degree. Thus, a high proportion of girls even before starting on their pregnancy are already anaemic, with pregnancy aggravating the pre-existing anaemia, which in turn contributes to high-risk pregnancy.

Iron deficiency anaemia is an important risk factor contributing to the high incidence of low birth weight deliveries in developing countries. Although the incidence of malaria and hookworm infestation have shown a substantial decline, a significant decrease in prevalence of anaemia has not been observed. Administration of iron/folate tablets to women during pregnancy may compensate for the poor availability of iron from cereal-based Asian diets.

Table 16.5. Prevalence of anaemia in rural India[8]

Age group (years)	Hyderabad (South India) %	Delhi (North India) %	Calcutta (East India) %
1–5	65.9	59.0	95.4
6–14	65.3	69.4	97.0
15–22	69.2	63.7	96.7
25–44	71.4	71.3	96.4
>45	47.6	59.3	92.4

MATERNAL ANTHROPOMETRIC STATUS

A recent report of the WHO[9], using secondary data analysis of the effect of maternal anthropometric status on low birth weight, has highlighted the adverse impact of maternal height and weight gain. Table 16.6 shows mean weight and height of women (post partum) from several countries of the Southeast Asian region. It clearly shows that the mothers in India rank the lowest amongst these countries in terms of body mass index (weight/height^2).

Table 16.6. Mean weights and heights of mothers (post partum)[9]

Country	Weight (kg)	Height (cm)
India	42.1 ± 4	150 ± 5
Indonesia	46.0 ± 6	149 ± 4
Myanmar	46.9 ± 8	151 ± 5
Nepal		
Rural	43.0 ± 5	150 ± 5
Urban	44.6 ± 6	150 ± 5
Sri Lanka	43.5 ± 7	150 ± 5
Thailand	49.9 ± 7	153 ± 5

On the basis of the observation that maternal body mass index shows a significant correlation with babies of low birth weight (Table 16.7), it has been suggested that measurement of body mass index, independent of age and parity, may be a useful index for identifying such mothers at risk.

Furthermore, nearly 24% of these adult women of reproductive age have a body weight less than 38 kg and 16% have heights less than 145 cm. According to generally accepted WHO criteria these women fall into a high-risk category as they are likely to suffer obstetrical complications and give birth to offspring of low birth weight, especially in a situation where antenatal care and obstetrical services are below par.

Table 16.7. Maternal body mass index and low birth weight[10]

Body mass index	Low birth weight (%)
< 16	53.1
16–17	41.4
17–18.5	35.9
18.5–20	27.7
20–25	26.4
25–30	14.7
> 30	20.0

AGE AT MARRIAGE

Teenage pregnancy in Western countries may be a consequence of ongoing social transformation, but in most of the developing countries like India it is due to tradition and culture. The average age of girls at marriage in India, according to the latest data, is 16.7 years. In most parts of North India, the average age has been found to be as low as 13.8 years, with consummation of marriage taking place at 15.3 years[11]. The average age at marriage in countries such as Thailand, Sri Lanka and Indonesia is higher. It is noteworthy that the state in India which records the highest mean birth weight and the lowest incidence of low birth weight, Kerala, is also the state where the mean age of girls at marriage is the highest.

ANTENATAL CARE

Obstetricians advise that antenatal care should begin at the latest six weeks after the last menstrual period. Most of the low income group women in both urban and rural areas do not avail themselves of the antenatal care facilities either because of ignorance or due to a lack of outreach of such services. Sushila Nayer[12], while evaluating existing health care systems in the Wardha district in Maharashtra, reported that only 40% of pregnant women were receiving antenatal care. An Indian multicentre task force (1990)[11] reported that 25% of pregnant women do not receive any antenatal checks, and only about a fifth of pregnant women receive adequate antenatal care.

Under these circumstances, a stunted woman who starts her pregnancy with a body weight of 38 kg or less and a haemoglobin level below 8 g/dl, and who may become a beneficiary of antenatal care only halfway through her pregnancy, is unlikely to achieve a body weight increase of more than 5–6 kg, or a haemoglobin level of 11 g by the end of pregnancy. It is in this context of a multifactorial constellation of risk factors, and the constraints on the outreach as well as quality of health care services in most of the developing countries, especially in the Southeast Asian region, that the screening, diagnosis and management of gestational diabetes must be viewed. Focusing on gestational diabetes in an isolated manner, as in the developed countries, is likely to be counterproductive.

SCREENING FOR GESTATIONAL DIABETES

IS SCREENING NECESSARY?

Pregnancy in women with pre-existing diabetes more often ends in perinatal death than does pregnancy in the non-diabetic population[13]. Furthermore the perinatal mortality in diabetic pregnancies is directly related to the degree of maternal hyperglycemia during the third trimester[14]. O'Sullivan[15] observed a four-fold increase in perinatal mortality in gestational diabetes when no treatment was administered during pregnancy. In addition to a higher perinatal mortality, the protagonists for screening and treatment of gestational diabetes also point to a greater perinatal morbidity, especially due to large-for-dates babies and a higher risk of Caesarean section[16]. In contrast, some more recent studies of gestational diabetes have shown a perinatal mortality similar to that in the general population[17], and any increase in maternofetal morbidity has been ascribed to maternal age or obesity[18], even questioning the distinct clinical entity of gestational diabetes.

Is it therefore justifiable to recommend screening of all pregnant women for glucose intolerance on the basis of these seemingly contradictory observations? The issues are further confounded in developing countries where perinatal mortality is influenced by a host of factors such as anaemia, toxaemia, urinary tract infection, poor antenatal and intranatal care, and the high incidence of low birth weight babies. The unresolved conceptual dichotomy has resulted in divergent recommendations even in the same country. While the American Diabetes Association[19] recommends screening of all pregnant women, the American College of Obstetricians and Gynecologists recommends screening only for women aged over 30 years[20].

Experience from several developing countries has recently become available. Chua *et al.*[21] in a study from Singapore recommended screening of all pregnant woman in a low-risk population defined as 'women without obstetric and historical risk factors for development of gestational diabetes mellitus', with a 50 g glucose load between 24 and 28 weeks gestation. However, in pregnant women with risk factors for gestational diabetes at the time of first antenatal visit a glucose tolerance test with a 75 g glucose load was recommended. Glucose tolerance screening during pregnancy has also been recommended for women in Soweto, South Africa, by Huddle *et al.*[22] where clinical screening criteria missed one-third of gestational diabetic cases. A high prevalence of gestational diabetes (9.1%) with increased rates of abortion and congenital anomalies in Benghazi, Libya, has been reported by Kadiki *et al.*[23], who have stressed the need to screen all pregnant women.

According to the guidelines on diabetic pregnancy suggested by the WHO Study Group on Diabetes in 1985, every pregnant woman should be screened for gestational diabetes between the 24th and 28th week of pregnancy[24]. A more recent WHO recommendation states that depending on local health priorities, resources and facilities, serious consideration should be given to screening all pregnant women for glucose intolerance at the beginning of the third trimester of pregnancy[25]. Clearly, well-designed studies need to be conducted to define generally acceptable guidelines.

In an effort to resolve some of the underlying issues, an international study, Hyperglycaemia and Adverse Pregnancy Outcome (HAPO), has been designed, to be undertaken in 25 field centres involving approximately 25 000 pregnant women. The general aim of the study is to achieve a major advance in knowledge on the levels of glucose during pregnancy that place the mother, fetus and neonate at increased risk. The study also aims to achieve the specific objective of arriving at an internationally acceptable set of criteria for the diagnosis and classification of hyperglycaemia in pregnancy based on the identification of specific adverse outcomes.

SCREENING FOR GESTATIONAL DIABETES IN DEVELOPING COUNTRIES: A POSSIBLE CONSENSUS

Having recognized the need for a 'multiscreen' for all locally and nationally relevant factors contributing to high-risk pregnancy, the issues related to screening and diagnosis of gestational diabetes in developing countries merit a consensus statement. Such a multiscreen must *a priori* include identification of pregnant women with a bad obstetric history in early pregnancy, recording body weight and height of the pregnant mother, checking blood pressure, detecting clinical evidence of anaemia or nutritional deficiency, measuring fundal height and abdominal girth, detection of obstetric problems like abnormal presentations, multiple pregnancy, toxaemia, and excluding cephalopelvic disproportion, followed by serial haemoglobin estimations and urinalysis. Based on the data thus generated, cases of high-risk pregnancy will be identified and so designated.

The authors would recommend that all such women with high-risk pregnancy be subjected to screening with a 50 g glucose load at 24–28 weeks of pregnancy. A blood glucose level of ≥ 7.8 mmol/l (140 mg/dl) at 1 h would necessitate further investigation by oral glucose tolerance test. For those developing countries where the financial resources and manpower are inadequate to fulfil the requirements of a protocol for screening all high-risk pregnant women, only those women with high-risk pregnancy who in addition have a previous history of gestational diabetes and/or a strong family history of diabetes should undergo the 75 g oral glucose tolerance test.

DIAGNOSIS OF GESTATIONAL DIABETES

Several attempts have been made to standardize criteria for the diagnosis of gestational diabetes, but the problem remains unresolved due to variability in the glucose load used for either screening or diagnosis, in the period of gestation at which diagnosis is made, on the methodology employed, and in the cut-off points used to separate diabetes from impaired glucose tolerance. Finally, there seems to be no 'gold standard' against which any of the diagnostic criteria may be validated. While some investigators have attempted to validate the criteria through clinical follow-up and possible correlation with either adverse pregnancy outcome or the later development of diabetes in the mother[15,26], others have adopted a purely statistical approach[27], defining gestational diabetes as the degree of hyperglycaemia two or three standard deviations above the mean observed in an unselected pregnant population.

There have been two major international efforts for standardization of criteria for the diagnosis of diabetes mellitus in pregnancy[28,29]. Both the US National Diabetes Data Group (NDDG) and the WHO Expert Committee have recommended the use of a 75 g glucose load for the oral glucose tolerance test; however, the NDDG have recommended the use of the criteria advocated by O'Sullivan[26] for the evaluation of carbohydrate tolerance during pregnancy. The inherent contradiction in this recommendation is due to the fact that the O'Sullivan criteria were originally developed using a 100 g glucose load. International agreement seems to be closer regarding the glucose load and the criteria to be adopted for the diagnosis of diabetes in a non-pregnant state, but the recommendations are divergent if the test has to be performed during pregnancy. This is further highlighted by the fact that while the WHO criteria made specific recommendations for the diagnosis of impaired glucose tolerance both during pregnant and non-pregnant states, the NDDG did not make any definitive recommendation, although several members of the Working Group recommended a 2 h post-glucose value between 120 and 164 mg/dl.

Keeping in view the recommendation made by the WHO Expert Committee in 1985[24] that the proposed diagnostic criteria be used as a guide to diagnosis until more detailed information becomes available on different populations, other diagnostic indices, and the development of complications, the authors have undertaken a study to validate diagnostic criteria of gestational diabetes and lesser degree, of carbohydrate tolerance in a North Indian population, with different anthropometric status and dietary habits. A total of 565 glucose tolerance tests were performed in 410 normal healthy pregnant women who reported consecutively to an antenatal clinic. Women with a known history of diabetes, a family history of diabetes or a bad obstetrical history were excluded, so as to select a homogeneous representative group of the normal population. The 75 g oral glucose tolerance tests were carried out by the method recommended by the WHO[28]. The study was blinded so as not to affect the clinical care which was provided to all subjects, following routine practice in the antenatal clinic. The results were decoded at the end of the study, and subsequently correlated with the clinical course regarding complications of pregnancy, fetal outcome and perinatal mortality.

Using WHO criteria, abnormal oral glucose tolerance tests were classified as either gestational diabetes or gestational impaired glucose tolerance. For every pregnancy complication that was used as an indicator there was a significantly higher prevalence in the group with gestational impaired glucose tolerance compared to normal, with a further increase for those graded as gestational diabetes (Figure 16.1).

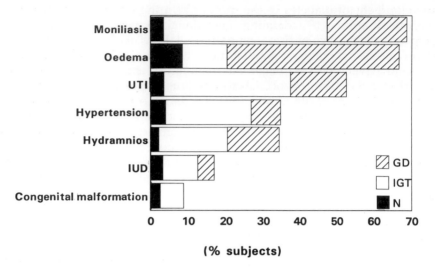

Figure 16.1. Complications of pregnancy. UTI, urinary tract infection; IUD, intrauterine death; GD, gestational diabetes; IGT, impaired glucose tolerance; N, normal

Labour was induced more frequently by artificial rupture of membranes and/or an oxytocin drip in both abnormal groups because of poly-hydramnios, pre-eclamptic toxaemia and intrauterine death (Table 16.8). A big baby with cephalopelvic disproportion formed a major indication for operative delivery either by forceps or by lower segment caesarean section.

Significantly higher birth weights, up to 3.89 + 0.06 kg, were observed in both the abnormal groups, compared to the mean birth weight of 2.89 + 0.02 kg in those with normal glucose tolerance ($p < 0.001$). Apgar scores observed at 1, 5, and 10 min intervals were lower in the newborns of mothers with abnormal glucose tolerance compared to the normal group ($p < 0.001$ for Apgar score at 5 min).

In view of these complications during pregnancy and labour, we

Table 16.8. Outcome of labour in 410 consecutive pregnancies related to result of 75 g oral glucose tolerance test[30]

OGTT	Spontaneous labour	Induced labour	Normal delivery	Forceps delivery	Caesarean Section
Normal	91.5%	8.5%	87.3%	7.2%	5.5%
IGT	84.2%	15.8%	26.3%	26.3%	47.4%
GD	50.0%	33.3%	16.7%	33.3%	50.0%

OGTT, oral glucose tolerance test; IGT, impaired glucose tolerance; GD, gestational diabetes.

suggested that impaired glucose tolerance during pregnancy carries a high risk of maternal fetal morbidity, and thus should be managed as a high-risk pregnancy on lines similar to gestational diabetes. The term gestational impaired glucose tolerance was introduced in 1985[30], although it was suggested that its association with high risk during pregnancy might be valid only in developing countries where additional factors like poor nutritional status and anaemia may interact with metabolic factors, and thus synergize or potentiate the possible risk to the mother and fetus. Over the years, supportive evidence for this concept has been obtained in several studies[26,31,32]. Taking cognizance of this, the WHO Study Group in 1994 adopted the terminology of gestational impaired glucose tolerance and recommended that during pregnancy these mothers should be treated in the same way as gestational diabetes[25].

MANAGEMENT

The twin objectives of management include maintenance of normoglycaemia and continuation of pregnancy to term while ensuring maternofetal safety. The principles and practice of management of gestational diabetes in developing countries are essentially similar to those practised elsewhere in the world[33], but the following specific issues need further deliberation.

DIET

Dietary advice to a woman with gestational diabetes should take into consideration her economic status, level of literacy, qualitative pattern of food consumption, and religious beliefs including vegetarianism. Any major departure from the usual pattern of staple food consumption should be avoided. Dietary instruction, especially for the illiterate or semiliterate, should be imparted with food models and diet menus using such models. To simplify the concept of weights and measures, the use of a handful (fist) which can hold about 30–35 g of uncooked cereal or pulses is preferable to the demonstration of a kitchen balance. 'Hands-on' experience has been validated as a mode of learning with enhancement of dietary compliance.

Essentially the daily dietary consumption in developing countries in Southeast Asia is of a fairly consistent and comparable pattern, providing about 75%, 12% and 14% of the total energy intake from carbohydrates, proteins and fats, respectively. Dietary compliance is ensured if there is no major deviation except for a minimal reduction in carbohydrate, and a corresponding increase in the protein intake[34].

INSULIN

The issue of continuous availability of insulin in developing countries is a crucial one. The WHO has recommended that 'in all countries, the availability of insulin as an essential life-saving drug should be ensured without imposition of taxes or restrictions regarding the transfer of technology for its manufacture'[25]. Its availability should be considered as 'right to life', and in gestational diabetes it is applicable equally both to the mother and to the growing fetus, with the right to be born alive and healthy. The technology of manufacture of insulin should be available in developing countries so that there is a uniform and uninterrupted supply of insulin at an affordable cost.

As in other developing countries, insulin storage was always considered a problem in rural areas of India where facilities of refrigeration are not generally available. It has been convincingly demonstrated that insulin can be stored for a period of up to four weeks in earthenware water pitchers or clay jars (approximate water temperature 23–27 °C) without loss of biological activity, as measured by glucose uptake by rat hemidiaphragm[35]. The cost of such jars is about 10 cents US!

EDUCATION

Because of low literacy rates in developing countries, especially in females, education of a woman with gestational diabetes poses a great challenge. Bold and imaginative approaches need to be designed to provide knowledge to the semi-literate and illiterate so as to bring a demonstrable change in their knowledge, attitude and practices. Such a change would favourably influence the course as well as the out-come of pregnancy. Regular antenatal check-up, self-monitoring of fetal movements, adherence to recommended diet and regular self-administration of insulin in the prescribed dose constitute the essential components of learning, to be reinforced periodically by community health workers.

In several developing countries, an appropriate mix of requisite health manpower is not available, with the result that nurses, dieticians, pharmacists and laboratory technologists are in short supply. In addition, communicable diseases, malnutrition and deficiency disorders pose priority demands on available health manpower. To augment human resources for health at grass root level, community health workers, following short courses of training, are entrusted with the responsibility of providing preventive and promotive services at the primary care level.

The role of such community workers, especially of village school teachers, following a period of adequate training including a range of learning activities and health-related team tasks, in the organization of integrated diabetes care approach, is being increasingly recognized. As the school teachers are well conversant with communication techniques and enjoy a close rapport with the families through their students, they constitute a significant human resource for maternal and child health care.

SERVICE DELIVERY SYSTEM

The quality and outreach of obstetrical care services depend upon the health care infrastructure, and the integration of such a programme within the total organizational framework of the national health system.

ORGANIZATION OF GESTATIONAL DIABETES CARE IN DEVELOPING COUNTRIES

Taking cognizance of the level of development, quality and outreach of health care systems in developing countries, and keeping in view the competing demands on health budgets and health manpower, it would be most appropriate to integrate gestational diabetes care into the maternal and child health programmes within the primary health care approach. With focus on high-risk pregnancy, screening and diagnosis of gestational diabetes becomes an achievable objective.

While first-contact antenatal care, including use of a 'multiscreen' protocol for identification of high-risk pregnancy, and screening for gestational diabetes should be a part of gestational diabetes care at primary level, the definitive management of pregnancy with diabetes would require an in-built system of referral from primary to secondary level (district or sub-district hospital, community health centre) where the specialist services of obstetrician, physician and paediatrician are generally available. To optimize gestational diabetes care, an essential prerequisite is to upgrade knowledge, skills and motivation through multiprofessional education with a problem-solving approach[36]. The health care professionals at the secondary level, in addition to providing continuing obstetrical care and neonatal care, are also expected to provide support and linkage to primary care workers, to ensure continuing education of such personnel. The maintenance and monitoring of metabolic control in the domiciliary setting, following a definitive prescribed management, is a critical input to be provided by primary care workers who also reinforce patient education through a close rapport with the families.

While further referral to tertiary care may be required on a case-to-case basis for specified indications, the major task of specialized diabetes centres is to prepare and update learning resource materials for use by gestational diabetes care providers at primary and secondary levels, to respond to the need of multiprofessional education, and to train the 'trainers' in education technology and communication skills. Finally, the development of appropriate diabetes care technology, as well as the monitoring and evaluation of gestational diabetes care programmes in coordination with health planners and administrators, are additional tasks at this level. The essential contours and contents of this model, also called the Kashmir model, are shown in Figure 16.2.

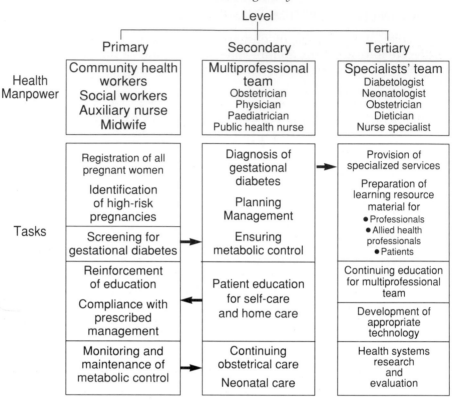

Figure 16.2. Gestational Diabetes Care Programme

As the efficiency and effectiveness of such a model must relate to a performance audit, measurable in terms of health impact and outcome, an evaluation was carried out with respect to: (1) functional organization of the health team; (2) task-related performance of the health team collectively and diabetes health care providers individually; (3) health care outcome measured as fetal and neonatal loss in pregnancy with diabetes in the project area, and compared with a control area; and (4) cost effectiveness[37]. A significant reduction in fetal and neonatal loss was demonstrable in the project area; such an outcome has received international attention and commendation[38]. The use of such a model in the National Diabetes Care and Control Programme in India has been rewarding. It may serve as a prototype for development of similar models elsewhere.

REFERENCES

1 Bajaj JS. Diabetes mellitus in developing countries. *Bull Int Diabetes Fed* 1988; **33**: 6.
2 Bajaj JS, Madan R. Diabetes in the tropics and developing countries. *Bull Int Diabetes Fed* 1993; **38**: 5.
3 Tandhanand S, Vannasaeng S. Diabetes in Asia. In: Krall LP (ed.), *World Book of Diabetes in Practice*. Elsevier, Amsterdam, 1988; 327–34.
4 Hadden DR. Geographic, ethnic and racial variation in the incidence of gestational diabetes mellitus. *Diabetes* 1985; **34**: 8–12.
5 Dornhorst A. Implications of gestational diabetes for the health of the mother. *Br J Obstet Gynaecol* 1994; **101**: 286–90.
6 *The Progress of Nations*. UNICEF, New York, 1994.
7 Ramachandran P. Need of organisation of antenatal and intrapartum care in India. *Demography India* 1992; **21**: 179–93.
8 Gopalan C. New dimensions of old problems. In: *Nutrition in Developmental Transition in South-East Asia*. SEARO. WHO, New Delhi, 1992; 34–48.
9 *The Use of Anthropometry for Women During the Reproductive Cycle and the Newborn Infant.* Report of the WHO Expert Committee, Geneva, 1993.
10 Naidu AN. Maternal body mass index and birth weight. *Nutr News* 1991; 12.
11 Indian Council of Medical Research. A National Collaborative Study of 'identification of high risk families mothers and outcome of their offsprings with particular reference to the problem of maternal nutrition, low birth weight perinatal and infant morbidity and mortality in rural and urban slums communities'. ICMR Task Force Study, 1990.
12 Sushila Nayar. Health Care Systems: an evaluation. Mahatma Gandhi Institute of Medical Sciences, Sevagram Wardha, 1985.
13 Gabbe SG. Management of diabetes in pregnancy: six decades of experience. In: Pitkin RM (ed.), *Yearbook of Obstetrics and Gynecology*. Yearbook Publishers, Chicago, 1980; 37.
14 Jovanovic L, Peterson CM. Management of the pregnant, insulin-dependent diabetic. *Diabetes Care* 1980; **3**: 63.
15 O'Sullivan JB, Charles D, Mahan CM *et al.* Gestational diabetes and perinatal mortality rate. *Am J Obstet Gynecol* 1973; **116**: 901.
16 Maresh M, Beard RW, Bray CS *et al.* Factors predisposing to an outcome of gestational diabetes. *Obstet Gynecol* 1989; **74**: 342–6.
17 Freinkel N. Summary and recommendations of the Second International Workshop-Conference on Gestational Diabetes Mellitus. *Diabetes* 1985; **34**: 123–6.
18 Jarret RJ. Gestational diabetes: a non entity? *Br Med J* 1993; **306**: 37–8.
19 American Diabetes Association Inc. Position statement on gestational diabetes mellitus. *Diabetes Care* 1991; **14**: 5–6.
20 American College of Obstetricians and Gynecologists. *Technical Bulletin: Management of Diabetes in Pregnancy* 1986; **91**: 1–5.
21 Chua S, Thai AC, Kek LP *et al.* The glucose challenge test: a screening test for gestational diabetes mellitus. *Singapore Med J* 1993; **34**: 303–5.
22 Huddle K, England M, Nagar A. Outcome of pregnancy in diabetes women in Soweto, South Africa 1983–1992. *Diabetic Med* 1993; **10**: 290–4.
23 Kadiki OA, Rama Subba Reddy M, Sahli MA *et al.* Outcome of pregnant diabetic patients in Benghazi (Libya) from 1984 to 1991. *Diabetes Res Clin Pract* 1993; **21**: 39–42.
24 Report of WHO Study Group on Diabetes Mellitus. *WHO Tech Rep Ser 727*. WHO, Geneva, 1985.
25 Report of WHO Study Group on Prevention of Diabetes Mellitus. *WHO Tech Rep Ser 844*. WHO, Geneva, 1994.
26 O'Sullivan JB, Mahan CM. Criteria for oral glucose tolerance test in pregnancy. *Diabetes* 1964; **13**: 278–85.
27 Lind T. A prospective multicentre study to determine the influence of pregnancy upon the 75 g oral glucose tolerance test: the Diabetes Pregnancy Study Group of the European Association for the Study of Diabetes. In: Sutherland HW, Stowers JM, Pearson DWM (eds), *Carbohydrate Metabolism in Pregnancy and the Newborn*, Vol. IV. Springer-Verlag, London, 1989; 209–26.

28 WHO Expert Committee on Diabetes Mellitus. Second Report. *WHO Tech Rep Ser 646.* WHO, Geneva, 1980.
29 National Diabetes Data Group. *Diabetes* 1979; **28**: 1039.
30 Madan R, Bajaj JS. Pregnancy and diabetes: problems and perspectives in developing countries. In: Serrano-Rios M, Lefebvre PJ (eds), *Diabetes, Proceedings of 12th Congress of International Diabetes Federation*, Excerpta Med Int Congr Series No 700, Amsterdam, 1985.
31 Pettit DJ, Knowler WC, Baird HR *et al.* Gestational diabetes: infant and maternal complications of pregnancy in relation to third-trimester glucose tolerance in Pima Indians. *Diabetes Care* 1980; **3**: 458.
32 Karlsson K, Kjellmer I. The outcome of diabetic pregnancies in relation to the mother's blood sugar level. *Am J Obstet Gynecol* 1972; **112**: 213.
33 Persson B, Hanson U, Lunell NO. Diabetes mellitus and pregnancy. In: Alberti KGMM, Defronzo RA, Keen H *et al.* (eds), *International Textbook of Diabetes Mellitus*. Wiley, Chichester, 1992; 1085–102.
34 Bajaj JS. Dietary management of diabetes mellitus in India and South East Asia. In Alberti KGM, Defronzo RA, Keen H *et al.* (eds), *International Textbook of Diabetes Mellitus*. Wiley, Chichester, 1992; 701–6.
35 Bajaj JS. Strategies for integration of diabetes in primary health care programs in developing countries. In: Luft R, Bajaj JS, Rosenqvist U (eds), *WHO Workshop on Diabetes Care as a Model for Primary Health Care*. Tryckeri Arne Lofgren, Stockholm, 1986; 28–37.
36 Bajaj JS. Multiprofessional education as an essential component of effective health services. *Med Educ* 1994; **28**: 86–91.
37 Madan R, Bajaj JS. Kashmir model: considering alternate health manpower sources. In: Luft R, Bajaj JS, Rosenqvist U (eds), *WHO Workshop on Diabetes Care as a Model for Primary Health Care*. Tryckeri Arne Lofgren, Stockholm, 1986; 54–62.
38 Hu Ching-Li. Mobilization against diabetes. In: Larkins RG, Zimmet PZ, Chisholm DJ (eds), *Diabetes 1988*. Excerpta Medica, Amsterdam, 1989; 873–6.

Part III

CHILDBIRTH

17

Labour and Delivery

JEREMY J.N. OATS

The Royal Women's Hospital Melbourne, Australia

The challenge to the team caring for the woman with diabetes mellitus is to conduct her labour and delivery in a manner that avoids unnecessary intervention but ensures the delivery of a healthy infant without causing unnecessary risk to both mother and child.

Traditionally women with diabetes were delivered prematurely in the belief that this minimized the risk of late fetal death *in utero*. This practice evolved simultaneously on both sides of the Atlantic. At King's College Hospital in London, Peel and Oakley in 1949[1] developed their protocol of delivering all pregnant diabetic women by 36 weeks gestation. This arose from their post-maturity theory in which they concluded that:' hyperglycaemia caused gross overdevelopment of the baby, which appeared to mature 3 to 4 weeks earlier than normal and we thought that it was post mature and poorly viable so that intrauterine death was frequent'[2].

This misconception was further reinforced because the perinatal mortality in their clinic was half that of comparable UK units which did not follow this practice. Prior to their management policy, the perinatal mortality at King's was 37%, a rate similar to that occurring in most units in the Northern Hemisphere. The principal reason for their improved perinatal results was due, however, to their close supervision of the pregnancy with careful control of maternal blood glucose levels, with diet and insulin, and admission to hospital at 32 weeks gestation where the mother remained until delivery. The neonatal death rate was, not surprisingly, higher than the other clinics. It is also salutary to note that the maternal mortality in 1949 was 2% (Table 17.1).

At the same time in Boston, White and colleagues[3] recommended that patients with class A diabetes be allowed to go to term, classes B and C to

Diabetes and Pregnancy: An International Approach to Diagnosis and Management.
Edited by A. Dornhorst and D. R. Hadden.
© 1996 John Wiley & Sons Ltd.

Table 17.1. Obstetric results prior to 1949. Diabetic pregnancy data from 26 teaching hospitals and from King's College Hospital, London[1]

	Total pregnancies	Died undelivered	Maternal mortality (%)	Intrauterine death (%)	Stillbirth (%)	Neonatal death (%)
Other units	458	3	2.2	18.7	10.7	10.7
King's	141	0	1.4	8.5	2.8	14.2

38 weeks and classes D, E and F should be delivered in the 35th week, because of the high incidence of intrauterine death in the 36th week.

These policies held sway for the next two decades. Amongst the first to question this protocol were Roversi and colleagues in Milan, Italy, who reported their experience for the years 1969–1975 in 1979[4]. Using a regimen of 'maximally tolerated insulin' to control blood glucose, 75% were delivered after 38 weeks gestation and 19% after 40 weeks. There were eight perinatal deaths (3.3%), two due to neural tube defects; the only late intrauterine death occurred at 37 weeks in a primigravida with White class F diabetes. Subsequently Drury and co-workers published their experience of 141 consecutive pregnancies managed at the National Maternity Hospital, Dublin[5]. Again the lynchpin of their protocol was close monitoring of blood glucose at home and allowing the pregnancy to go to term regardless of the severity of the diabetes, provided no obstetric complications developed. Ninety-nine (85%) delivered after 38 weeks gestation; a third of these went into spontaneous labour. Overall, spontaneous labour occurred in 57%. The caesarean section rate was 20% and the induction rate was 34%. In 1992, the Dublin National Maternity Hospital experience was updated by Rasmussen *et al.*[6]. The mean gestation at delivery of the 276 pregnancies delivered between 1981 and 1990 was 39 weeks, 83% delivering at 38 or more weeks and 41% at or beyond 40 weeks. The induction rate was 27% and the elective caesarean section rate 19%. The outcome of the 112 patients who delivered at or after 40 weeks gestation is detailed in Table 17.2.

The perinatal mortality rate was 5.8%, seven of the 16 deaths being due to lethal malformations. All of the five deaths of normally formed infants born after 37 weeks gestation had been preceded by clinically apparent polyhydramnios, macrosomia or poor control (Table 17.3).

Kjos and colleagues[7] from Los Angeles have questioned this policy of allowing uncomplicated diabetic pregnancies to go to full term. They randomly allocated 200 such pregnancies whose fetuses were judged to be appropriate for gestational age at 38 weeks gestation either to active induction of labour within five days, or to expectant management which entailed monitoring with twice-weekly cardiotocography and amniotic

Table 17.2. Onset, mode of delivery and pregnancy outcome in 276 diabetic pregnancies, National Maternity Hospital, Dublin, 1981–1990

Onset of labour	Spontaneous	55%
	Induced	32%
	Elective caesarean section	13%
Mode of delivery following spontaneous or induced onset of labour	Normal vaginal delivery	82%
	Forceps	8%
	Caesarean section	9%
Neonatal outcome	Birth weight > 90th centile	28%
	Admission to neonatal nursery	21%
	Respiratory distress syndrome	0%
	Neonatal jaundice	5%
	Neonatal hypoglycaemia	7%
Perinatal mortality	See Table 17.3	0.9%

Adapted with permission from Rasmussen *et al.*[6]

Table 17.3. Factors associated with perinatal deaths in 5 normally formed infants born after 37 weeks gestation, National Maternity Hospital Dublin, 1981–1990

White Class	Antenatal complications	Gestation	Birth weight g
C	Polyhydramnios Poor control	NND 37 weeks	3820
A	Macrosomia Poor control	FDIU 37 weeks	4700[a]
B	Polyhydramnios Macrosomia Poor control	FDIU 38 weeks	4480[a]
D	Macrosomia	FDIU 39 weeks	5180[a]
C	Polyhydramnios	FDIU 41 weeks	4360[a]

NND, Neonatal death; FDIU, Fetal death *in utero*.
[a]Birthweight > 90th centile for gestational age.
Adapted with permission from Rasmussen *et al.*[6].

fluid volume assessment and weekly clinical examination. The gestation of the group managed expectantly was increased by one week, but 49% required induction of labour for obstetric indications, and the caesarean section rate was in fact greater (31% vs 25%). Moreover, even after controlling for gestational age, maternal age and maternal body weight the percentage of macrosomic infants in the expectantly managed group was significantly greater (23% vs 10%). It was concluded that delivery should be contemplated at 38 weeks, and if not completed, close monitoring of the fetus should be maintained.

TIMING OF DELIVERY

Until further confirmation of the findings from Los Angeles, it would seem reasonable to follow the current widely followed practice of allowing uncomplicated diabetic pregnancies to continue to full-term providing that:

1. there has been tight metabolic control;
2. there is no clinical and/or ultrasonic evidence of fetal macrosomia;
3. there is no clinical and/or ultrasonic evidence of polyhydramnios;
4. there is no evidence of impaired fetoplacental function;
5. there are no other obstetric complications such as proteinuric hypertension (severe pre-eclampsia), major placenta praevia or intra-uterine growth retardation, which would themselves indicate the need for delivery.

This policy has been shown to result in a low risk of perinatal mortality and of neonatal and maternal morbidity. Furthermore it helps to reduce the maternal perception that the fact that she happens to have uncomplicated diabetes automatically means that she is destined to have a pregnancy that will inevitably end in caesarean section or induction of labour.

MODE OF DELIVERY

Prior to the current policy of not routinely delivering all women with diabetes by 37–38 weeks gestation, caesarean section was the mode of delivery for almost half of those with diabetes established before the pregnancy, with rates varying from 19% to 83%. The reaons for these high rates were suggested to be failed induction, obstructed labour secondary to fetal macrosomia, and fetal distress[9]. Shoulder dystocia with its long-term consequence of permanent brachial plexus palsy has also been a factor in the readiness to resort to abdominal delivery in the presence of perceived fetal macrosomia[8]. The dilemma confronting the obstetrician is the poor predictability of the likely occurrence of significant shoulder dystocia. Using birth weight alone as a predictor is quite unsatisfactory. The incidence of shoulder dystocia in infants weighing between 4000 and 4500 g is 3% and for those over 4500 g is 10–14%. Consequently if elective caesarean section is employed in the latter group to avoid shoulder dystocia, 90% or more will have been delivered by this route unnecessarily[10]. Keller and colleagues[11], in a study of 210 patients with gestational diabetes whose offspring weighed more than 3500 g, reported that 15 of the 120 vaginal deliveries were complicated by shoulder dystocia. Of these 15 infants, seven weighed less than 4000 g and only one (7%) had a permanent brachial plexus palsy. Furthermore ultrasonic estimation of fetal weight is at best ± 10%, so that an estimated weight of 4000 g could in reality range from 3600 to 4400 g, and if the estimate is 4500 g, from 4050 to 4950 g[8]. In a recent study Chauhan *et al.*[12] reported that intrapartum sonography was not significantly more accurate in predicting macrosomia than clinical assessment.

Thus the fact that the woman has diabetes, either established prior to the pregnancy or gestational, should not influence the decision on how she should be delivered; the same obstetric factors that prevail in any pregnancy should determine this decision. If the woman does require delivery by caesarean section, the risk of neonatal respiratory distress syndrome is reduced by preventing neonatal hypoxia. The use of an epidural anaesthetic is therefore the preferred method, and if a general anaesthetic is required then a short induction–delivery interval minimizes the Apgar score[13].

INDUCTION OF LABOUR

Before prostaglandin E_2 became available to effect effacement of the unfavourable cervix, a common practice was to administer an oxytocic infusion over a one-to three-day period[14]. This practice carried a significant risk of maternal hyponatraemia, due to oxytocin-induced antidiuresis, and interfered with the woman's normal food intake and consequently disturbed her diabetic control. After inserting the prostaglandin gel it is important to monitor the fetal heart and uterine contractions as prostaglandin-induced uterine hypertonia can cause significant fetal distress, resulting in fetal death[15].

CONDUCT OF LABOUR

Following spontaneous onset or induction the management of the labour, with the exception of the medical management of the woman's diabetes which is discussed below, is similar to that of any high-risk pregnancy. Likewise the assessment of the progress of the first stage of labour (judged by cervical dilatation and descent of the presenting part) or the second stage does not differ from any other high-risk labour. Consequently the same factors used to determine the need for operative delivery do not have to be influenced by the fact that the woman has diabetes.

Although the debate on the efficacy of continuous electronic fetal heart rate monitoring has yet to be conclusively resolved[16], it is important to stress that women with diabetes exemplify all the recognized risk factors for intrapartum fetal hypoxia, fetal acidosis and low Apgar scores[14]. In a matched controlled study of 46 women with diabetes, Olofsson *et al.*

reported that the incidence of ominous fetal heart rate patterns and low fetal scalp pH values (< 7.26) was more common in women with diabetes (17%) than the control group (11%) although this did not reach statistical significance.

If continuous auscultation can be guaranteed, then electronic monitoring could possibly be dispensed with, but most units do not have the available staff to provide such meticulous surveillance, and until superior means of intrapartum monitoring become available cardiotocography will remain the mainstay.

MEDICAL MANAGEMENT OF LABOUR

The principal objective is to maintain maternal euglycaemia as maternal hyperglycaemia can cause neonatal hypoglycaemia[18]. Jovanovic and Peterson[19] in 1983 demonstrated that many women with insulin-dependent diabetes do not need any insulin to maintain euglycaemia during the active phase of labour, whether the labour was induced or had a spontaneous onset. The latter group did, however, require insulin during the second stage of labour. Others, including Golde *et al.*[20] and Moore[14], found that about half of their patients did require insulin throughout labour. Those most likely to need more insulin were patients whose insulin-dependent diabetes has been poorly controlled, and obese women with non-insulin-dependent diabetes associated with marked insulin resistance. The basic protocol used by Moore is detailed in Table 17.4 (see also pages 130 and 262).

Table 17.4. Guidelines for insulin infusion during labour and delivery in insulin-dependent diabetes and non-insulin-dependent diabetes

Capillary blood glucose (mmol/l)	Insulin infusion rate (units/h)
< 4.4	0.0
4.4–5.5	0.5
5.6–7.7	1.0
7.8–10.0	1.5
10.1–12.2	2.0
> 12.2	2.5

Notes
1. Constant infusion of 5% dextrose and 0.5% saline at 125 ml/h.
2. Guidelines will need to be adjusted for individual patients.
3. The capillary blood glucose should be measured hourly.
Adapted with permission from Moore[14].

If the woman is being induced, the morning insulin should be withheld and an intravenous infusion of 5% dextrose commenced as early as possible, particularly if she has been given medium- or long-acting insulin the evening before. For those being delivered by elective caesarean section, the operation should ideally be scheduled first thing in the morning to minimize unnecessary maternal metabolic disturbance which may flow on to the fetus.

Post delivery the mother's insulin requirements drop rapidly and usually return to her pre-pregnancy regimen within the first couple of days[21]. However, there can be quite marked swings in the maternal glucose levels especially if the mother is breastfeeding, so that close supervision is required until stabilization is achieved.

CONCLUSION

Meticulous antenatal management of maternal blood glucose, thus reducing fetal hyperinsulinism and its consequent associated complications which include macrosomia, chronic hypoxia and polyhydramnios, should minimize the need for premature induction of labour in women with established insulin-dependent or non-insulin-dependent diabetes, and especially those with gestational diabetes. The increased likelihood of spontaneous onset of labour will reduce the possibility of requiring delivery by caesarean section. Avoiding unnecessary energy intake during labour helps maintain maternal blood glucose within the normoglycaemic range, and again reduces neonatal metabolic complications. Because women with diabetes are in a high-risk category, close fetal monitoring is important.

REFERENCES

1 Peel J, Oakley WG. *Transactions of the 12th British Congress of Obstetrics and Gynaecology*, 1949; 161.
2 Peel J. A historical review of diabetes and pregnancy: *J Obstet Gynaecol Br Common* 1972; **79**: 385–95.
3 White P, Koshy P, Duckers J. The management of pregnancy complicated by diabetes and of children of diabetic mothers. *Med Clin North Am* 1953; **37**: 1481–96.
4 Roversi GD, Gargiulo M, Nicolini U *et al*. A new approach to the treatment of diabetic pregnant women. *Am J Obstet Gynecol* 1979; **135**: 567–76.
5 Drury MI, Stronge JM, Foley ME, MacDonald DW. Pregnancy in the diabetic patient: timing and mode of delivery. *Obstet Gynecol* 1983; **62**: 279–82.
6 Rasmussen MJ, Firth R, Foley M, Stronge JM. The timing of delivery in diabetic pregnancy: a 10-year review. *Aust N Z J Obstet Gynaecol* 1992; **32**: 313–17.
7 Kjos SL, Henry OA, Montoro M *et al*. Insulin requiring diabetes in pregnancy: a randomised trial of active induction of labor and expectant management. *Am J Obstet Gynecol* 1993; **169**: 611–15.
8 Coustan DR. Delivery: timing, mode and management. In: Reece EA, Coustan DR (eds), *Diabetes Mellitus in Pregnancy. Principles and Practices*. Churchill Livingstone, Edinburgh, 1988; 525–33.

9 Cousins L. Pregnancy complications among diabetic women: review 1965–1985. *Obstet Gynecol Survey* 1987; **42**: 140–9.

10 Neye RL. Infants of diabetic mothers: a quantitative morphological study. *Pediatrics* 1965; **35**: 980–8.

11 Keller JD, Lopez-Zeno JA, Dooley SL, Socol ML. Shoulder dystocia and birth trauma in gestational diabetes: a five-year experience. *Am J Obstet Gynecol* 1991; **165**: 928–30.

12 Chauhan SP, Cowan BD, Magann EF *et al.* Intrapartum detection of a macrosomic fetus: clinical versus 8 sonographic models. *Aust N Z J Obstet Gynaecol* 1995; **35**: 266–70.

13 Mountain KR. The infant of the diabetic mother. *Bailliere's Clin Obstet Gynaecol* 1991; **5**: 413–42.

14 Moore TR. Intrapartum management of labor and delivery. In: Hollingsworth DR (ed.), *Pregnancy, Diabetes and Birth*, 2nd edn. Williams & Wilkins, Baltimore, 1992; 226–37.

15 Quinn MA, Murphy AJ. Fetal death following extraamniotic prostaglandin gel: report of two cases. *Br J Obstet Gynaecol* 1981; **88**: 650–5.

16 Freeman R. Editorial. Intrapartum fetal monitoring: a disappointing story. *N Engl J Med* 1990; **322**: 624–6.

17 Olofsson P, Ingemarsson I, Solum T. Fetal distress during labour in diabetic pregnancy. In: Olofsson P (ed.), *Improved Care in Diabetic Pregnancy*, Vol. VII. Lund, 1986; 1–12.

18 Light IJ, Keenan WJ, Sutherland JM. Maternal intravenous glucose administration as a cause of hypoglycemia in the infant of the diabetic mother. *Am J Obstet Gynecol* 1972; **113**: 345–50.

19 Jovanovic L, Peterson CM. Insulin and glucose requirements during the first stage of labor in insulin-dependent women. *Am J Med* 1983; **75**: 607–12.

20 Golde SH, Good-Anderson B, Montoro M, Artal R. Insulin requirements during labor: a reappraisal. *Am J Obstet Gynecol* 1982; **144**: 556–9.

21 Hadden DR. Medical management of diabetes in pregnancy. *Bailliere's Clin Obstet Gynaecol* 1991; **5**: 369–94.

18

Neonatal Complications, Including Hypoglycaemia

JANE M. HAWDON[1] and ALBERT AYNSLEY-GREEN[2]
[1]University College Hospital, London, UK and
[2]Institute of Child Health, London, UK

Perinatal mortality rates for infants of diabetic mothers have reduced 10-fold in the last 40 years. In the 1940s the rate was approximately 40%. Now it does not differ significantly from that of infants of non-diabetic mothers and, in one single centre, rates have fallen from 26% in 1966 to 2–3% in 1990[1,2]. This reduction in mortality has thrown more emphasis on the need to address the neonatal morbidity associated with maternal diabetes. Although it is anticipated that careful attention to diabetic control in pregnancy and obstetric management will be associated with a reduction in the severity of neonatal complications to the extent that most babies may be cared for just as their counterparts who are not infants of diabetic mothers, some problems may persist. These problems may be related to obstetric factors such as preterm delivery, independently related to the presence of maternal diabetes, or arise as a result of both of these factors (e.g. respiratory distress syndrome).

HYPOGLYCAEMIA

UNDERLYING MECHANISMS AND PREVALENCE

Despite much previous and current interest, there is still considerable controversy regarding the management of neonatal hypoglycaemia in all at-risk groups, including infants of diabetic mothers, particularly with regard to the neurological implications of low blood glucose concentrations

Diabetes and Pregnancy: An International Approach to Diagnosis and Management.
Edited by A. Dornhorst and D. R. Hadden.
© 1996 John Wiley & Sons Ltd.

in the absence of fits or other clinical signs of hypoglycaemia[3]. Therefore, although there is much information regarding the pathogenesis of hypoglycaemia in the infant of the diabetic mother, there is as much uncertainty regarding its clinical significance as there is in other groups of neonates.

Neonatal hypoglycaemia in the infants of diabetic mothers has been recognized for many years[4]. It is thought to be secondary to neonatal hyperinsulinism, which is the result of fetal hyperglycaemia. The hypoglycaemic action of insulin is via the suppression of glycogenolysis and of gluconeogenesis[5]. However, infants of diabetic mothers have been shown to mount a counterregulatory hormone response which may curtail hypoglycaemia[6-8]. The prevalence of hypoglycaemia in infants of diabetic mothers varies between studies. This is not surprising in the light of the variations in diagnostic methods, in the levels of blood glucose concentration used to define hypoglycaemia, in the clinical management of pregnant diabetic women between centres and over time, in practices of glucose administration to mothers in labour, and in neonatal management, particularly feeding (Table 18.1). Even within individual studies, neonatal hypoglycaemia is not a universal finding. For example, in the study of Andersen *et al.*[9], despite the withholding of enteral or intravenous

Table 18.1. Prevalence of hypoglycaemia in published studies

Author	Date	Definition hypoglycaemia (mmol/l)	Age	Clinical details	Prevalence (%)
Karlsson and Kjellmer[14]	1972	<1.1		1961–1970	11
Francois et al.[44]	1974	<1.7	<5 days		61
Brans et al.[15]	1982	<2.2	<4h		52
Andersen et al.[9]	1982	<1.9	<24h	No i.v./enteral feeds	25
Andersen et al.[10]	1985	<1.8	<2h	Glucose in labour	21
Landon et al.[85]	1987	<1.7	<2h	Well controlled in preg. Poor control in preg.	19 41
Miodovnik et al.[47]	1987	<1.7	<4h	CS—no labour CS—labour SVD	43 36 23
Berk et al.[40]	1989	<2.2	<4h	Macrosomic Non macrosomic	60 50
Hanson and Persson[31]	1993	<1.7			8
Knip et al.[23]	1993	<1.7	<2h 4h	Pre feed Post feed	60 0

CS, caesarean section; SVD, spontaneous vaginal deliveries.

nutrition until 24 h of age, only 25% of the infants of diabetic mothers were hypoglycaemic. This suggests that each infant has a different susceptibility to hypoglycaemia.

The risk of neonatal hypoglycaemia has been related to various maternal factors. For example, early postnatal blood glucose concentrations have been negatively related to the maternal blood glucose concentration at delivery and to the cord plasma insulin concentration. Neonatal hypoglycaemia did not occur when the maternal blood glucose concentration at delivery was less than 7.1 mmol/l[10,11]. Early postnatal hypoglycaemia has also been described in infants whose non-diabetic mothers received intravenous glucose during labour[12]. These findings support the Pedersen hypothesis that maternal hyperglycaemia results in the sequence of fetal hyperglycaemia, fetal hyperinsulinaemia and neonatal hypoglycaemia[13]. However, no relationship has been demonstrated between longer-term maternal diabetic control, e.g. blood glucose concentration during pregnancy, haemoglobin A_{1c} (HbA$_{1c}$) level and the intensity of diabetic management, and the presence of neonatal hypoglycaemia[14-16]. Finally, neonatal hypoglycaemia has also been related to the passage of insulin antibodies across the placenta, but the clinical importance of this has waned with the increased use of human insulin[17].

Many studies fail to differentiate between transient low blood glucose concentrations shortly after birth, and hypoglycaemia which persists despite the introduction of enteral feeds. An early postnatal fall in blood glucose concentrations is an almost universal finding in neonates and is unlikely to be of pathological significance. Low blood glucose levels may even persist after this period in term, breastfed infants of non-diabetic mothers but such infants mount an effective counterregulatory ketogenic response, thus providing alternative fuels for cerebral metabolism[18,19]. Therefore, the diagnosis of hypoglycaemia as a pathological entity in the infant of the diabetic mother requires the demonstration of its persistence beyond the first few postnatal hours associated with a failure to mount a lipolytic and ketogenic response. Normal neonatal insulin/glucose relationships differ from those of adults in that insulin release is not totally suppressed at low blood glucose levels and circulating insulin concentrations may be higher than expected when compared to adult data[20,21]. Therefore, in order to demonstrate the postnatal persistence of hyperinsulinism in infants of diabetic mothers, their insulin/glucose relationships should be compared with similarly aged infants of non-diabetic mothers. Moreover, a highly specific insulin assay should be used to avoid cross-reaction with insulin propeptide molecules, which are abundant in neonatal plasma[21]. Such data relating to postnatal concentrations of glucose and alternative fuels and insulin/glucose relationships are not yet available for infants of diabetic mothers but it is likely that they have blood glucose and plasma insulin concentrations which revert to normal over the first postnatal day[8,22,23] (Hawdon, unpublished data, Table 18.2).

Table 18.2. Blood glucose and plasma insulin concentrations (median, range, number of subjects) in preterm neonates of non-diabetic mothers and neonates of variable gestation of diabetic mothers who attended combined diabetic–antenatal clinics. Although the infants of diabetic mothers had lower blood glucose concentrations and higher plasma insulin concentrations on the first postnatal day, ranges for insulin were wide in both groups of neonates and no differences were seen after 24 h of age. Note the absence of high cord blood glucose concentrations in the infants of diabetic mothers, suggesting that intrapartum diabetic control was good

	Infants of non-diabetic mothers		Infants of diabetic mothers	
Plasma insulin concentration (pmol/l)				
Cord	64 (8–166)	(9)	187 (8–567)	(5)
<2 h	50 (8–133)	(13)	68 (17–201)	(7)
2–24 h	46 (11–122)	(12)	91 (57–389)	(7)*
Day 2	52 (17–178)	(9)	84 (33–311)	(8)
Day 3	29 (13–192)	(15)	46 (8–306)	(6)
Day 4	52 (5–199)	(9)	111 (23–497)	(5)
Day 5	52 (13–191)	(8)	61 (14–271)	(5)
Birth–5 days	50 (5–199)	(75)	70 (8–567)	(43)**
Blood glucose concentration (mmol/l)				
Cord	4.7 (2.3–11)	(9)	4.1 (2.4–5.7)	(6)
<2 h	2.9 (1.5–13.9)	(14)	1.6 (1.5–4.0)	(7)
2–24 h	5.3 (1.9–15.0)	(12)	3.1 (1.6–4.7)	(9)*
Day 2	4.1 (2.3–6.8)	(10)	4.0 (1.5–4.8)	(8)
Day 3	4.0 (2.5–9.7)	(15)	4.1 (3.0–6.3)	(6)
Day 4	4.4 (2.0–8.8)	(11)	3.8 (3.7–10.5)	(5)
Day 5	4.1 (2.1–9.2)	(8)	4.0 (3.1–5.0)	(5)
Birth–5 days	4.2 (1.5–15.0)	(79)	3.8 (1.5–10.5)	(46)*

*$p < 0.05$; **$p < 0.01$.
Hawdon *et al.* (unpublished data).

ALTERNATIVE FUELS

If hypoglycaemia is secondary to hyperinsulinism, then there is additional concern regarding the availability of alternative fuels such as free fatty acids and ketone bodies, which are thought to be important in postnatal metabolic adaptation in term infants of non-diabetic mothers[20]. Although it has been reported that one-day-old infants of diabetic mothers, especially those who were hypoglycaemic, had lower free fatty acid concentrations than infants of non-diabetic mothers, recent stable isotope turnover studies have failed to demonstrate a difference between these two groups in terms of fatty acid and ketone body concentrations and rates of lipolysis[9,24]. Further studies are required to document ketone body/glucose relationships in infants of diabetic mothers beyond the first postnatal day and to compare these relationships with infants of non-diabetic mothers.

NEUROLOGICAL IMPLICATIONS

The major clinical concern relating to neonatal hypoglycaemia is the risk of neurological damage[25]. There are no adequate prospective controlled studies, even in infants of non-diabetic mothers, which have investigated the acute and long-term effects of hypoglycaemia, nor any which have determined whether transient self-limiting hypoglycaemia is less harmful than persistent hypoglycaemia. However, it is of interest to note that the fetuses of diabetic rats and dogs have a higher brain glycogen content than controls, and thus may be protected from the potential neurological sequelae of low blood glucose concentrations by local mobilization of glucose from glycogen[26,27]. Although neonatal hypoglycaemia has not been independently implicated in any adverse outcome for the infant of the diabetic mother, in order to provide complete reassurance for clinicians and parents the neurological implications must be investigated with a large enough cohort to define outcome in relation to neonatal hypoglycaemia after controlling for other perinatal risk factors, and by collecting antenatal data to examine the effect of maternal hypoglycaemia which may result in fetal hypoglycaemia[22,28]. It is of greater concern that lower intelligence in childhood has been related to raised maternal non-esterified fatty acid and β-hydroxybutyrate concentrations in the third trimester, after correcting for other perinatal and social influences[29].

CLINICAL MANAGEMENT

In view of the potential adverse neurological effects of neonatal hypoglycaemia and hypoketonaemia, many clinicians choose to screen for hypoglycaemia in infants of diabetic mothers. However, it is not known whether all such infants are at risk and should have blood glucose monitoring or whether severe hypoglycaemia is restricted to a small number who could be identified for screening by clinical parameters, such as the quality of maternal intrapartum diabetic control. It is now widely accepted that glucose reagent strips are insufficiently accurate for the diagnosis of hypoglycaemia and low readings should be confirmed by accurate blood glucose analysis[3]. The question regarding the blood glucose level at which treatment should be commenced cannot be satisfactorily determined until further studies of neurological function and the counterregulatory response are made in infants of diabetic mothers[3].

It is likely that hyperinsulinism and hypoglycaemia are transient phenomena in most infants of diabetic mothers (Hawdon, unpublished data, Table 18.2). Therefore, the initial management of the otherwise healthy infant of a diabetic mother should consist of early and regular enteral feeds, with particular emphasis on the establishment of breastfeeding. Blood glucose concentrations may be monitored in infants who are most at risk of hypoglycaemia (such as those whose mothers had poor diabetic control or were hyperglycaemic in labour), for the first 24 h starting before the second feed and consideration should be given to formula feed supplementation of breast feeds if blood glucose concentrations are low (less than 2.0–2.5 mmol/l).

If blood glucose concentrations remain low in two consecutive pre-feed measurements despite optimizing enteral intakes, or if the baby has signs of hypoglycaemia (fits or reduced level of consciousness), intravenous glucose may be commenced, initially at a rate of 5 mg/kg per minute (3 ml/kg per hour of 10% dextrose) and increased according to blood glucose concentrations. If neonatal hyperinsulinism results in excessively high glucose requirements (greater than 10 mg/kg per minute), glucose solutions of strengths greater than 10% may be required and the insertion of a percutaneous silastic long line will be required because of the risk of extravasation injury when concentrated glucose solutions are used. Enteral feeds should not be discontinued or reduced when intravenous glucose is commenced, unless the baby has other complications placing it at risk of fluid overload, such as congenital heart disease. As the baby spontaneously recovers its own glucose control, the intravenous glucose rate may be gradually reduced in stages to minimize the risk of rebound hypoglycaemia. Accurate blood glucose monitoring is essential for the management of the infant of the diabetic mother who is receiving intravenous glucose.

As with any other baby undergoing neonatal intensive care, blood glucose monitoring and treatment of hypoglycaemia are important aspects of clinical management of the infant of the diabetic mother who has other major clinical problems, such as respiratory distress or perinatal asphyxia.

If hypoglycaemia proves to be a transient self-limiting entity in most infants of diabetic mothers, it will be unnecessarily meddlesome to perform frequent blood glucose estimations on otherwise healthy babies and to deny mothers the opportunity for exclusive breastfeeding. However, many authors have described practices, such as elective admission to neonatal units and intravenous glucose infusions for infants of diabetic mothers, which are sure to compromise successful breastfeeding and will increase the workload of neonatal units[2]. Therefore, it is of major importance to establish the significance of neonatal hypoglycaemia in infants of diabetic mothers so that scientifically based management policies may be established. Until such studies are performed our pragmatic recommendations are to carry out pre-feed blood glucose monitoring of such infants on the first postnatal day, to supplement early breast feeds with formula milk if blood glucose levels are low, and to consider intravenous glucose therapy if blood glucose levels are persistently low despite optimizing enteral milk intake. Not all infants of diabetic mothers will become hypoglycaemic and if early blood glucose levels are satisfactory monitoring should be discontinued[30].

MACROSOMIA

Like other complications of being the infant of a diabetic mother, lower incidences of macrosomia appear to be related to improved maternal diabetic management. Twenty per cent of infants of diabetic mothers born in Sweden in 1982–1985 had birth weights above the 97th centile but in an Italian study of strict maternal diabetic control only 8% of infants had birth weights above the 90th centile[31,32]. However, neonatal birth weights above the 97th centile, and macrosomia involving mainly heart, liver and spleen, still occur in some infants after pregnancies complicated by diabetes[22]. It has even been suggested that there is a unimodal right shift in the population of infants of diabetic mothers when compared to infants of non-diabetic mothers so that all the former, irrespective of their position on centile charts, may have birth weights greater than their 'genetic potential'[33].

Macrosomia may be secondary to increased substrate availability, to the somatotrophic action of insulin via its binding to insulin-like growth factor 1 (IGF-I) receptors, or to insulin-induced increases in circulating IGF-I concentrations[34,35]. Studies in experimental animals have demonstrated that there is increased protein synthesis in selected tissues (brain, heart, liver) as well as increased adiposity in young animals born after diabetic pregnancy[36]. Infants of diabetic mothers usually have 'normal' body measurements by six months of age, but have an increased risk of obesity in adolescence[37]. This may represent another example of 'programming', whereby the intrauterine environment manifests its effects even in adult life[38].

The presence of macrosomia has been related to elevated cord C-peptide concentrations but it is of interest that macrosomia is not independently associated with increased risk of other neonatal complications of diabetic pregnancies such as hypoglycaemia[15,22,39,40]. Many neonatologists choose to screen for neonatal hypoglycaemia in macrosomic infants of diabetic mothers (and even in large babies who are not infants of diabetic mothers). Prospective studies are required to establish whether the macrosomic infant of the diabetic mother really is at greater risk of persistent hypoglycaemia.

Labour and delivery may be prolonged and complicated when babies are macrosomic, thus increasing the risk of perinatal asphyxia and birth trauma[16]. However, the risks of caesarean section to mother and baby, for example anaesthetic risks to the mother and increased incidence of respiratory morbidity in the infant, must also be considered in the decision regarding mode of delivery.

It must not be forgotten that occasionally infants of diabetic mothers have experienced intrauterine growth retardation and will be small for gestational age[41]. This may be because of maternal diabetic vasculopathy leading to placental insufficiency, or because antenatal blood glucose concentrations have been maintained at too low a level[42]. On the other hand, studies in animals suggest that hyperglycaemia in a narrow interval early in pregnancy may impair fetal development and that the growth retardation may be secondary to reduced IGF-II expression, but this has not been explored in human subjects[43]. Small-for-gestational age infants of diabetic mothers present different clinical problems from those who are macrosomic in that their body energy stores will be diminished and they are at greater risk for perinatal asphyxia. They should be managed in the same way as other small-for-gestational age babies with early and frequent enteral feeds or intravenous nutrition[3].

RESPIRATORY COMPLICATIONS

Earlier studies showed that the respiratory distress syndrome was a major contributor to the high mortality rate of infants of diabetic mothers. The relative risk of this occurring was 5.6 times greater in infants of diabetic mothers, and the syndrome was more common when maternal diabetic control was poor[14,44–46]. Although mortality in infants of diabetic mothers has improved, more recent studies have confirmed that they are still at greater risk of the respiratory distress syndrome and transient tachypnoea of the newborn, especially after caesarean section. The incidence of the respiratory distress syndrome after caesarean section without labour was 20%, compared to 10% after vaginal delivery in one study[47]. Others have reported lower incidences; for example, in Sweden between 1982 and 1985 the incidence of the respiratory distress syndrome was 1.6% in infants of diabetic mothers compared to 0.6% in infants of non-diabetic mothers, and of transient tachypnoea of the newborn 3.3% in infants of diabetic mothers compared to 0.8%[31].

Studies of fetal rat and rabbit type II pneumocytes have shown that insulin inhibits cortisol-induced lecithin synthesis, probably by inhibiting the production of fibroblast–pneumocyte factor which promotes phosphatidylcholine synthesis[48,49]. Other studies of fetal rat lung explants have demonstrated that high glucose concentrations inhibit the incorporation of choline into phosphatidylcholine and that butyrate inhibits the transcription of mRNA for surfactant proteins[50,51]. These mechanisms may combine to result in surfactant deficiency and the increased incidence of the respiratory distress syndrome in infants of diabetic mothers[52,53].

Some authors still recommend the assessment of lung maturation by determining lecithin:sphingomyelin ratios in amniotic fluid prior to planned delivery but this is not commonly practised in the UK and will not rule out delayed development of the surfactant-associated proteins[1,22,41]. Recent evidence suggests that the respiratory distress syndrome and transient tachypnoea of the newborn occur in a substantial number of infants of non-diabetic mothers when delivery (especially by caesarean section) is before term[54]. To minimize respiratory complications in infants of diabetic mothers, obstetricians should aim to deliver each infant as close to term as possible, to allow delivery to occur after spontaneous onset of labour, and to prescribe antenatal steroid treatment for mothers who may deliver before term in order to enhance fetal lung maturity. There is no published evidence that administration of steroids to diabetic mothers disrupts diabetic control. Postnatal management of the infant of the diabetic mother does not differ from that of the infants of non-diabetic mothers in terms of investigation and treatment of respiratory distress.

HYPOCALCAEMIA

Recent texts suggest that this is a frequent biochemical complication for the infant of the diabetic mother[22], but its significance in terms of serious clinical manifestations has not been documented. It has been suggested that maternal urinary magnesium loss and the resulting magnesium deficiency in the diabetic mother and her fetus inhibit the recovery of parathyroid hormone levels (which fall and then rise in the normal neonate after birth) resulting in neonatal hypocalcaemia[55,56]. Hypocalcaemia ($<2\,mmol/l$ in term infants and $<1.75\,mmol/l$ in preterm infants) and hypomagnesaemia ($<0.66\,mmol/l$) were found in 17.6% and 9.8% respectively of neonates whose mothers had strict diabetic control, and in 31.7% and 15.1% of neonates whose mothers were less well controlled[55]. In this study, the serum calcium concentration was inversely related to maternal HbA_{1c} level at delivery, suggesting that third trimester diabetic control influences maternal magnesium concentrations and the development of neonatal hypocalcaemia.

However, none of the studies which document hypocalcaemia in infants of diabetic mothers indicates whether hypocalcaemia was transient or prolonged or whether it was associated with clinical signs or complications. Hypocalcaemia is usually self-limiting and very rarely presents with clinical signs. Management may be expectant and routine monitoring of plasma calcium concentrations is not necessary in the otherwise healthy infant of the diabetic mother. If clinical signs are seen, hypocalcaemia and hypomagnesaemia should be corrected according to standard protocols[57].

POLYCYTHAEMIA

Only a few studies have commented on this complication, with variation in reported incidence from 7% in non-macrosomic infants of diabetic mothers to 24% in those who were macrosomic. It is thought to be more common after vaginal delivery than after caesarean section[40,47]. Lysis of this red cell load may explain the higher than usual incidence of hyperbilirubinaemia in infants of diabetic mothers[31].

The mechanism for polycythaemia is thought to be the high cellular metabolic rate for glucose as a result of insulin-stimulated glucose entry, resulting in increased cellular oxygen uptake, relative hypoxaemia and stimulation of erythropoietin[58,59]. Evidence for the presence of fetal hypoxaemia and cellular hypoxia comes from studies of experimental animals whose fetuses were rendered hyperinsulinaemic or hyperglycaemic and from human cordocentesis studies which have demonstrated that blood lactate concentrations in third trimester fetuses of diabetic mothers are higher than those of controls and are inversely proportional to blood partial pressures of oxygen[22,59,60].

It is unlikely that clinically significant sequelae result from mild polycythaemia and hyperbilirubinaemia in most infants of diabetic mothers but monitoring and management should be according to routine local neonatal practice and partial plasma exchange should be carried out if a venous haematocrit is greater than 70%.

CONGENITAL MALFORMATIONS

The increased incidence of congenital abnormalities has been documented by many authors (varying from 5% to 11%, compared to 1–2% in infants of non-diabetic mothers), and appears to be related to the quality of maternal diabetic control particularly in early pregnancy[11,14,22]. Lower incidences have been reported in one study of strict diabetic control during pregnancy (1.6%) and in another group who received specialized antenatal diabetic management within 21 days of conception (4.9%)[32,61]. A further study from Denmark documented a decline in the malformation rate in an unselected population of diabetic mothers from 7.2% in the years 1967–1981 to 3.1% in the years 1981–1986, with a particularly low incidence (1%) in those who had planned pregnancy and pre-pregnancy counselling[62]. Many diverse abnormalities have been described and some have a much greater incidence in infants of diabetic mothers than in the normal population (Table 18.3). It should be noted that data are taken from studies performed more than a decade ago and there are no recent large studies of the incidence of congenital malformations in infants of diabetic mothers.

Although the precise nature of the teratogen is not known, maternal hyperglycaemia in the first trimester, at the time of organogenesis, is a poor prognostic factor[63]. Infants of diabetic mothers with major non-central nervous system malformations were found to have lower IQ measures than those without malformations at follow-up to three years, and infants of mothers with less good diabetic control had smaller head circumferences and impaired language development than those with good diabetic control or non-diabetic controls[64]. The same factors which are teratogenic in terms of somatic malformations may also adversely affect brain development at a critical stage. This emphasizes the importance of optimal diabetic control, even before conception, as the critical period may occur very early in

Table 18.3. The incidence and relative risk of those congenital malformations in infants of diabetic mothers thought to be of significantly greater incidence than in infants of non-diabetic mothers

Malformation	Incidence/1000 births	Relative risk cf. infants of non-diabetic mothers
Cardiac	10	4
Anencephaly	3	5
Arthrogryphosis	0.3	28
Ureteral duplication	0.7	23
Cystic kidney	0.6	4
Renal agenesis	0.3	5
Anorectal atresia	0.3	4
Caudal regression	1.3	212
Pseudohermaphroditism	0.6	11

From Combs and Kitzmiller[86].

pregnancy. Increased antenatal surveillance should detect many of the congenital malformations so that termination of pregnancy may be discussed or appropriate plans made for delivery and neonatal management. Nowadays it is usual and desirable for neonatologists to become involved in the counselling of parents and the planning of postnatal management, and the delivery of affected infants should take place in obstetric units where comprehensive neonatal and surgical support is available.

CARDIAC ABNORMALITIES

In addition to the increased incidence of structural congenital heart disease, infants of diabetic mothers are at risk of reversible cardiac abnormalities such as cardiomyopathy and asymmetric septal hypertrophy[65-67]. The prevalences reported in one study were 8.2% for structural heart defects and 31% for asymmetric septal hypertrophy. Cardiomyopathy may be more common in macrosomic infants of diabetic mothers (8.3% compared to 1.8% in normal-sized infants)[2,68].

Septal hypertrophy may be a consequence of high fetal insulin levels acting on insulin or IGF-II receptors which are present in high density particularly in the interventricular septum[69,70]. Studies in adults have demonstrated that prolonged hyperinsulinaemia results in pathological changes in arterial smooth muscle which are associated with the development of atherosclerosis, and that hyperinsulinism is independently associated with hypertension[71,72]. It is not known whether these processes occur in the presence of prolonged fetal hyperinsulinaemia, but it has been shown that hyperinsulinaemic fetal sheep have altered proportions of vasoconstricting and vasodilating prostaglandins, and this may contribute to fetal cardiovascular disease[73].

Most cases of cardiomyopathy and asymmetric septal hypertrophy resolve spontaneously over the first few postnatal weeks and few compromise the infant's clinical condition. Severe cases may present with cardiac failure and signs of respiratory distress such as tachypnoea, increased oxygen requirements and poor feeding. The long-term effects of perinatal hyperinsulinism in terms of adult cardiovascular disease have not yet been defined. The advice of paediatric cardiologists should be sought for the assessment and management of babies who have symptomatic cardiomyopathy.

PERINATAL MORTALITY

Although perinatal mortality rates in infants of diabetic mothers are falling, most studies still report them to be higher than normal (19% in one study of babies born in 1958–1971, and 3.1% (four times the national average) in infants of diabetic mothers born in Sweden in 1982–1985)[5,31,44]. An early study demonstrated that perinatal mortality rate was related to maternal diabetic control (good control 3.8%, poor control 24%; intensive management 9.4%, non-intensive management 21.4%)[14]. Few studies have differentiated between the perinatal mortality associated with congenital abnormalities and that arising as a result of perinatal complications such as perinatal asphyxia, which may occur in up to 27% of infants of diabetic mothers and is most common when there is maternal nephropathy or maternal hyperglycaemia prior to delivery[74]. The identification of fetuses at risk of treatable causes of death would allow closer monitoring in pregnancy and labour and the delivery of the infant at a centre where neonatal intensive care is available.

GESTATIONAL DIABETES

The above discussion relates mainly to infants of mothers who were insulin dependent prior to pregnancy. The complications for infants of gestational diabetes are less clearly defined. There is some debate as to whether these babies have greater morbidity than infants of non-diabetic mothers but, as with the infant of the insulin-dependent diabetic mother, obstetricians and neonatologists should be aware that the infant of the gestational diabetic mother may be at risk of macrosomia and complications of delivery, depending on the degree of antenatal perturbation and blood glucose concentrations[42,75]. It has been reported that morbidity is less when mothers with gestational diabetes receive insulin treatment rather than dietary management[76-81]. In truth, there is probably a continuum of glucose tolerance in pregnancy, as blood glucose levels and glucose disposal rates after a glucose tolerance test are distributed unimodally in non-diabetic mothers, and the frequencies of the characteristic manifestations of fetal hyperinsulinism have continuous relationships with the degree of glucose intolerance[82,83].

CONCLUSION

It is anticipated that pre-conceptional counselling, close attention to maternal diabetic control in pregnancy, reduction in preterm delivery and caesarean section rates, and avoidance of maternal hyperglycaemia in labour will further reduce the prevalence of complications in infants of diabetic mothers so that ultimately their postnatal management need not differ from that of any other healthy baby. However, some mothers do not receive such intensive antenatal care whilst others have diabetes which is particularly difficult to control. Paediatricians should be alert for adverse sequelae in the infants of these mothers, but at the same time should endeavour to nurse the baby and mother together and minimize invasive treatments. Prospective studies are required to investigate the exact perinatal morbidity associated with maternal diabetes in the current era, particularly with respect to the incidence and clinical significance of hypoglycaemia, hypocalcaemia and polycythaemia. In addition, in the light of recent studies which have raised the concept of 'programming' of the human fetus and neonate by the intrauterine and early postnatal environments, the long-term sequelae for the offspring of maternal diabetics should be investigated[38,84].

REFERENCES

1 Hunter DJS. Diabetes in pregnancy. In: Chalmers I, Enkin M, Keirse MJNC (eds), *Effective Care in Pregnancy and Childbirth*. Oxford University Press, Oxford, 1992; 579–94.
2 Mountain KR. The infant of the diabetic mother. *Clin Obstet Gynaecol* 1991; **5**: 413–42.
3 Hawdon JM, Ward Platt MP, Aynsley-Green A. Prevention and management of neonatal hypoglycaemia. *Arch Dis Child* 1994; **70**: 60–5.
4 Komrower CM. Blood sugar levels in babies born of diabetic mothers. *Arch Dis Child* 1954; **29**: 28–33.
5 Jame P, Ktorza A, Bihoreau MT *et al*. Impaired hepatic glycogenolysis related to hyperinsulinaemia in newborns from hyperglycaemic pregnant rats. *Pediatr Res* 1990; **28**: 646–51.
6 Artal R, Doug N, Wu P, Sperling MA. Circulating catecholamines and glucagon in infants of strictly controlled diabetic mothers. *Biol Neonate* 1988; **53**: 121–5.
7 Broberger U, Hansson U, Lagercrantz H, Persson B. Sympathoadrenal activity and metabolic adjustment during the first 12 hours after birth in infants of diabetic mothers. *Acta Paediatr Scand* 1984; **73**: 620–5.
8 Hestel J, Kuhl C. Metabolic adaptations during the neonatal period in infants in diabetic mothers. *Acta Endocrinol* (Suppl.) 1986; **277**: 136–40.
9 Andersen GE, Hestel J, Kuhl J, Molsted-Pederson L. Metabolic events in infants of diabetic mothers during the first twenty four hours after birth. II. Changes in plasma lipids. *Acta Paediatr Scand* 1982; **71**: 27 32.
10 Andersen O, Hestel J, Scholonker L, Kuhl C. Influence of the maternal plasma glucose concentration at delivery on the risk of hypoglycaemia in infants of insulin dependent diabetic mothers. *Acta Paediatr Scand* 1985; **74**: 268–73.

11 Plehwe WE, Storey CN, Sharman RP, Turtle JR. Outcome of pregnancy complicated by diabetes: experience with 232 patients in a 4 year period. *Diabetes Res* 1984; **1**: 67–73.
12 Philipson EH, Kalhan SC, Rika MM, Pimental R. Effects of maternal glucose infusion on fetal acid–base status in human pregnancy. *Am J Obstet Gynecol* 1987; **157**: 866–73.
13 Pedersen J, Bojsen-Moller B, Poulsen H. Blood sugar in newborn infants of diabetic mothers. *Acta Endocrinol* 1954; **15**: 33.
14 Karlsson K, Kjellmer I. The outcome of diabetic pregnancies in relation to the mother's blood sugar level. *Am J Obstet Gynecol* 1972; **112**: 213–20.
15 Brans YW, Huff RW, Shannon DC, Hunter MA. Maternal diabetes and neonatal macrosomia. I. Post partum neonatal maternal haemoglobin A1c levels and neonatal hypoglycaemia. *Pediatrics* 1982; **70**: 576–81.
16 McFarland KF, Himayu E. Neonatal morbidity in infants of diabetic mothers. *Diabetes Care* 1985; **8**: 333–6.
17 Murata K, Toyoda N, Sugigama U. The effects of insulin antibodies during diabetic pregnancy on newborn infants. *Asia Oceania J Obstet Gynecol* 1990; **16**: 115–22.
18 Srinivasan G, Pildes RS, Cattamanchi G *et al*. Plasma glucose values in normal neonates: a new look. *J Pediatr* 1986; **109**: 114–17.
19 Hawdon JM, Ward Platt MP, Aynsley-Green A. Patterns of metabolic adaptation for preterm and term infants in the first neonatal week. *Arch Dis Child* 1992; **67**: 357–65.
20 Hawdon JM, Aynsley-Green A, Alberti KGMM, Ward Platt MP. The role of pancreatic insulin secretion in neonatal glucoregulation. I. Healthy term and preterm infants. *Arch Dis Child* 1993; **68**: 274–9.
21 Hawdon JM, Hubbard M, Hales CN, Clark P. The use of a specific immunoradiometric assay to determine preterm neonatal insulin–glucose relationships. *Arch Dis Child* 1995; **73**: F166–9.
22 Cornblath M, Schwartz R. Infant of the diabetic mother. In: Cornblath M, Schwartz R (eds), *Disorders of Carbohydrate Metabolism in Infancy*. BSP, Boston, 1991; 125–74.
23 Knip M, Kaapa P, Koivisto M. Hormonal enteroinsular axis in newborn infants of insulin treated diabetic mothers. *J Clin Endocrinol Metab* 1993; **77**: 1340–4.
24 Patel D, Kalhan S. Glycerol metabolism and triglyceride-fatty acid cycling in the human newborn: effect of maternal diabetes and intrauterine growth retardation. *Pediatr Res* 1992; **31**: 52–8.
25 Cornblath M, Schwartz R, Aynsley-Green A, Lloyd JK. Hypoglycaemia in infancy: the need for a rational definition. A Ciba Foundation discussion meeting. *Pediatrics* 1990; **85**: 834–7.
26 Brennan WA, Wees BA, Swierczynski SL. The effect of maternal diabetes on glycogen metabolism in the embryonic rat. *Biochem Inst* 1991; **23**: 769–77.
27 Kliegman RM, Miettinen EC, Campbell G. Enhanced cerebral substrate pools in the fetus and neonate of the diabetic canine mother. Diabetes 1985; 34: 129–34.
28 Persson B, Gentz J. Follow-up of children of insulin-dependent and gestational diabetic mothers: neuropsychological outcome. *Acta Paediatr Scand* 1984; **73**: 349–58.
29 Rizzo T, Metzger BE, Burns WJ, Burns K. Correlations between antepartum maternal metabolism and child intelligence. *N Engl J Med* 1991; **825**: 911–16.
30 Hawdon JM, Aynsley-Green A. Hypoglycaemia in the newborn. *Curr Pediatr* 1994; **4**: 168–73.
31 Hanson U, Persson B. Outcome of pregnancies complicated by type I insulin dependent diabetes in Sweden: acute pregnancy complications, neonatal mortality and morbidity. *Am J Perinatol* 1993; **10**: 330–3.
32 Roversi GD, Garguilo M, Nicolini U *et al*. A new approach to the treatment of diabetic pregnant women. *Am J Obstet Gynecol* 1979; **135**: 567–76.
33 Bradley RJ, Nicolaides KH, Brudenell JM. Are all infants of diabetic mothers 'macrosomic'? *Br Med J* **297**: 1583–4.
34 Delmis J, Drazannsic A, Ivanisevic M, Suchanek E. Glucose, insulin, HGH and IGFI levels in maternal serum, amniotic fluid and umbilical venous serum: a comparison between late normal pregnancy and pregnancies complicated with diabetes and fetal growth retardation. *J Perinat Med* 1992; **20**: 47–56.
35 Milner RDG, Hill DJ. Fetal growth control: the role of insulin and related peptides. *Clin Endocrinol* 1984; **21**: 415–33.

36 Johnson JD, Dunham T, Wogenisch FJ *et al*. Fetal hyperinsulinaemia and protein turnover in fetal rat tissues. *Diabetes* 1990; **39**: 541–8.

37 Anon. Hyperinsulinaemia and macrosomia. *N Engl J Med* 1990; **323**: 340–2.

38 Barker DJP. *Fetal and Infant Origins of Adult Disease*. British Medical Journal, London, 1992.

39 Stenninger E, Schollin J, Aman J. Neonatal macrosomia and hypoglycaemia in children of mothers with insulin treated gestational diabetes mellitus. *Acta Paediatr Scand* 1992; **80**: 1014–18.

40 Berk MA, Mimoumi F, Miodovnik M *et al*. Macrosomia in infants of insulin dependent mothers. *Pediatrics* 1989; **83**: 1029–34.

41 Cordero L, Landon MB. Infant of the diabetic mother. *Clin Perinatol* 1993; **20**: 635–48.

42 Langer O, Levy J, Brustman C. Glycemic control in gestational diabetes mellitus. How tight is tight enough: small for gestational age versus large for gestational age? *Am J Obstet Gynecol* 1989; **161**: 646–53.

43 Chernicky CL, Redline RW, Tan HQ *et al*. Expression of insulin-like growth factors I and II in conceptuses from normal and diabetic mice. *Mol Reprod Dev* 1994; **37**: 382–90.

44 Francois R, Picaud JJ, Ruitton-Ugliengo A *et al*. The newborn of diabetic mothers. *Biol Neonate* 1974; **24**: 1–31.

45 Robert M, Neff R, Hubbel J *et al*. Association between maternal diabetes and the respiratory distress syndrome in the newborn. *N Engl J Med* 1976; **294**: 357–60.

46 Usher RH, Allen AC, McLean FH. Risk of respiratory distress syndrome related to gestational age, route of delivery and maternal diabetes. *Am J Obstet Gynecol* 1971; **111**: 826–32.

47 Miodovnik M, Mimoumi F, Tsang RC *et al*. Management of the insulin dependent diabetic during labor and delivery: influences on neonatal outcome. *Am J Perinatol* 1987; **4**: 106–14.

48 Smith BT, Giroud CJP, Robert M, Avery ME. Insulin antagonism of the cortisol action on lecithin synthesis by cultured fetal lung cells. *J Pediatr* 1975; **87**: 953–5.

49 Carlson KS, Smith BT, Pool M. Insulin acts on the fibroblast to inhibit glucocorticoid stimulation of lung maturation. *J Appl Physiol* 1984; **57**: 1577–9.

50 Gewolb IH. High glucose causes delayed fetal lung maturation in vitro. *Exp Lung Res* 1993; **19**: 619–30.

51 Peterec SM, Nichols KV, Dynia DW *et al*. Butyrate modulates surfactant protein m RNA in fetal rat lung by altering mRNA transcription and stability. *Am J Physiol* 1994; **267**: L9–15.

52 Bourbon JR, Farrell PM. Fetal lung development in the diabetic pregnancy. *Pediatr Res* 1985; 19: 253–67.

53 Stubbs WA, Stubbs SM. Hyperinsulinism, diabetes mellitus and respiratory distress of the newborn: a common link? *Lancet* 1978; **i**: 308–9.

54 Morrisson JJ, Rennie J, Milton PJD. Neonatal respiratory morbidity and timing of elective caesarean section at term. *Br J Obstet Gynaecol* 1995; **102**: 101–6.

55 Demaini S, Mimouni F, Tsang RC *et al*. Impact of metabolic control of diabetes during pregnancy on neonatal hypocalcaemia: a randomized study. *Obstet Gynecol* 1994; **83**: 918–22.

56 Mimouni F, Tsang RC, Hertzberg VS *et al*. Parathyroid hormone and calcitriol changes in normal and insulin dependent diabetic pregnancies. *Obstet Gynecol* 1989; **74**: 49–54.

57 Barnes ND. Endocrine disorders. In: Roberton NRC (ed.), *Textbook of Neonatology*. Churchill Livingstone, Edinburgh, 1992; 806–7.

58 Widness JA, Susa JB, Garcia JF *et al*. Increased erythropoiesis and elevated erythropoietin in infants born to diabetic mothers and in hyperinsulinaemic rhesus fetuses. *J Clin Invest* 1981; **67**: 637–42.

59 Phillipps AF, Dubin JW, Malty PJ, Raye JR. Anetanatal hypoxaemia and hyperinsulinaemia in the chronically hyperglycaemic fetal lamb. *Pediatr Res* 1982; **16**: 653–8.

60 Bradley RJ, Brudenell JM, Nicolaides KH. Fetal acidosis and hyperlacticaemia diagnosed by cordocentesis in pregnancies complicated by maternal diabetes mellitus. *Diabetes Med* 1991; **8**: 464–8.

61 Mills JL, Knopp RH, Simpson JL *et al*. Lack of relation of increased malformation rates in infants of diabetic mothers to glycemic control during organogenesis. *N Engl J Med* 1988; **318**: 671–6.

62 Damm P, Molsted-Pedersen L. Significant decrease in congenital malformations in

newborn infants of an unselected population of diabetic mothers. *Am J Obstet Gynecol* 1989; **161**: 1163–7.

63 Miller E, Hare JW, Cloherty JP *et al.* Elevated maternal hemoglobin A1c in early pregnancy and major congenital anomalies in infants of diabetic mothers. *N Engl J Med* 1981; **304**: 1331–4.

64 Sells CJ, Robinson NM, Brown Z, Knopp RH. Long term developmental follow up of infants of diabetic mothers. *J Pediatr* 1994; **125**: S9–17.

65 Gutgessell HP, Spur ME, Rosenberg HS. Characterization of the cardiomyopathy in infants of diabetic mothers. *Circulation* 1980; **61**: 441–9.

66 Veille J-C, Sivakoff M, Hanson R, Fanaroff AA. Interventricular septal thickness in fetuses of diabetic mothers. *Obstet Gynecol* 1992; **79**: 51–4.

67 Wolfe RR, Way GL. Cardiomyopathies in infants of diabetic mothers. *Johns Hopkins Med J* 1977; **140**: 177–80.

68 Cooper MJ, Enderlein MA, Tarsoff H, Roge CL. Asymmetric septal hypertrophy in infants of diabetic mothers: fetal echocardiography and the impact of maternal diabetic control. *Am J Dis Child* 1992; **146**: 226–9.

69 Breitwesser JA, Meyer RA, Sperling MA *et al.* Cardiac septal hypertrophy in hyperinsulinaemic infants. *J Pediatr* 1980; **96**: 535–9.

70 Geffner ME, Santulli TV, Kaplan SA. Hypertrophic cardiomyopathy in total lipodystrophy: insulin action in the face of insulin resistance. *J Pediatr* 1987; **110**: 161.

71 Stout RW. Insulin and atheroma: 20 year perspective. *Diabetes Care* 1990; **13**: 631–54.

72 Reaven GM, Hoffman BB. Hypertension as a disease of carbohydrate and lipoprotein metabolism. *Am J Med* 1989; **87**: 2s–6s.

73 Stonestreet BS, Ogburn PI, Goldstein M *et al.* Effects of chronic fetal hyperinsulinaemia on plasma arachidonic acid and prostaglandin concentrations. *Am J Obstet Gynecol* 1989; **161**: 894–9.

74 Mimouni F, Miodovnik M, Siddiqi TA *et al.* Perinatal asphyxia in infants of insulin dependent diabetic mothers. *J Pediatr* 1988; **113**: 345–53.

75 Coustan DR. Screening and diagnosis of gestational diabetes. *Clin Obstet Gynecol* 1991; **5**: 293–313.

76 Diamond MP, Salyer SC, Vaugh WK *et al.* Continuing neonatal morbidity in infants of women with class A diabetes. *South Med J* 1984; **77**: 1386–8, 1392.

77 Dicker D, Feldberg D, Yoskaya A *et al.* Pregnancy outcome in gestational diabetes with preconceptual counselling. *Aust NZ J Obstet Gynecol* 1987; **27**: 184–7.

78 Jarrett RJ. Gestational diabetes. *Matern Child Health* 1993; 374–7.

79 Jarrett RJ. Gestational diabetes: a non-entity? *Br Med J* 1993; **306**: 37–8.

80 Weiner CP. Effect of varying degrees of normal glucose metabolism on maternal and perinatal outcome. *Am J Obstet Gynecol* 1988; **159**: 862–70.

81 Weiss PAM. Prophylactic insulin in gestational diabetes. *Obstet Gynecol* 1988; **71**: 951–2.

82 Farmer G, Russell G, Hamilton-Nicol DR *et al.* The influence of maternal glucose metabolism on fetal growth, development and morbidity in 917 singleton pregnancies in non-diabetic women. *Diabetologia* 1988; **31**: 134–41.

83 Herman G, Raimondi B. Glucose tolerance, fetal growth and pregnancy complications in normal women. *Am J Perinatol* 1988; **5**: 168–71.

84 Dorner G, Plagemann A. Perinatal hyperinsulinism as possible predisposing factor for diabetes mellitus, obesity and enhanced cardiovascular risk in later life. *Horm Metab Res* 1994; **26**: 213–21.

85 Landon MB, Gabbe SG, Piana R *et al.* Neonatal morbidity in pregnancy complicated by diabetes mellitus: predictive value of maternal glycaemic profiles. *Am J Obstet Gynecol* 1987; **156**: 1089–95.

86 Combs CA, Kitzmiller JC. Spontaneous abortion and congenital malformation in diabetes. *Clin Obstet Gynaecol* 1991; **5**: 315–31.

Part IV

LONG-TERM IMPLICATIONS OF A DIABETIC PREGNANCY

19

Contraception and Future Pregnancies

HEULWEN MORGAN

Whittington Hospital, London, UK

Planning one's family with appropriate spacing of childbearing such that control of pre-existing diabetes is optimum, is vital to reduce morbidity and complications in such pregnancies. High glucose concentrations *in vitro* cause abnormal embryos by altering prostaglandin metabolism and by generation of free oxygen radicals[1,2]. Glycated haemoglobin assays were introduced in the late 1970s. Miller *et al.*[3] showed *in vivo* that women whose haemoglobin HbA_{1c} was less than 8.5% before 14 weeks gestation had a 3.4% risk of malformation whereas those whose HbA_{1c} was over 8.5% had a 22.4% risk. In Denmark 75% of pregnancies were 'planned' in diabetic women between 1982 and 1986, the frequency of congenital malformations being much lower in planned than in unplanned pregnancies[4]. The abnormality rate was close to that of the non-diabetic population.

Similarly, those attending pre-pregnancy clinics have a lower rate of congenital abnormality in their offspring than that of non-attenders (relative risk 7.4, 95% confidence interval 1.7–33.2)[5]. Non-attenders, however, were of poorer social status, were more likely to smoke and their glycaemic control was worse in early pregnancy. Poor first trimester glycaemic control is significantly associated with congenital abnormalities, maternal vasculopathy being another risk factor. Kitzmiller's study[6] indicated that women seen before conception for a median of 17 weeks had a congenital abnormality rate of 1.2% in their infants as compared with 10.9% in mothers who presented late in pregnancy. Mean blood glucose levels of 3.3–7.8 mmol/l were obtained in half the women before pregnancy occurred. The purpose of pre-pregnancy counselling is to educate not only

Diabetes and Pregnancy: An International Approach to Diagnosis and Management.
Edited by A. Dornhorst and D. R. Hadden.
© 1996 John Wiley & Sons Ltd.

regarding the adverse outcomes that can be reduced by meticulous diabetic control such as to encourage the latter, but also to advise regarding medical suitability for pregnancy and suggest contraceptive methods appropriate to the individual woman and her partner.

In an ideal world, therefore, contraceptive methods should be used in diabetic women until the metabolic control is as near perfect as is possible. A Japanese study[7] found major congenital malformations in none of the infants of insulin-dependent diabetic mothers, but in 5.8% of infants of non-insulin-dependent diabetic mothers, and related this to the poor management of their diabetes before pregnancy. Certainly, it is advocated that these women should convert from oral hypoglycaemics to insulin and aim for precise control when trying to conceive. Indeed, in an audit study at the Whittington Hospital (unpublished data) the congenital abnormalities occurred exclusively in the non-insulin-dependent diabetic pregnancies (Table 19.1).

Table 19.1. Congenital abnormalities

Congenital abnormality	Pre-existing IDDM	Pre-existing NIDDM	Gestational DM diet	Gestational DM insulin	Diabetes not recorded	Total
Cardiac	0	0	0	0	0	0
Neural tube defects	0	2	0	0	0	2
Sacral agenesis	0	0	0	0	0	0
Renal abnormalities	0	0	0	0	0	0
Hypoplastic leg	0	1	0	0	0	1
None	22	8	36	29	1	96
Total	22	11	36	29	1	99

NB: Above calculated on the number of actual babies delivered.
IDDM, insulin-dependent diabetes mellitus; NIDDM, non-insulin-dependent diabetes mellitus; DM, diabetes mellitus.

What advice should one give regarding contraception and future pregnancy in this population? Various methods of contraception will be dealt with in turn, attitudes and knowledge discussed and the implications of future pregnancy outlined.

CONTRACEPTION

The compliant use of contraception necessitates motivation on the part of the user and user friendliness on the part of the contraceptive. The gates have opened for diabetic women and their partners in that the oestrogen dosage in the combined pill has lowered, and newer less androgenic progestogens have been introduced. The intrauterine contraceptive device (IUCD) is an option, with innovations such as the levonorgestrel/IUCD providing help with coincident gynaecological problems. Depot preparations have been introduced that are reversible by removal and permanent methods are suitable for those who have completed their families or for those who decide to do so after balancing the risk analysis scales. The choice of using barrier methods, in particular the condom, may be made because of an increased awareness of the need for protection against sexually transmitted diseases and the wish to reduce exposure to HIV. Many diabetic subjects will have religious convictions and conscientious use of natural family-planning methods is to be encouraged in the group who are not prepared to use other methods. Specific method usage can be modified or changed by the transmission of appropriate individual advice regarding diabetic control prior to pregnancy.

An audit of women attending a diabetic antenatal clinic between 1988 and 1994 (Whittington Hospital, unpublished data) revealed a large 'did not arrive' rate for postnatal glucose tolerance testing for women who had had gestational diabetes. This highlights a need for improvement in this area and closure of the audit loop will clarify whether this is occurring. This emphasizes the need to use the antenatal period to discuss future contraceptive issues and prepare the path for its effective use.

NATURAL FAMILY PLANNING

The World Health Organization multicentre trial of the ovulation method of natural family planning was undertaken in 1975–1979[8-10]. The main conclusions were as follows:

1. Irrespective of cultural, educational or economic background, over 95% of fertile women can, and are willing to, recognize the mucus signs of fertility.
2. In this fertile group of women having regular intercourse without use of barrier or chemical methods the fertility rate was 22.6 pregnancies per 100 women years.
3. The preovulatory and postovulatory days designated by the ovulation method of natural family planning rules as infertile were indeed infertile, as the pregnancies in this phase were four per 1000 acts of intercourse.
4. The designated fertile phase was indeed fertile, as intercourse during this phase resulted in conception, with increasing frequency the nearer to ovulation the intercourse occurred.

Studies so far reported in the 1990s conducted in the Moslem, Hindu, Chinese and Christian cultures reports a pregnancy rate per 100 women years between 1.7 (Belgium), 2.0 (India) and 10.6 (Europe)[11]. Clearly, a stable relationship is essential for success with this method. The complicating factor may be irregular cycling although good diabetic control will mostly regulate menstruation and it is the cervical mucus signs, not the calendar dates, that are used in this method. Other methods should also be discussed with the group of couples wishing to use natural family planning as adequate teaching and understanding of cervical mucus assessment is paramount to its success.

BARRIER METHODS

A couple may wish to use both natural family planning and a barrier method in order to lower the failure rate. British women under 35 years using the diaphragm and spermicide have a reported pregnancy rate range of 2.3–12.2 per 100 women years[12,13]. Several studies have shown protection from cervical gonorrhoea[14] and hospitalization for pelvic inflammatory disease[15] among diaphragm users. Young diabetic women should indeed protect themselves from sexually transmitted diseases to avoid tubal damage as a causation of infertility and to avoid the alteration of diabetic control inherent in an infective process.

Latex condoms provide an impervious barrier *in vitro* to most sexually transmitted disease pathogens, including HIV. For effectiveness in use, condoms must be applied prior to genital contact and used consistently. Protection of both males and females against gonorrhoea, urethritis, pelvic inflammatory disease and HIV seroconversion has been shown by the use of condoms[16]. Obviously, user motivation is vital – health education has been shown to be effective even in poorly educated and impoverished communities[17]. To maximize protection from pregnancy a spermicide should also be used.

INTRAUTERINE DEVICES

Kronmals *et al.*[18] reanalysed the data from the American Women's Health Study[19] to find that the relative risk of pelvic inflammatory disease for IUCD users versus no contraception was 1.02 (CI 0.86–1.21) – neither a significant decrease nor an increase in risk. Multiple sexual partners and the prevalence of causative organisms in a community are of much greater importance in the causation of pelvic inflammatory disease than is the use of an IUCD. Thus, in a mutually monogamous relationship the IUCD is a safe method in this respect.

Although there is no convincing case for the IUCD promoting pelvic inflammatory disease there is evidence for the introduction of infection at insertion. Should antibiotic cover be given for the procedure? Two African studies[20,21] randomly allocated women to receive 200 mg doxycycline or placebo. Prior to insertion microbiological testing occurred. This did not influence randomization. One study found a reduction in abdominal pain and/or bleeding which reached significance, whilst the other found no significant differences between the treated and placebo groups. The pelvic inflammatory disease rates were lower overall than anticipated, and 15 out of 21 developing infection did so within a month of insertion. Thus, it does not seem justified to cover with prophylactic antibiotics even in a high prevalence area for this condition.

The risk of infection in a diabetic woman is of promoting ketoacidosis. Should one screen for infection prior to insertion, therefore? A study[22] comparing one group of patients screened for *Chlamydia* and treated, if positive, with doxycycline 100 mg twice daily for two weeks and then rechecked, and a control group who had not been screened or treated, showed a significant reduction in pelvic inflammatory disease in the study group; in particular, in those using their first IUCD. Screening would seem a sensible recommendation in diabetic patients.

Conventional teaching advises the use of IUCD in parous women. To reduce the risk of heavy periods and infection in nulliparous patients a short Multiload® and mini-Gravigard® were introduced. However, no significant difference has been found between standard devices and the smaller ones[23]. Continuation rates in nulliparous women have been shown to be higher with the standard devices. The risk of pelvic inflammatory disease is in the sexual behaviour and not in age or parity and therefore a careful history is important in young nulliparous women. The young insulin-dependent diabetic woman with vascular disease can avoid the possible metabolic effects of hormonal contraception by use of an IUCD but, as above, cases should be carefully selected.

The specific use of the Copper 7 IUCD in diabetic women was looked at by Gosden *et al.*[24]. These Edinburgh workers found that 11 of 30 diabetic patients became pregnant within one year. They examined 21 coils from insulin-dependent diabetic women to find that they, as well as devices from pregnant non-diabetic patients, had more sulphur and chloride in the deposit on the coil and less calcareous deposit. This article was followed by several letters refuting this high failure rate[25] in diabetic women. Subsequent work by Skouby *et al.*[26] compared the use of the Copper T device between insulin-dependent diabetic women and controls, the latter being older and of increased parity. No difference in corrosion was found in the devices between the groups, and the continuation rate was 87–88% at one year. The pregnancy rates were similar in the diabetic subjects and the controls, but the time span was only one year.

The pregnancy rate was approximately one per 100 women years in Skouby's study; in Kimmerle's[27] evaluation in 1993 it was 1.7 per 100 in insulin-dependent diabetic patients. Kimmerle compared diabetic and non-diabetic women over three years but there were only 59 insulin-dependent diabetic women. Continuity and effectiveness were comparable in both his groups.

More recently Kjos *et al.*[28] conducted a prospective observational study of the Cu T 380A IUCD in women with non-insulin-dependent diabetes. These women tend to be older, parous and overweight. An IUCD might be considered the ideal contraceptive. The patients were well selected, screened prior to insertion, and routine antibiotic prophylaxis was not used. Of the 176 in the study, 131 women had had gestational diabetes. The continuation rate at one year was 93%, and 70% at three years. The pregnancy rate was 1.57 per 100 women years. The cumulative pregnancy rate at three years was 4%. The Copper T 380A has been reported to have a failure rate of 1.4% after 72 months of use[29]. Is the higher pregnancy rate due to small numbers in the diabetic studies or is the reduced fibrinolytic activity[30] in the endometrium of diabetic users the cause of this increased pregnancy rate?

In all these studies there is no evidence to support an increased incidence of acute salpingitis associated with IUCD use in diabetic women. The advent of the Copper T 380 Ag (with addition of silver) with lower pregnancy rates of around 1.4%[31] should allow this method to be acceptable to a large number of diabetic women.

CONTRACEPTION USING PROGESTOGENS

Progestogens are given for contraceptive purposes by depot injections, implants, in IUCDs and orally. Traditional teaching advises the use of the progesterone-only oral contraceptive pill in women with diabetes. The most recent exciting development is labelled 'contraception for the twenty-first century'[32] – the Mirena® levonorgestrel intrauterine contraceptive, available for use in the UK since April 1995, after extensive trials of its use in Finland. The basic NHS price is in the region of £100 (1996). The prescribing information mentions 'severe arterial disease' as a contraindication and precaution should be observed when there are multiple risk factors for arterial disease, blood glucose concentration needing to be monitored in diabetic users. Diabetes should in any case be kept under close control and treatment modified accordingly.

The advantages in comparative trials with other IUCDs[33,34] have been highlighted as being a lower pregnancy rate; a reduction in heavy menstruation leading to oligo- or amenorrhoea; fewer ectopic pregnancies, estimated as being an 80–90% reduction in ectopic pregnancy rate compared with women using no contraception; and a lower incidence of fibroid formation. Also, in the levonorgestrel device users the incidence of pelvic inflammatory disease was low regardless of age, whereas in the comparative group using the Copper IUCD NovaT there was a significantly increased rate ($p < 0.01$) amongst the youngest women. The trials mentioned used levonorgestrel coils containing 46 mg (five years) and 60 mg (seven years) of steroid. The marketed product in the UK contains 52 mg levonorgestrel BP[32], and has been licensed for three years' effective use. The failure rate for Mirena® is 0.14/100 women years, comparable with male sterilization and lower than all other methods according to Pearl Index data[35]. This IUCD is revolutionary perhaps in its ability to treat gynaecological problems such as endometriosis, fibroids and irregular vaginal bleeding, to the extent of avoiding surgical treatments in these cases (Professor A. Singer, personal communication). It may also help premenstrual tension and with its extremely low failure rate is very attractive.

Are there disadvantages? Clearly, in a woman who has either insulin-dependent or non-insulin-dependent diabetes, or indeed those who may develop diabetes after having gestational diabetes, the metabolic effects of the hormone content and its effect on progression of disease have to be assessed. Secondly, the Mirena® coil is slightly thicker, and it may be necessary to use local anaesthetic for insertion, particularly in nulliparous women. Thirdly, during the first few months irregular bleeding can occur prior to development of oligo- or amenorrhoea, so patients need to be warned of this[33]. In the initial months of treatment ovarian follicular enlargement or cysts can develop in the ovary; expectant management is advocated[32]. The device releases 20 μg of steroid daily. Circulatory levels that are reached after it has been in place for a few months (steady state levels) are lower than those for a levonorgestrel implant, the progesterone-only oral contraceptive, and are very much lower than the levels reached using combined oral contraception[32].

To consider the effect on diabetes of taking the progesterone-only oral contraceptive, compliance is a potential problem as the pill must be taken each day, although those on oral hypoglycaemics and insulin take it with their medication. The tendency to decreased glucose tolerance seems essentially related to the dosage and type of progestogen[36]. The mechanism of decreased glucose tolerance seems related partially to increased peripheral insulin resistance that is potentially caused by a post-receptor defect in insulin action. Insulin resistance may induce not only glucose intolerance but also hypertension, obesity and dyslipoproteinaemia (high very low-density lipoprotein and low high-density lipoprotein values). All these variables add to the risk of coronary heart and arterial disease.

Contraceptives containing a low daily dose of levonorgestrel or gestodene are associated with a significantly lower risk of impaired glucose tolerance, even in women with previous gestational diabetes[37]. The newer 19-nortestosterone gonane progestogens are very selective and have low affinity to the androgen receptor, resulting in higher sex hormone binding globulin levels and thus a reduction in free testosterone, so are of low androgenicity. These progestogens (desogestrel, norgestimate and gestodene) are also more 'lipid friendly'. Gestodene is also the most potent, thus a lower dose can be used.

Adverse serum lipids are associated with both increased cardiovascular risk and atherosclerosis. Accelerated atherosclerosis has been implicated in the pathophysiology of microvascular and macrovascular disease in diabetes. In a dose- and potency-related fashion, synthetic progestogens decrease high-density lipoprotein (HDL) cholesterol and increase low-density lipoprotein (LDL) cholesterol[38]. Therefore, the ideal progesterone-only contraceptive would be made of a daily low dose of the new generation of progestogens mentioned above.

A consensus view is that the effects of the already available progesterone-only oral contraceptives on carbohydrate metabolism are minimal. Some long-term users have shown a slight deterioration in glucose tolerance and a tendency to hyperinsulinism. It may be that the subjects looked at were in any case prone to develop these effects. The reduced level of circulating steroid with the levonorgestrel IUCD, approximately equivalent to taking two levonorgestrel progesterone-only pills per week, implies a very small change in carbohydrate metabolism, although interestingly in the Andersson study[34] there was a significantly higher incidence of acne, breast tenderness, headache, weight change and depression, said to be hormonal side effects. Further studies should be performed within the diabetic and post-gestational diabetic population. Progesterone-only pills are not absolutely contraindicated in a diabetic woman with evidence of arteriopathy but obviously use of the most lipid-friendly progestogen would be more satisfactory[39].

The progesterone-only oral contraceptive has little effect on hepatic secretion of plasma proteins. It affects cervical mucus, maybe protecting the user against pelvic infection, and does not cause a change in blood pressure. Current ischaemic heart disease and severe hereditary lipid abnormalities would be contraindications to its use and established hypertension a relative one. Irregular vaginal bleeding can occur as well as functional ovarian cysts, which resolve spontaneously. Many will have anovulation or deficient luteal function. This method does seem a good choice particularly in the older diabetic woman, the failure rate being 0.3–4 per 100 women years[35].

Norplant® consists of six flexible closed capsules for subdermal implantation designed to release the progestogen levonorgestrel over a period of five years. It is placed subcutaneously in a fan-like manner in the upper arm and has low pregnancy rates of 0.7 per 100 women years at four years of use. The effect of this preparation on clotting factors and plasma lipids has been inconsistent. A statistically significant increase in glucose and insulin levels during glucose tolerance testing has been shown in non-diabetic users, thus its use is not advised in either previously gestational diabetic women or in currently diabetic women[40].

Depot doses of medroxyprogesterone acetate 150 mg given three monthly, or norethisterone enanthate 200 mg every 8–10 weeks are suitable for those with non-compliance problems. Studies with the depot preparation have shown a deterioration in glucose tolerance and lowered serum triglyceride and HDL cholesterol levels[41]. These preparations also, unlike the levonorgestrel device, have a delayed effect on the return of fertility after cessation of use. They should be used with caution and close monitoring in diabetic women.

Vaginal rings to deliver the steroid have the advantage of being removed and inserted by the woman[42]. Rings with constant low release of 20 μg per day levonorgestrel and 20 μg 3-ketodesogestrel have been developed. Plasma levels are steady and the 'first-pass effect' on the liver is also eliminated by the vaginal route. The 3-ketodesogestrel ring has been found to be more effective as a contraceptive than the progesterone-only pill[43]. This may well be an option for diabetic or potentially diabetic women provided it is fully explained and patient acceptability is high. Studies have not been undertaken in such a population to date.

Irregular vaginal bleeding affects a proportion of women using progestogen-only methods, a full explanation being mandatory before starting.

COMBINED HORMONAL CONTRACEPTION

Once again this can be administered as a local delivery of oestrogen and progestogen to the vagina using a ring. A two-compartment approach has been used. The dose is 12 μg of ethinyloestradiol and 120 μg of 3-ketodesogestrel. Continuation rates are high – the devices are removed for seven days (the seven-day gap in oral combined contraceptive use). The ring lasts three months in total. As a newer progestogen (see previous comments) is used this may well be suitable for a diabetic population. The effects of progestogens have already been outlined. A 19-nortestosterone gonane progestogen should be chosen, which is of low androgenicity.

The average serum lipid changes that occur in non-insulin-dependent diabetes with a combined oral contraceptive pill, are an increase in triglycerides, an increase in very low-density lipoprotein (VLDL) triglyceride and a normal or lower than normal level of HDL cholesterol. Cholesterol and LDL cholesterol remain normal. These women also tend to be obese. Some women with gestational diabetes will continue to have abnormal glucose tolerance post pregnancy. About 5% will develop insulin-dependent diabetes within five years of pregnancy – these women are under 30 years of age, slim and do not have a family history of diabetes. The non-insulin-dependent group often have a family history, are obese, and required insulin in pregnancy[44]. Gestational diabetic women need to be regularly investigated (yearly) as once they develop impaired glucose tolerance their lipid profile changes to that outlined for non-insulin-dependent diabetes[45]. It is vital therefore for these women to avoid the other risk factors of obesity and smoking, and to receive early treatment for any hypertension to avoid coronary heart disease and progression of diabetic vasculopathy. The average changes in insulin-dependent diabetes are that triglycerides increase or remain normal, cholesterol is normal or reduced, VLDL triglycerides are increased or normal, LDL cholesterol is normal or reduced and HDL cholesterol is increased or normal. The lipid changes that occur with the combined oral contraceptive pill are less with the new lower-dose combined oral contraceptive pills – they cause a smaller increase in LDL cholesterol and a variable but smaller decrease in HDL cholesterol than higher-dosage pills. Also, with decreasing progestogen dose and change of type, the development of insulin resistance is virtually non-existent. The use of triphasic formulations[46] and the lowest-dose pills have a failure rate of 0.2 per 100 women years[35].

Modern low-dose preparations are responsible for a rise in systolic blood pressure of around 5 mmHg and a rise in diastolic blood pressure of around 2 mmHg. This would be expected to increase the low relative risk of cerebral haemorrhage, cerebral infarction and coronary heart disease to 1.7, 1.5 and 1.2 respectively[47]. Against this background one can understand the relative contraindication of combined oral contraception in diabetic women.

The possibility of prolonged exposure to oral contraceptives leading to an increased risk of developing diabetes mellitus has been refuted in the Royal College of General Practitioners and the Oxford/Family Planning Association cohort studies[48]. Combined oral contraceptives, due to the oestrogen component, increase coagulability by increasing levels of factor VIIc and fibrinogen. The effect of preparations on coagulation, fibrinolysis and platelet function has been shown to be less with 30 μg of oestrogen than with 50 μg[49]. The Northwick Park Heart Study showed gradation of increasing factor VIIc and fibrinogen from non-users, users of 30 μg oestrogen pills and 50 μg oestrogen preparations[50].

Oestrogens raise HDL cholesterol and triglycerides. Changes are dependent, therefore, on the balance of oestrogen and progestogen. In biphasic and triphasic pills the dosages change and Mercilon® provides a pill with a daily dose of 20 μg oestrogen. Combined oral contraceptives containing the new-generation progestogens tend to raise HDL cholesterol and lower LDL cholesterol[51,52]. The concomitant increase in triglycerides seen may be potentially adverse although some experts believe that atherogenicity is expressed only against a background of reduced HDL cholesterol.

The use of combined oral contraceptives in insulin-dependent diabetes mellitus has been looked at in several studies. Petersen *et al.*[53] used the tissue plasminogen activator (t-PA) and inhibitor (PA-1) system and von

Willebrand factor as indirect indicators of vascular endothelial function, and urine albumin excretion rate as a clinically important marker of glomerular endothelial function. Thirteen women with insulin-dependent diabetes were followed prospectively whilst on ethinyloestradiol 30 μg and gestodene 75 μg for one year. They were compared with 13 women also with uncomplicated diabetes not on oral contraception. None of the subjects developed increased renal albumin excretion. There was, however, an increase in plasma levels of thrombin–antithrombin III complexes and D dimer during treatment but their ratio remained unchanged. No change in insulin requirements or HbA_{1c} occurred. Antigen concentrations of t-PA and PAI-1 in plasma decreased proportionally during hormonal treatment. Again insulin needs did not change. The levels of von Willebrand factor increased on oral contraception. This suggests that the coagulation system of diabetic women may be more sensitive to sex hormones, but the unchanged ratio implies a compensated procoagulant response and establishment of a new equilibrium. Longer studies are needed to see if the increased von Willebrand factor does over time predispose to nephropathy as increases have been found in non-diabetic women using other oral contraceptives[54].

Garg *et al.*[55] have looked at renal and retinal complications in a retrospective case–control assessment. There were 43 women in each arm followed for a mean of 3.4 years (range one to seven years). A mixture of oral contraceptives were used containing 50 μg or less of ethinyloestradiol or mestranol with various progestogens. Their outcome measures of HbA_{1c} levels, albumin excretion rates and mean retinopathy scores were no different between the study group and controls during the time period observed.

Petersen *et al.*[56] using the same monophasic contraceptive (30 μg ethinyloestradiol and 75 μg gestodene) as previously quoted, found that after one year of use total cholesterol and HDL cholesterol were unchanged, and LDL cholesterol was decreased in the treatment group of insulin-dependent diabetic women without serious vascular complications.

In conclusion, insulin-dependent diabetic patients need close medical supervision if prescribed low-dose combined oral contraceptives. Longer prospective trials need to be conducted and one would recommend as low as possible an oestrogen dose, 20–30 μg, as well as greater-potency, low-dose, new-generation progestogens. Blood pressure, weight and HbA_{1c} should be measured approximately four monthly, with lipids assessed every 6–12 months. Precise glucose monitoring should occur.

There is little data available on non-insulin-dependent diabetic women and combined oral contraceptive use. This group, frequently obese, need to be advised regarding diet and exercise with the aim of losing weight. The same recommendation regarding the kind of combined oral contraceptive should be made as above. If hypertension develops or there is deteriorating lipid metabolism, use of the pill should be curtailed. Attention, as is usual, must be paid to good glycaemic control.

Evaluation has been made in the literature of women with previous gestational diabetes mellitus and use of the combined oral contraceptive pill. The same principles apply as to the previous two categories of women. A controlled, randomized, prospective study by Kjos *et al.*[57] randomized women into one of two low-dose combined oral contraceptive groups (one had norethindrone 0.4 mg and ethinyloestradiol 35 μg and the other levonorgestrel 0.050–0.125 mg with ethinyloestradiol 30–40 μg). The control group had also had gestational diabetes – they were older, heavier and of increased parity. Body mass index was raised in the three groups. One hundred and fifty-six completed 6–13 months of treatment. There was no significant difference in the area under the glucose tolerance test curve with different methods but within groups there was an increase in area under the curve over time. This was significant in both oral contraceptive groups ($p < 0.04$) and not significant in the non-oral contraceptive group. All women diagnosed as diabetic postnatally were excluded. The prevalence of impaired glucose tolerance and diabetes was not significantly different between groups at 6–13 months. Seventeen per cent of the non-oral contraceptive group had impaired glucose tolerance and 17% had diabetes; 11% of the monophasic group had impaired glucose tolerance and 15% diabetes; 14% of the triphasic group had impaired glucose tolerance with 20% being diabetic. There was a significant increase in HDL cholesterol in the monophasic group.

All these women should, in any event, have their diabetic status tested annually. Use of the potent gonane progestogens is associated with a substantial reduction and even a lack of adverse effects on carbohydrate metabolism. Ethinyloestradiol 30 μg with desogestrel 150 μg daily in 21 women over one year showed borderline increases in blood glucose and increased insulin responses, with C-peptide increased. In other studies with this combination over six months no change was found, in particular no change with a combined oral contraceptive using 20 μg ethinyloestradiol and 150 μg desogestrel. In comparing ethinyloestradiol 30 μg and gestodene 75 μg with triphasic ethinyloestradiol 32 μg and gestodene 79 μg mean daily dose, the monophasic compound slightly increased glucose and insulin levels in the oral glucose tolerance test, with none developing impaired glucose tolerance, but in the triphasic subjects' responses were unchanged over 12 months[36].

Gosland *et al.*[58] stresses the need to pay attention to statistical power in future studies and that a wide range of metabolic changes such as changes in lipoproteins and measures of haematosis need to be fully evaluated. Clearly, there is no room for complacency but the impact of the most modern combined oral contraceptives is to reduce the complications associated with their use in diabetic and potentially diabetic women, using a triphasic or a 20 μg oestrogen regimen.

STERILIZATION

For those couples who have completed their families, or after realizing the high risks of future pregnancies when retinopathy and nephropathy are severe, permanent contraception is the answer. The male partner is easier to sterilize but the implications for future pregnancies rest with the female. Individual couples make their choice. Obesity adds to the risk of the procedure, most using laparoscopic techniques to apply a clip or ring to the isthmus of the Fallopian tube. Thus, a warning should occur regarding the possibility of the increased chance of a laparotomy occurring, with its morbidity and hospital stay. The couple should also be warned of the failure rate of 0–0.2 per 100 women years for male sterilization and 0–0.5 per 100 women years for the female procedure[35].

FUTURE PREGNANCIES

The decision to use permanent or temporary contraception is dependent on the couple's social and emotional needs and the inherent morbidity in embarking on a further pregnancy. Pre-conception counselling is discussed in an earlier chapter. A group of medical students under the supervision of Helen Lunt in New Zealand[59] assessed the attitude and knowledge regarding contraception and pregnancy counselling in insulin-dependent diabetes. One hundred and twenty-four women, 86% of those eligible, underwent an interview; 85 were using contraception, 35% the combined oral contraceptive pill, 12% the progesterone-only pill, 24% condoms, 12% of the partners had had a vasectomy and 12% of the women were sterilized. All of them were aware of the importance of good glucose control during pregnancy. Thirty-nine per cent had avoided the combined pill because of concerns regarding metabolic and vascular side effects. Only half were aware of a figure for genetic risk of passing insulin-dependent diabetes to an offspring (1.3%)[60]. Sufficient specific advice should be given regarding appropriate contraceptive use – there is awareness of the risk of future pregnancies for the mother but not necessarily for the future well-being of the infant.

Preparing for a future pregnancy includes avoidance of smoking, which may lead to intrauterine growth retardation; weight loss, if obese, to reduce the risk of a macrosomic infant; and exemplary blood glucose control to provide the fetus with a normal fuel mixture to avoid teratogenicity. It is also recommended that folic acid 0.04 mg is taken daily before pregnancy. Whilst on reversible contraception the first three aims should be achieved.

There should be a continuum of care with early first-trimester attendance at the antenatal clinic to enable ultrasonographic assessment of gestation. The HbA$_{1c}$ should have been normal prior to pregnancy, the aim being to maintain this level. Strict adherence to a pregnancy diabetic diet is encouraged, ideally a body mass index within the normal range (19.8–26 kg/m^2) being achieved before pregnancy to avoid an unduly large baby.

When there is pre-existing impaired renal function and hypertension a further decline in renal function during pregnancy has been found[61], the long-term effect being an earlier requirement for renal replacement than would have been expected without pregnancy. Age and desire for pregnancy is a factor in counselling. Recent studies suggest that pregnancy may be less harmful to the retina than previously thought. Nevertheless, some women experience a worsening of retinopathy as a result of pregnancy[62]. Thus, before embarking on a further pregnancy women who have complicated insulin-dependent diabetes should be reviewed by an interested renal physician and ophthalmologist.

Rosenn and co-workers[63] prospectively studied 55 insulin-dependent diabetic patients seen before nine weeks gestation in two consecutive pregnancies. A control group of 55 insulin-dependent women were matched with the others by maternal age and year of pregnancy. Glycaemic control in early pregnancy, earlier week of entry, and lower HBA$_{1c}$ at nine and 14 weeks occurred in the study group undergoing their second pregnancy with the carers as compared with their first pregnancy and with the control group. There was a decreased spontaneous abortion rate and major malformation rate in the study group during their second pregnancies. Progression of disease had occurred, however, between pregnancies, with 65% having advanced diabetic complications as compared with 46% in their previous pregnancies, and 44% in the controls. Education and good glucose control had overcome many of the obstetric issues.

Physical training is associated with increased sensitivity to insulin in skeletal muscle and adipose tissue of women with non-insulin-dependent diabetes[64]. Thus exercise in addition to diet in preventing weight gain and promoting weight loss should be advised in this group of patients prior to and during future pregnancy.

What of future pregnancies subsequent to a gestational diabetic pregnancy? Gaudier *et al.*[65] found a 52% recurrence of the diabetes in women with raised body mass index (>35 kg/m^2) who had delivered large-for-dates babies. More of the recurrent group had needed insulin in pregnancy and had a higher fasting blood glucose. Such pregnancies should be managed by an obstetric/diabetic team approach. In another study, glucose tolerance testing before 24 weeks gestation in subsequent pregnancies, repeated at 26–30 weeks if normal, gave a 49.4% recurrence, two thirds being positive before 24 weeks[66]. Those testing positive in early pregnancy had a higher perinatal mortality rate.

Buchanan compared 87 women who had a second pregnancy with women who did not and found a 3.3-fold relative risk of developing non-insulin-dependent diabetes after gestational diabetes[68].

When the female partner in a relationship has diabetes of any type they must be aware that timing of pregnancy during optimum control of the metabolic derangement will give the best outcome for both mother and baby.

ADDENDUM

On 18 October 1995 the Committee on Safety of Medicines in the UK advised doctors of evidence from three epidemiological research papers, awaiting publication, of different excess risk of venous thromboembolism for women taking combined oral contraceptives containing the progestogens gestodene and desogestrel, in comparison to those containing levonorgestrel, norethisterone or ethynodiol diacetate[67]. Evidence was not present to know if combined pills containing norgestimate is associated with an altered risk of thromboembolism. The advice given was that women with risk factors for venous thromboembolic disease – obesity (body mass index $> 30 \, kg/m^2$), varicose veins or a previous history of thrombosis – should avoid brands containing gestodene or desogestrel if they are to continue with the combined pill. Some women with diabetes, particularly non-insulin-dependent diabetes, fall into the obesity category.

The change in risk that was found was around a two-fold increase over the excess risk of 5–10 cases per 100 000 women per annum found for women taking oral contraceptives containing levonorgestrel, norethisterone or ethynodiol diacetate. It was also stated that the risks associated with unwanted pregnancies are far greater than the risks of continuing the third-generation progestogen pills.

The Family Planning Association and the Faculty of Family Planning and Reproductive Health Care issued a response to the Committee of Safety of Medicines letter[68]. This stated that a previous personal history of venous thrombosis is a contraindication to any combined oral contraceptive and that a change of brand is also advised for other women using gestodene or desogestrel based pills except those who are, or might, predictably be, intolerant of other brands.

The risk of venous thromboembolism was also outlined and expressed as:

Healthy women not taking hormones	5 of 100 000 each year
Women in the year of a pregnancy	60 of 100 000 each year

Women taking combined pills containing
gestodene and desogestrel   30 of 100 000 each year

Women taking combined pills containing
levonorgestrel, norethisterone, ethynodiol
diacetate   15 of 100 000 each year

The mortality of venous thrombosis was quoted as 2%.

The figures take into account the worst case of risks currently understood and help in presenting the significance of the epidemiological research findings to women.

REFERENCES

1 Eriksson UJ, Borg LA, Forsberg H, Styrud J. Diabetic embryopathy: studies with animal and in vitro models. *Diabetes* 1991; **40** (Suppl. 2): 94–8.
2 Eriksson UJ, Borg LA. Protection by free oxygen radicals scavenging enzymes against glucose-induced embryonic malformations in vitro. *Diabetologia* 1991; **34**: 325–31.
3 Miller E, Hare JW, Cloherty JP *et al.* Elevated maternal haemoglobin A_{1c} in early pregnancy and major congenital anomalies in infants of diabetic mothers. *N Engl J Med* 1981; **304**: 1331–4.
4 Damm P, Mølsted-Pedersen L. Significant decrease in congenital malformations in newborn infants of an unselected population of diabetic women. *Am J Obstet Gynecol* 1989; **161**: 1163–7.
5 Steel JM, Johnstone FD, Hepburn DA, Smith AF. Can pre-pregnancy care of diabetic women reduce the risk of abnormal babies? *Br Med J* 1990; **301**: 1070–4.
6 Kitzmiller JL, Gavin LA, Gin GD *et al.* Preconception care of diabetes: glycaemic control prevents congenital anomalies. *JAMA* 1991; **265**: 731–6.
7 Omori Y, Minei S, Testuo T *et al.* Current status of pregnancy in diabetic women: a comparison of pregnancy in IDDM and NIDDM mothers. *Diabetes Res Clin Pract* 1994; **24** (Suppl.): 273–8.
8 World Health Organization. A prospective multicentre trial of the ovulation method of natural family planning. I. The teaching phase. *Fertil Steril* 1981; **36**: 152–8.
9 World Health Organization. A prospective multicentre trial of the ovulation method of natural family planning. II. The effectiveness phase. *Fertil Steril* 1981; **36**: 591–8.
10 World Health Organization. A prospective multicentre trial of the ovulation method of natural family planning. III. Characteristics of the menstrual cycle and of the fertile phase. *Fertil Steril* 1983; **40**: 773–8.
11 Ryder B, Campbell H. Natural family planning in the 1990s. *Lancet* 1995; **346**: 233–4.
12 Vessey M, Lawless M, Yeates D. Efficiency of different contraceptive methods. *Lancet* 1982; i: 841–2.
13 Bounds W, Guillebaud J. Randomised comparison of the use effectiveness and patient acceptability of the collatex (Today) contraceptive sponge and the diaphragm. *Br J Fam Plan* 1984; **10**: 69–75.
14 Austin H, Law WC, Alexander J. A case control study of spermicides and gonorrhoea. *JAMA* 1984; **251**: 2822–4.
15 Kelleghan J, Rubin GL, Ory WH, Layde PM. Barrier method contraceptives and pelvic inflammatory disease. *JAMA* 1982; **248**: 184–7.
16 Grimes DA, Cates W Jr. Family planning and sexually transmitted disease. In: Haues KK, Mandh P, Sparling PF, Weisner PJ (eds), *Textbook of Venereology*. McGraw-Hill, New York, 1990; 1087–94.

17 Ngugi EN, Plummer FA, Simonsen JN *et al.* Prevention of transmission of human immunodeficiency virus in Africa: effectiveness of condom promotion and health education among prostitutes. *Lancet* 1988; **ii**: 887–90.

18 Kronmals RA, Whitney CW, Muniford SD. The intrauterine device and pelvic inflammatory disease: the women's health study reanalysed. *J Clin Epidemiol* 1991; **44**: 109–22.

19 Burkman RT. Association between intrauterine device and pelvic inflammatory disease. *Obstet Gynecol* 1981; **57**: 269–76.

20 Sinci SK, Schulz KF, Lamptey PR *et al.* Preventing IUCD related pelvic infection: the efficacy of prophylactic doxycycline at insertion. *Br J Obstet Gynaecol* 1990; **97**: 412–19.

21 Lapido OA, Farr G, Otolorin E *et al.* Prevention of IUD related pelvic infection: the efficacy of prophylactic doxycycline at IUD insertion. *Adv Contracept* 1991; **7**: 43–54.

22 Sprague D, Bullough C, Rashid S, Roberts S. Screening for and treating *Chlamydia trachomatis* and *Neisseria gonorrhoea* before contraceptive use and subsequent pelvic inflammatory disease. *Br J Fam Plan* 1990; **16**: 54–8.

23 Petersen KR, Brooks L, Jacobson B, Skouby SO. Intrauterine devices in nulliparous women. *Adv Contracept* 1991; **7**: 333–8.

24 Gosden C, Steel J, Ross A, Springbett A. Intrauterine contraceptive devices in diabetic women. *Lancet* 1982; **i**: 530–5.

25 Thiery M, Vanketz H, Kurz K *et al.* Intrauterine contraceptive devices for diabetic women. *Lancet* 1982; **ii**: 883.

26 Skouby SO, Mølsted-Pedersen L, Kosonen A. Consequences of intrauterine contraception in diabetic women. *Fertil Steril* 1984; **42**: 568–73.

27 Kimmerle R, Weiss R, Berger M, Kurz KH. Effectiveness, safety and acceptability of a copper intrauterine device (Cu safe 300) in type I diabetic women. *Diabetes Care* 1993; **16**: 1227–30.

28 Kjos SL, Ballagh SA, La Cour M *et al.* The Copper T380A intrauterine device in women with type II diabetes mellitus. *Obstet Gynecol* 1994; **84**: 1006–9.

29 Population Information Program. IUDs – a new look. *Population Reports Series* 1988; B5.

30 Larsson B, Karlsson K, Liedholm P *et al.* Fibrinolytic activity of the endometrium in diabetic women using Cu IUDs. *Contraception* 1977; **15**: 711–14.

31 Sivin I, Stern J, Diez J *et al.* Two years of intrauterine contraception with levonorgestrel and with copper: a randomised comparison of the T Cu 380Ag and levonorgestrel 20 mcg/day devices. *Contraception* 1987; **3**: 245–55.

32 *Prescribing Information Data Sheet and Summary of Product Characteristics: Mirena®.* Leiras OY, Pansiatic 47, FIN 20210 Turku, Finland. Distributed by Phamacia-Lurias Ltd. Milton Keynes.

33 Sivin I, Stern J. Health during prolonged use of levonorgestrel 20 mcg/day and the copper T Cu 380 Ag intrauterine contraceptive devices: a multicenter study. *Fertil Steril* 1994; **61**: 70–6.

34 Andersson K, Odlind V, Rybo G. Levonorgestrel-releasing and copper releasing (Nova T) IUDs during five years of use. *Contraception* 1994; **49**: 56–71.

35 Guillebaud J. The population explosion and importance of fertility control. In: *Contraception: Your Questions Answered.* Churchill Livingstone, Edinburgh, 1993; 11.

36 Gaspard UJ, Lefebure PJ. Clinical aspects of the relationship between oral contraceptives, abnormalities in carbohydrate metabolism and the development of cardiovascular disease. *Am J Obstet Gynecol* 1990; **163**: 334–43.

37 Harvengt C. Effect of oral contraceptive use on the incidence of impaired glucose tolerance and diabetes mellitus. *Diabetes Metab* 1992; **18**: 71–7.

38 Wahl P, Walden C, Knopp R *et al.* Effect of oestrogen/progestin potency on lipid/lipoprotein cholesterol. *N Engl J Med* 1981; **308**: 862–7.

39 Guillebaud J. Oestrogen-free hormonal contraception. In: *Contraception: Your Questions Answered.* Churchill Livingstone, Edinburgh, 1993; 246–51.

40 Konje JC, Otolorin EO, Ladipo AO. The effect of continuous subdermal levonorgestrel (Norplant) on carbohydrate metabolism. *Am J Obstet Gynecol* 1992; **166**: 15–19.

41 Liew DFM, Ng CSA, Yong YM *et al.* Long term effects of depo-provera on carbohydrate and lipid metabolism. *Contraception* 1985; **31**: 51–64.

42 Newton J. Long acting methods of contraception. In: Drife JO, Baird DT (eds), *British Medical Bulletin: Contraception.* 1993; 40–62.

43 Jackson R, Newton JR. Pharmacodynamics of a contraceptive vaginal ring. *Contraception* 1989; **39**: 653–66.

44 Dornhorst A, Bailey PC, Anyaoku V *et al.* Abnormalities of glucose tolerance following gestational diabetes. *Q J Med* 1990; **284** (New Series 77): 1219–28.

45 Kjos SL, Buchanan TA, Montoro M *et al.* Serum lipids within 36 months of delivery in women with gestational diabetes. *Diabetes* 1991; **40** (Suppl. 2): 142–6.

46 Gaspard UJ. Metabolic effects of oral contraceptives. *Am J Obstet Gynecol* 1987; **157**: 1029–41.

47 Prentice RL. On the ability of blood pressure effects to explain the relation between oral contraceptives and cardiovascular disease. *Am J Epidemiol* 1988; **127**: 213–19.

48 Grice D, Villard-Mackintosh L, Yeates D, Vessey M. Oral contraceptives and diabetes mellitus. *Br J Fam Plan* 1991; **17**: 39–40.

49 Bonnar J, Coagulation effects of oral contraception. *Am J Obstet Gynecol* 1987; **157**: 1042–8.

50 Cecily C, Kelleher MD. Clinical aspects of the relationship between oral contraceptives and abnormalities of the haemostatic system: relation to the development of cardiovascular disease. *Am J Obstet Gynecol* 1990; **163**: 392–5.

51 Gosland IF, Crook D, Simpson R *et al.* The effects of different formulations of oral contraceptive agents on lipid and carbohydrate metabolism. *N Engl J Med* 1990; **323**: 1375–81.

52 Eyong E, Elstein M. Clinical update on a new progestogen – gestodene. *Br J Fam Plan* 1989; **15**: 18–22.

53 Petersen KR, Skouby SO, Sidelmann J, Jespersen J. Assessment of endothelial function during oral contraception in women with insulin dependent diabetes mellitus. *Metabolism* 1994; **43**: 1379–83.

54 David JL, Gaspard UJ, Gillian D *et al.* Hemostasis profile in women taking low dose oral contraceptives. *Am J Obstet Gynecol* 1990; **163**: 20–3.

55 Garg SK, Chase PH, Marshall G *et al.* Oral contraceptives and renal and retinal complications in young women with insulin dependent diabetes mellitus. *JAMA* 1994; **271**: 1099–102.

56 Petersen KR, Skouby SO, Sidelmann J *et al.* Effects of contraceptive steroids on cardiovascular risk factors in women with insulin dependent diabetes mellitus. *Am J Obstet Gynecol* 1994; **171**: 400–5.

57 Kjos SL, Shoupe D, Douyan S *et al.* Effect of low dose oral contraceptives on carbohydrate and lipid metabolism in women with recent gestational diabetes: results of a controlled randomised prospective study. *Am J Obstet Gynecol* 1990; **163**: 1822–7.

58 Gosland IF, Crook D, Wynn V. Low dose oral contraceptives and carbohydrate metabolism. *Am J Obstet Gynecol* 1990; **163**: 348–53.

59 Gibb D, Hockey S, Brown LJ, Lunt H. Attitudes and knowledge regarding contraception and prepregnancy counselling in insulin dependent diabetes. *NZ Med M* 1994; **107**: 484–6.

60 Hagay Z, Reece EA. Diabetes mellitus in pregnancy and periconceptional genetic counselling. *Am J Perinatol* 1992; **9**: 87–93.

61 Biesenbach G, Stoger H, Zazgornik J. Influence of pregnancy on progression of diabetic nephropathy and subsequent requirement of renal replacement therapy in female type I diabetic patients with impaired renal function. *Nephrol Dial Transplant* 1992; **7**: 105–9.

62 Elman KD, Welch RA, Frank RN *et al.* Diabetic retinopathy in pregnancy: a review. *Obstet Gynecol* 1990; **75**: 119–27.

63 Rosenn B, Miodovnik M, Mimouni F *et al.* Patient experience in a diabetic program project improves subsequent pregnancy outcome. *Obstet Gynecol* 1991; **77**: 87–91.

64 Horton ES. Exercise in the treatment of NIDDM: applications for GDM? *Diabetes* 1991; **40** (Suppl. 2): 175–8.

65 Gaudier FL, Hauth JC, Poist M *et al.* Recurrence of gestational diabetes. *Obstet Gynecol* 1992; **80**: 755–8.

66 Dong ZG, Beischer NA, Wein P, Sheedy MT. Value of early glucose tolerance testing in women who had gestational diabetes in their previous pregnancy. *Aust NZ J Obstet Gynecol* 1993; **33**: 350–7.

67 Combined oral contraceptives and thromboembolism. Committee on Safety of Medicines. Letter to all doctors, 18 October 1995.
68 Bromham D, O'Brien T. Information for Health Professionals further to the Committee on Safety of Medicines, Advice on the Safety of Oral Contraceptives dated 18 October 1995. Letter from Faculty of Family Planning and Reproductive Health Care and the Family Planning Association, 26 October 1995.

20

Diabetes Following Gestational Diabetes Mellitus

PETER DAMM

Rigshospitalet, Copenhagen, Denmark

DIABETES AND IMPAIRED GLUCOSE TOLERANCE IN WOMEN WITH PREVIOUS GESTATIONAL DIABETES

During a normal pregnancy glucose tolerance deteriorates gradually, but in the majority of women glucose tolerance stays within the normal range[1]. However, 1–3% of all women will develop gestational diabetes mellitus, defined as a carbohydrate intolerance of varying severity with onset or first recognition during pregnancy irrespective of the glycaemic status after delivery[2-4]. Gestational diabetes is a heterogeneous disorder which in the majority of cases can be managed satisfactorily by dietary treatment alone, while insulin treatment is required in other cases. Glucose tolerance returns to normal post partum in the majority of women with gestational diabetes[1,5].

This condition has short-term implications for the pregnant woman and her fetus/newborn infant, but also long-term significance for both the mother and the infant. This chapter describes the long-term consequences for women with gestational diabetes with respect to development of abnormal glucose tolerance (diabetes mellitus or impaired glucose tolerance) later in life.

Although glucose tolerance normalizes shortly after pregnancy with gestational diabetes in the majority of women, the risk of developing overt diabetes or impaired glucose tolerance later in life is markedly increased[6]. Incidences of diabetes between 3% and 65% have been reported with varying follow-up periods after an index pregnancy. Table 20.1 summarizes

Diabetes and Pregnancy: An International Approach to Diagnosis and Management.
Edited by A. Dornhorst and D. R. Hadden.
© 1996 John Wiley & Sons Ltd.

Table 20.1. Follow-up studies of women with previous gestational diabetes

Reference	City	No.	Diagnostic OGTT in pregnancy	Length of follow-up	Diagnostic OGTT at follow-up (diagnostic criteria)	Abnormal glucose tolerance (DM + IGT)	Control group
Mestman[31]	Los Angeles, USA	89	100 g	12–18 years	interview	65% DM	
O'Sullivan[12]	Boston, USA	615	100 g	22–28 years	100 g (WHO)	36% DM	+ (5.5% DM)
Dornhorst et al.[8]	London, UK	56	50 g	6–12 years	75 g (WHO)	64% (39% DM, 25% IGT)	
Ali and Alexis[24]	Trinidad	60	75 g	3–7 years	75 g (WHO)	(62% DM, 17% IGT)	
Kjos et al.[40]	Los Angeles, USA	246	100 g	5–8 weeks	75 g (NDDG)	19% (10% DM, 9% IGT)	
Henry and Beischer[19]	Melbourne, Australia	881	50 g	Up to 17 years	75 g (WHO)	27% (12% DM, 16% IGT)	+ (1% DM)
Catalano et al.[11]	Vermont, USA	103	100 g	7 weeks	75 g (NDDG)	22% (3% DM, 4% IGT)[a]	
Persson et al.[9]	Stockholm, Sweden	145	50 g	3–4 years	75 g (WHO)	25% (3.4% DM, 22% IGT)	+ (4% IGT)
Damm et al.[20]	Copenhagen, Denmark	241[b]	50 g	2–11 years	75 g (WHO)	34% (3.7 IDDM, 13.7% NIDDM, 17% IGT)	+ (5.3% IGT)
Coustan et al.[10]	Providence, USA	350	100 g	up to 10 years	75 (NDDG)	11% (7% DM, 4% IGT)	
Metzger et al.[13]	Chicago, USA	274	100 g	up to 5 years	100 g (NDDG)	57% (41% DM, 16% IGT)	
Kjos et al.[14]	Los Angeles, USA	671	100 g	up to 7 years	75 g (NDDG)	22% DM	
Greenberg et al.[15]	San Diego, USA	94	100 g	6 weeks	75 g (NDDG)	34% (16% DM, 18% IGT)	

DM, diabetes mellitus; IDDM, insulin-dependent diabetes mellitus; NIDDM, non-insulin-dependent diabetes mellitus; IGT, impaired glucose tolerance; OGTT, oral glucose tolerance test.
[a]15% non-diagnostic.
[b]Only diet-treated gestational diabetic women.

some of the follow-up studies on former gestational diabetic women published during the last decade. Comparison of the published studies produces difficulties due to the heterogeneity of both the patient populations and of gestational diabetes itself[7], and will be discussed.

DIAGNOSTIC TESTS AND CRITERIA FOR GESTATIONAL DIABETES AND FOLLOW-UP

A major problem is that different diagnostic tests and different criteria for gestational diabetes have been used. The same diagnostic criteria have only been applied pairwise in the studies of Dornhorst *et al.*[8] and Persson *et al.*[9]; the studies of Coustan *et al.*[10] and Catalano *et al.*[11], and in the four studies of O'Sullivan[12], Metzger *et al.*[13], Kjos *et al.*[14] and Greenberg *et al.*[15]. It is obvious that the higher the blood glucose levels needed to fulfil the criteria for the diagnosis of gestational diabetes, the higher risk of subsequent development of diabetes is to be expected.

At the follow-up examination the majority of the studies applied to a 75 g oral glucose tolerance test evaluated by World Health Organization (WHO)[16] or National Diabetes Data Group (NDDG)[17] criteria. These two sets of criteria are very similar but the NDDG criteria might be expected to give slightly lower rates of diabetes and impaired glucose tolerance[18]. Both WHO and NDDG criteria have also been applied to a 100 g oral glucose tolerance test[12,13], a procedure that tends to slightly overestimate the incidence of diabetes if correction for the increased glucose load is not made.

Not all women who had gestational diabetes during a specific period are able to participate in a follow-up examination years later. It is important, however, that the women investigated at follow-up constitute a representative and large subset of the initial population to be sure not to select the material in any way that can bias the results. If women treated with insulin during pregnancy are overrepresented at follow-up compared to diet-treated women, as in the study by Catalano *et al.*[11], one would expect a higher incidence of abnormal glucose tolerance at follow-up. This kind of bias could very likely occur since it might well be that these women, due to more severe disease, will be more compliant with respect to medical follow-up examinations. It has been documented that mothers with gestational diabetes with significantly increased fasting plasma glucose, and therefore treated with insulin, have a significantly higher risk of developing overt diabetes later in life than those treated with diet only[10,11,13,19]. However, the plasma glucose level at which insulin therapy is initiated varies between different studies, and insulin treatment is instituted at a lower glucose level in North America than in Scandinavia[11,20]. According to the current definition of gestational diabetes[4] a subset of the insulin-treated mothers will be women with insulin-dependent diabetes with onset during pregnancy. In a Danish population, these women have been shown to have nearly 100% incidence of subsequent development of diabetes[21], although the majority could be discharged from the hospital after delivery without insulin treatment. A high incidence of diabetes later in life has also been reported in women treated with oral hypoglycaemic agents during pregnancy[22]. To compare different follow-up studies it is therefore important to know the treatment and metabolic status during the index pregnancy. The current definition of gestational diabetes also allows women with undiagnosed diabetes antedating the pregnancy to be so categorized. The proportion of these women will tend to be increased in populations where the social security system and health system are inadequately developed, which will consequently give high rates of abnormal glucose tolerance after pregnancy.

Since the incidence of overt diabetes in the general population as well as in women with previous gestational diabetes increases with age, it is important to consider the time span between the index pregnancy and follow-up examination when comparing various studies. Life-table analysis has been used to estimate the cumulative incidence rate of diabetes in some studies[13,14,19,23], giving markedly higher values than the crude incidence rates. Although previous studies report that some of the women with a history of gestational diabetes, who have developed diabetes by the time of follow-up, were then being treated with insulin[8,9,11,13,14,24,25], few have tried meticulously to distinguish between insulin-dependent diabetes and non-insulin-dependent diabetes. It has generally been assumed that gestational diabetes is associated only with an increased risk for later development of the latter.

GEOGRAPHIC AND ETHNIC DIFFERENCES

Another very important factor when comparing different studies is the ethnic mixture of populations. It is well known that the background incidence of diabetes and the relative proportion of insulin-dependent and non-insulin-dependent diabetes vary among different populations. Pima Indians in Arizona and Hispanics in Los Angeles are often very obese and have a very high prevalence of non-insulin-dependent and a low incidence of insulin-dependent diabetes, whereas Scandinavian Caucasians in Denmark, a less obese population, have a lower total incidence of diabetes, but a significantly higher incidence of insulin-dependent and relatively lower incidence of non-insulin-dependent diabetes. Also, it has been shown that African Americans have a higher incidence of diabetes than white Caucasians[26]. Different rates of gestational diabetes have also been shown within studies among various ethnic groups[27,28].

This underlines the importance of the inclusion of an appropriate control group of women with normal glucose tolerance during pregnancy in follow-up studies of women with previous gestational diabetes, which has only been taken into consideration in a few studies[9,12,19,20]. These found that the net excess of diabetes was respectively 3%[9], 30%[12], 11%[19] and 17%[20].

COPENHAGEN STUDIES

We evaluated glucose tolerance 2–11 years after pregnancy in an ethnically homogeneous group (90% white Caucasians) of former diet-treated gestational diabetic women. A clear distinction between insulin-dependent and non-insulin-dependent diabetes was made by means of clinical criteria as well as an intravenous glucagon test. After a six-year median observation time since the index pregnancy, 34% of 241 women with previous diet-treated gestational diabetes had developed abnormal glucose tolerance; 3.4% were classified as insulin-dependent, 13.4% as non-insulin-dependent and 17.0% as impaired glucose tolerance. In four women (three insulin-dependent, one non-insulin-dependent diabetes) diabetes was diagnosed two to three months post partum, but more than half of the non-insulin-dependent diabetic women were diagnosed for the first time at the follow-up examination 2–11 years after their pregnancy[20,29]. Among the controls 5.3% had impaired glucose tolerance. Women who developed insulin-dependent diabetes were younger and leaner during the index pregnancy than those women who did not. A high prevalence was found of the HLA-DR types DR3 and DR4 typical of insulin-dependent diabetes, as well as of islet cell antibodies, in the women who developed insulin-dependent diabetes[29]. Insulin-dependent diabetes tended to be diagnosed closer to pregnancy than non-insulin dependent (14 (3–52) vs 48 (2–117) months, median (range)). We found that even women with previous 'mild' gestational diabetes have a significantly increased risk of subsequent development of all forms of diabetes. The finding of a 34% incidence of abnormal glucose tolerance is in agreement with another study from Scandinavia[9], allowing for the shorter observation time in that study; others have found considerably higher incidences of abnormal glucose tolerance[6,8,13,14,19,30,31]. These other studies have studied a broader spectrum of women with gestational diabetes, including insulin-treated women, and the ethnic composition of the populations studied was different from our own.

Despite very different incidences in different studies it is concluded that women with gestational diabetes have a considerably increased risk of developing diabetes (primarily non-insulin-dependent) or impaired glucose tolerance in the years following pregnancy. It is likely that the incidence of abnormal glucose tolerance will increase with increasing follow-up time since pregnancy. Nevertheless around 20% of previous gestational diabetic women developing overt diabetes will, in a Danish population, develop insulin-dependent diabetes, a fact which has been underestimated in some of the previous studies. As we found a trend for insulin-dependent diabetes to be diagnosed sooner after the pregnancy than non-insulin-dependent diabetes[20], we expect that the relative proportion of insulin-dependent diabetes among women developing diabetes will decrease when the population is followed for a longer period of time after the index pregnancy.

PREDICTIVE FACTORS FOR DEVELOPMENT OF OVERT DIABETES IN WOMEN WITH PREVIOUS GESTATIONAL DIABETES

Acknowledging that women with gestational diabetes are at risk for subsequent development of overt diabetes it is important to identify high-risk women. Many potential predictive factors such as plasma glucose, plasma insulin, and maternal relative weight for age are associated with each other, and it is therefore necessary to control for covariance and confounding factors in the analysis of predictive factors, which has not always been taken into consideration in previous studies.

In our own study[20] three significant independent predictor variables for development of diabetes were identified: high fasting plasma glucose level at diagnosis, preterm delivery and an oral glucose tolerance test two months post partum which still fulfilled the criteria for gestational diabetes. The finding of a high fasting glucose (odds ratio 3.4, 95% confidence interval 1.8–6.1, high vs low quartile) as a predictive variable is consistent with previous studies[10,11,14,32]. Studies in non-gestational diabetes populations have also reported that high fasting glucose predicts development of non-insulin-dependent diabetes[33]. As shown by Lam[32], the majority of gestational diabetic women who in the postpartum period still have an abnormal glucose tolerance will improve and return to normal glucose tolerance within one year. Nevertheless it is to be expected that these women, having a relatively more profound deterioration of glucose tolerance, will have a higher incidence of diabetes later in life. In agreement with this, we found that an abnormal outcome of the postpartum oral glucose tolerance test predicts the later development of overt diabetes (odds ratio 4.9, 95% confidence interval 2.1–11.2)[20], a finding later confirmed by Kjos *et al.*[14], who found that an abnormal postpartum oral glucose tolerance test was the best predictor of the future development of non-insulin-dependent diabetes.

Preterm delivery was also a predictive factor (odds ratio 3.6, 95% confidence interval 1.1–11.6) which has not previously been reported. Preterm delivery was not necessarily caused by iatrogenic intervention, and it is well known that pregnant women with insulin-dependent diabetes have a considerably increased risk of preterm delivery, which increases with poor metabolic control[34]. It could be speculated that the gestational diabetic women who delivered preterm in some way might have had a more serious glucose intolerance than the remainder.

In contrast to some of the previous studies[10,12,13] no association between the development of diabetes and maternal overweight or age was found in our population. When the analysis was carried out without the women who later developed insulin-dependent diabetes, relative maternal overweight (body mass index $\geq 25 \text{ kg/m}^2$) did predict non-insulin-dependent diabetes. Some studies have used diabetes[14,23] and others abnormal glucose tolerance (both diabetes and impaired glucose tolerance)[10,11,32] as the endpoint in the analysis of predictive factors, and this might contribute to the different results of different studies. In our own data, undertaking multivariate analysis with abnormal glucose tolerance (diabetes or impaired glucose tolerance) as the dependent variable, the following independent predictive factors were identified: fasting glucose level at diagnosis (odds ratio 2.2, 95% confidence interval 1.4–3.3), early diagnosis (<32 completed weeks, odds ratio 2.3, 95% confidence interval 1.2–4.3) and an abnormal outcome of the postpartum oral glucose tolerance test (odds ratio 4.9, 95% confidence interval 2.5–9.4). Early diagnosis of gestational diabetes has also been found to predict development of diabetes[14].

Other factors that have been shown to be predictive for the later development of diabetes or abnormal glucose tolerance are the 2 h glucose level or the glucose area under the curve at the diagnostic oral glucose tolerance test[14,20,23,32]. The 2 h glucose during the oral glucose tolerance test has previously been reported to predict development of diabetes in non-gestational diabetes populations[33]. In our studies[20,35], plasma insulin was measured during the oral glucose tolerance test at the time of diagnosis, and postpartum, in 91 women, enabling an evaluation of the predictive value of fasting and post-glucose insulin levels for subsequent development of overt diabetes. In accord with the findings of Metzger *et al.*[13] we found that low insulin secretion during the oral glucose tolerance test at diagnosis was a significant predictor of the later development of diabetes. A recent study in Los Angeles of Latino women showed that a single pregnancy, independent of the effect of weight gain, accelerated the development of non-insulin-dependent diabetes in a group of women with a high prevalence of pancreatic beta-cell dysfunction[35a]. This implies that episodes of pregnancy-associated insulin resistance may contribute to the decline in beta-cell function.

IMMUNOLOGICAL MARKERS

Islet cell antibodies and insulin autoantibodies are well-known predictive markers for insulin-dependent diabetes. In Copenhagen[29] three out of four islet cell antibody-positive gestational diabetic subjects developed insulin-dependent diabetes 3–52 months after pregnancy, giving a 75% predictive value of a positive titre at diagnosis, with sensitivity and specificity 50% and 99% respectively. The relative risk of development of insulin-dependent diabetes in islet cell antibody positive subjects was 34 (95% confidence interval 10–118) compared to antibody-negative subjects. Our results are in concordance with studies in other populations[13,36–38]. Insulin autoantibodies were not useful as a predictor of insulin-dependent diabetes in our study due to the fact that none of the mothers were positive during pregnancy, in accord with Metzger *et al.*[13]. The presence of serum antibodies against glumatic acid decarboxylase (GAD65) has also been found to predict development of insulin-dependent diabetes and recently we have found that a positive GAD65 autoantibody titre at the diagnosis of gestational diabetes was highly predictive[39]. The predictive value was similar to that obtained from islet cell antibody studies, since three of 139 women were GAD65 autoantibody positive and all three had insulin-dependent diabetes at follow-up examination 4–11 years after pregnancy. In the future, GAD65 autoantibodies might be of clinical use as a supplement or alternative to islet cell autoantibodies to identify pre-insulin-dependent diabetic subjects as candidates for preventive treatment. However, such prophylactic treatment is still experimental, and it seems not yet advisable to screeen all women with gestational diabetes for any of these autoantibodies.

In conclusion, substantial evidence indicates that every woman with gestational diabetes should be examined with an oral glucose tolerance test about two months post partum. A high frequency of abnormal glucose tolerance is found at this time[11,13–15,20,32,40], and the result of the test has been shown in very different populations[14,20] to be highly predictive for the development of later overt diabetes. Although a relatively decreased pancreatic beta cell function in women with gestational diabetes predicts the development of diabetes, measurement of plasma insulin during the diagnostic oral glucose tolerance test will in many centres be inconvenient for other than scientific purposes. Testing for islet cell and GAD65 antoantibodies might be relevant in the future. It is important for regular assessment of glucose tolerance in women with previous gestational diabetes to secure an early diagnosis of diabetes or impaired glucose tolerance, especially if the oral glucose tolerance test in the postpartum period was abnormal.

REFERENCES

1 Kühl C. Glucose metabolism during and after pregnancy in normal and gestational diabetic women. I. Influence of normal pregnancy on serum glucose and insulin concentration during basal fasting conditions and after a challenge with glucose. *Acta Endocrinol* 1975; **79:** 709–19.
2 Gabbe SG. Gestational diabetes mellitus. *N Engl J Med* 1986; **315:** 1025–6.
3 Guttorm E. Practical screening for diabetes mellitus in pregnant women. *Acta Endocrinol* 1974; **75:** 11–24.
4 Summary and recommendations of the Third International Workshop-Conference on Gestational Diabetes Mellitus. *Diabetes* 1991; **40** (Suppl. 2): 197–201.
5 Kühl C, Hornnes PJ, Andersen O. Etiology and pathophysiology of gestational diabetes mellitus. *Diabetes* 1985; **34** (Suppl. 2): 66–70.
6 O'Sullivan JB. Diabetes mellitus after GDM. *Diabetes* 1991; **29** (Suppl. 2): 131–5.
7 Freinkel N, Metzger BE, Phelps RL *et al.* Gestational diabetes mellitus: heterogeneity of maternal age, weight, insulin secretion, HLA-antigens, and islet cell antibodies and the impact of maternal metabolism on pancreatic B-cell somatic development in the offspring. *Diabetes* 1985; **34** (Suppl. 2): 1–7.
8 Dornhorst A, Bailey PC, Anyaoku V *et al.* Abnormalities of glucose tolerance following gestational diabetes. *Q J Med* 1990; **284:** 1219–28.

9   Persson B, Hanson U, Hartling SG, Binder C. Follow-up of women with previous GDM. Insulin, C-peptide, and proinsulin responses to oral glucose load. *Diabetes* 1991; **40** (Suppl. 2): 136–41.
10 Coustan DR, Carpenter MW, O'Sullivan PS, Carr SR. Gestational diabetes: Predictors of subsequent disordered metabolism. *Am J Obstet Gynecol* 1993; **168:** 1139–45.
11 Catalano PM, Varno KM, Bernstein IM, Amini SB. Incidence and risk factors associated with abnormal postpartum glucose tolerance in women with gestational diabetes. *Am J Obstet Gynecol* 1991; **165:** 914–19.
12 O'Sullivan JB. The Boston gestational diabetes studies: review and prospectives. In: Sutherland HW, Stowers JM, Pearson DWM (eds), *Carbohydrate Metabolism in Pregnancy and the Newborn.* Springer-Verlag, Berlin, 1989; 287–94.
13 Metzger BE, Cho NH, Roston SM, Radvany R. Prepregnancy weight and antepartum insulin secretion predict glucose tolerance five years after gestational diabetes mellitus. *Diabetes Care* 1993; **16:** 1598–605.
14 Kjos SL, Peters RK, Xiang A *et al.* Predicting future diabetes in Latino women with gestational diabetes: utility of early post partum glucose tolerance testing. *Diabetes* 1995; **44:** 586–91.
15 Greenberg LR, Moore TR, Murphy H. Gestational diabetes mellitus: antenatal variables as predictors of postpartum glucose intolerance. *Obstet Gynecol* 1995; **86:** 97–101.
16 World Health Organization Study Group. Diabetes Mellitus. *World Health Organization Technical Report Series 727*, Geneva, 1985.
17 National Diabetes Data Group. Classification of diagnosis of diabetes mellitus and other categories of glucose intolerance. *Diabetes* 1979; **28:** 1039–57.
18 Motala AA, Omar MAK. Evaluation of WHO and NDDG criteria for impaired glucose tolerance. *Diabetes Res Clin Pract* 1994; **23:** 103–9.
19 Henry OA, Beischer NA. Long-term implications of gestational diabetes for the mother. In: Oats JN (ed.), *Baillière's Clinical Obstetrics and Gynaecology.* Baillière Tindall, London, 1991; 461–83.
20 Damm P, Kühl, C, Bertelsen A, Mølsted-Pedersen L. Predictive factors for the development of diabetes in women with previous gestational diabetes mellitus. *Am J Obstet Gynecol* 1992; **167:** 607–16.
21 Buschard K, Hougaard P, Mølsted-Pedersen L, Kühl C. Type 1 (insulin-dependent) diabetes mellitus diagnosed during pregnancy: a clinical and prognostic study. *Diabetologia* 1990; **33:** 31–5.
22 Mølsted-Pedersen L, Damm P, Buschard K. Diabetes diagnosed during pregnancy. In: Sutherland HW, Stowers JM, Pearson DWM (eds), *Carbohydrate Metabolism in Pregnancy and the Newborn.* Springer-Verlag, Berlin, 1989; 277–86.
23 O'Sullivan JB. Gestational diabetes: factors influencing the rates of subsequent diabetes. In: Sutherland HW, Stowers JM (eds), *Carbohydrate Metabolism in Pregnancy and the Newborn.* Springer-Verlag, Berlin, 1979; 425–35.
24 Ali Z, Alexis SD. Occurrence of diabetes mellitus after gestational diabetes in Trinidad. *Diabetes Care* 1990; **13:** 527–9.
25 O'Sullivan JB. Subsequent morbidity among gestational diabetic women. In: Sutherland HW, Stowers JM (eds), *Carbohydrate Metabolism in Pregnancy and the Newborn.* Churchill Livingstone, Edinburgh, 1984; 174–80.
26 Harris MI, Hadden WC, Knowler WC, Bennett PH. Prevalence of diabetes and impaired glucose tolerance and plasma glucose levels in U.S. population aged 20–74 yr. *Diabetes* 1987; **36:** 523–34.
27 Dornhorst A, Paterson CM, Nicholls JSD *et al.* High prevalence of gestational diabetes in women from ethnic minority groups. *Diabetes Med* 1992; **9:** 820–5.
28 Dooley SL, Metzger BE, Cho NH. Gestational diabetes mellitus: influence of race on disease prevalence and perinatal outcome in a U.S. population. *Diabetes* 1991; **40** (Suppl. 2): 25–9.
29 Damm P, Kühl C, Buschard K *et al.* Prevalence and predictive value of islet cell antibodies and insulin antoantibodies in women with gestational diabetes. *Diabetes Med* 1994; **11:** 558–63.
30 Metzger BE, Bybee DE, Freinkel N *et al.* Gestational diabetes mellitus: correlations between the phenotypic and genotypic characteristics of the mother and abnormal glucose tolerance

during the first year post partum. *Diabetes* 1985; **34** (Suppl. 2): 111–15.

31 Mestman JH. Follow-up studies in women with gestational diabetes mellitus: the experience at Los Angeles Country/University of Southern California Medical Center. In: Weiss PAM, Coustan DR (eds), *Gestational Diabetes*. Springer-Verlag, Vienna, 1988; 191–8.

32 Lam KSL, Li DF, Lauder IJ *et al*. Prediction of presistent carbohydrate intolerance in patients with gestational diabetes. *Diabetes Res Clin Pract* 1991; **12:** 181–6.

33 Stern MP, Morales PA, Valdez RA *et al*. Predicting diabetes: moving beyond impaired glucose tolerance. *Diabetes* 1993; **42:** 706–14.

34 Mimouni F, Miovdovnik M, Siddiqi TA *et al*. High spontaneous premature labor rate in insulin-dependent diabetic pregnant women: an association with poor glycemic control and urogenital infection. *Obstet Gynecol* 1988; **72:** 175–80.

35 Damm P, Kühl C, Hornnes PJ, Mølsted-Pedersen L. A longitudinal study of plasma insulin and glucagon in women with previous gestational diabetes. *Diabetes Care* 1995; **18:** 654–65.

35a Peters RK, Kjos SL, Xiang A, Buchanan TA. Long-term diabetogenic effect of single pregnancy in women with previous gestational diabetes mellitus. *Lancet* 1996; **347:** 227–30.

36 Catalano PM, Tyzbir ED, Sims EAH. Incidence and significance of islet cell antibodies in women with previous gestational diabetes. *Diabetes Care* 1990; **13:** 478–82.

37 Mauricio D, Corcoy RM, Codina M *et al*. Islet cell antibodies identify a subset of gestational diabetic women with higher risk of developing diabetes mellitus shortly after pregnancy. *Diabetes Nutr Metab* 1992; **5:** 237–41.

38 Steel JM, Irvine WJ, Clark BF. The significance of pancreatic islet cell antibody and abnormal glucose tolerance during pregnancy. *J Clin Lab Immunol* 1980; **4:** 83–5.

39 Damm P, Peterson JS, Dyrberg T *et al*. Prevalence and predictive value of GAD65 autoantibodies in women with gestational diabetes. *Diabetologia* 1995; **38** (Suppl. 1): A70 (Abstract).

40 Kjos SL, Buchanan TA, Greenspoon JS *et al*. Gestational diabetes mellitus: the prevalence of glucose intolerance and diabetes mellitus in the first two months post partum. *Am J Obstet Gynecol* 1990; **168:** 93–8.

21

Prevention of Diabetes Following Gestational Diabetes

MICHELA ROSSI and ANNE DORNHORST
Royal Postgraduate Medical School, London, UK

THE CASE FOR PRIMARY PREVENTION

The prevalence of non-insulin-dependent diabetes and impaired glucose tolerance is increasing worldwide, reaching epidemic proportions in many countries[1]. As death rates from communicable disease fall, those from non-communicable disease rise. Diabetes is now amongst the five leading causes of death from disease for most countries. The cost of managing diabetic complications, both microvascular (retinopathy, nephropathy and neuropathy), and macrovascular (coronary heart disease, stroke and peripheral vascular disease), has been estimated to be 5% of the total health care expenditure for the UK[2].

At present, primary prevention of diabetes is not widely practised. Instead, the treatment of diabetes is centred on preventing the development of diabetic complications (secondary prevention) and minimizing the morbidity from established complications (tertiary prevention). The proven benefits of secondary and tertiary prevention have formed the basis of the annual diabetic outpatient review, which is advocated for all patients. During this diabetic complications are systematically screened for (retinopathy, nephropathy, neuropathy and vascular disease) and education on lifestyle modification given to lessen morbidity and mortality. Unfortunately the late diagnosis of non-insulin-dependent diabetes all too frequently results in active management of diabetes only being introduced after complications have developed. It is now recognized that if the human and monetary cost of diabetes are to be effectively reduced, preventive

Diabetes and Pregnancy: An International Approach to Diagnosis and Management.
Edited by A. Dornhorst and D. R. Hadden.
© 1996 John Wiley & Sons Ltd.

strategies need to begin earlier, through a combination of delaying the onset of diabetes (primary prevention), making the diagnosis earlier and instituting treatment sooner (secondary prevention)[3]. It has been estimated that if the onset of non-insulin-dependent diabetes is delayed by six years and effective treatment commenced at the time of disease onset, sight-threatening diabetic retinopathy would be halved.

To date, there have been no long-term controlled clinical studies confirming the benefits of primary prevention programmes on the development of diabetes. Studies have, however, reported a reduced progression of impaired glucose tolerance to non-insulin-dependent diabetes following the introduction of primary prevention programmes[4]. Longitudinal observational rather than interventional studies, on men and women, have consistently shown that weight control, physical activity and a low-fat diet reduce the risk of diabetes. A common finding of these studies is that the individual at greatest perceived risk appears to benefit most when these lifestyle changes are introduced. The potential for primary prevention programmes has arisen from observational epidemiology data performed predominantly on non-diabetic populations.

The persuasive theoretical argument for the primary prevention of diabetes has resulted in the European section of the World Health Organization (WHO) and the International Diabetic Federation endorsing primary preventive strategies, which are summarized in the 1995 Acropolis Affirmation[5]. Special mention is made of targeting high-risk groups for primary prevention, including women with a history of gestational diabetes, as well as individuals with impaired glucose tolerance or a first-degree relative with diabetes[6]. The present chapter examines the likely benefits of providing health education and structured follow-up to women with a history of gestational diabetes. The chapter concentrates on the prevention of non-insulin-dependent diabetes and its associated cardiac morbidity.

SCREENING VERSUS TARGETING

Preventive health care aims to reduce contributory risk factors, in the case of diabetes, obesity, physical inactivity and a high-fat diet. This can be implemented through a population strategy (screening) or by identifying high-risk groups (targeting)[7]. Screening aims to reach all members of a population in an attempt to reduce the prevalence of risk factors. To date no demonstrable benefit has been shown for population screening for diabetes mellitus.

Targeting is based on identifying high-risk persons for supervised interventional management, be it behavioural lifestyle modification or pharmaceutical. By focusing on the most vulnerable individual and avoiding unnecessary disturbance and expense to those not at increased risk, targeting offers an efficient use of resources. However, the identification of high-risk groups can itself be problematic, usually requiring some measure of population screening. Blood glucose values, both fasting and postprandial, are a poor predictor of future risk of diabetes. Unlike blood pressure and plasma cholesterol concentration, which have a linear relationship with the risk of stroke or coronary vascular disease, respectively, there is no such relationship for plasma glucose concentration (within the normal distribution curve) with future risk of diabetes. It is only when the plasma glucose has risen outside the normal range and glucose intolerance is present that a relationship is found. Therefore the use of blood glucose to select at-risk groups for targeting falls short of the prerequisite of sensitivity, specificity and cost effectiveness for a screening programme, making the use of historic data to identify at-risk groups for diabetes more attractive. Identifying individuals with a family member with non-insulin-dependent diabetes or those with an obstetric history suggestive of gestational diabetes has been shown to be an effective way of selecting at-risk individuals[8].

PREVIOUS GESTATIONAL DIABETIC WOMEN: AN AT-RISK GROUP

Gestational diabetic women have a well-documented risk of future diabetes. At the time of diagnosis they are pre-menopausal and therefore unlikely to have already developed significant macrovascular disease. As housewives they are likely to be in control of buying and preparing the family meals and are therefore in a position to implement lifestyle dietary changes. These women will also have an understanding of their risk and have received basic diabetic education during pregnancy. In addition, as a majority of women become pregnant the screening for gestational diabetes provides an opportunity of identify a large proportion of women at risk of diabetes, at an age when lifestyle modification hopefully may reduce both the development of diabetes and cardiovascular disease (see below). Another separate but important reason for considering these women an at-risk group requiring follow-up is to lessen the risk of future pregnancies occurring in women with undiagnosed diabetes.

RISK FACTORS FOR NON-INSULIN-DEPENDENT DIABETES FOLLOWING A PREGNANCY COMPLICATED BY GESTATIONAL DIABETES

The progression to diabetes following a pregnancy complicated by gestational diabetes is known to be influenced by both unmodifiable risk factors, such as ethnicity, age, family history and degree of hyperglycaemia in pregnancy, as well as potentially modifiable risk factors which include obesity and future weight gain. Population studies would also predict that physical activity and the composition of the diet represent other modifiable risk factors. Preventive programmes need to focus on the modifiable risk factors, using the unmodifiable factors to further highlight those women most at risk.

UNMODIFIABLE RISK FACTORS

Both ethnicity and age are important risk factors for the development of gestational diabetes and the rate of progression to non-insulin-dependent diabetes following the pregnancy. The influence of ethnicity reflects the prevalence of non-insulin-dependent diabetes within a given population. A wide variation in prevalence rates of both impaired glucose tolerance and non-insulin-dependent diabetes in women of childbearing age have been reported from different countries[9]. The WHO has collected data from 29 different female populations which shows that while prevalence rates for non-insulin-dependent diabetes in the lowest tertile are below 1% those in the highest tertile are in excess of 6%. Populations at particular risk include native Americans and South Pacific islanders. Similar data exist for impaired glucose tolerance, where prevalence varies from 0 to 18%, with a third of the female populations studied having a prevalence greater than 7%.

A knowledge of the background age-related prevalence of non-insulin-dependent diabetes and impaired glucose tolerance for a given ethnic group is important when planning follow-up programmes for women with gestational diabetes. Knowledge of the usual age of onset of that population for non-insulin-dependent diabetes predicts the time over which preventive programmes would need to be implemented to see a reduction in its prevalence. In ethnic groups with very high progression rates (~50% within five years), such as women from the Indian subcontinent[10] or American Hispanic women[11], follow-up management should be geared as much to the early detection and treatment of diabetes (secondary prevention) as to primary prevention. The progression to non-insulin-dependent diabetes in white populations is considerably slower, being less than 10% by the end of the first decade but increasing to more than 20% by the end of the second decade from the index pregnancy[12]. O'Sullivan's data on a predominantly white and black population suggests this progression to non-insulin-dependent diabetes continues to rise in the third decade after a gestational diabetes pregnancy, the progression rate being highest in obese women[13]. It is therefore likely that preventive programmes would need to be reinforced over a period of 20–30 years in populations whose onset of diabetes is usually in the fifth and sixth decades of life.

POTENTIAL MODIFIABLE RISK FACTORS

Obesity

Obesity is the most important modifiable risk factor in the development of non-insulin-dependent diabetes. Obesity appears an especially important risk factor in women. Of the 1800 newly diagnosed patients enrolled in the UK Prospective Diabetic study, 41% of the women were above their ideal body weight compared with 21% of the men[14]. In the American Nurses Health Study[15] 61% of newly diagnosed non-insulin-dependent diabetic women between the ages of 30 and 64 years had a body mass index in excess of 29 kg/m^2.

Women with previous gestational diabetes are metabolically vulnerable, having already shown their inability to maintain glucose tolerance when their insulin sensitivity falls in pregnancy[16], the restoration of glucose tolerance post partum being dependent on their insulin sensitivity returning to pre-pregnancy values. Post partum, even when glucose tolerant, these women have evidence of impaired beta cell secretion[17]; many are also insulin insensitive due to coexisting obesity or other factors[18]. It is the combination of this impaired insulin response in the presence of obesity which makes the previous gestational diabetic women so much at risk of diabetes. In an American multi-ethnic follow-up study obese women with an insulin response to glucose in the lowest tertile had an eight-fold increased risk of developing diabetes after five years over non-obese women with higher insulin responses[19]. Long-term maintenance of glucose tolerance depends on ensuring that insulin sensitivity does not fall to that critical level encountered in pregnancy. Obesity and weight gain are important factors influencing insulin sensitivity. Weight loss in women improves insulin sensitivity, especially when associated with a decrease in abdominal fat distribution and waist–hip ratio[20]. The association of abdominal fat mass with reduced insulin sensitivity and risk of non-insulin-dependent diabetes is well documented in both men and women[21,22].

Weight gain and obesity are important contributing factors for the development of non-insulin-dependent diabetes following a pregnancy complicated by gestational diabetes[13,17,19]. In O'Sullivan's original follow-up study of women with previous gestational diabetes those who were obese or gained weight subsequent to their pregnancy had an approximately two-fold greater frequency of diabetes by 16 years[13]. Many women with gestational diabetes are obese at presentation, and while normalization of body weight post partum is perhaps unrealistic, emphasis on modest weight reduction and prevention of future weight gain is realistic. Significant metabolic improvement has been documented with modest weight loss, including improvement of glycaemic control, lipid profile and blood pressure. It has been estimated that a 10 kg weight loss would lessen the reduction in life expectancy associated with non-insulin-dependent diabetes by as much as 35%[23]. However, the benefits of weight loss are likely to be dependent on the degree of obesity present[24]. Weight loss in obese (body mass index $>29 \, kg/m^2$) non-insulin-dependent diabetic subjects was associated with a modest decrease in mortality in a 10-year multinational WHO study involving 1544 diabetic women; however, there was a three-fold increased mortality rate in the non-obese (body mass index $<26 \, kg/m^2$) who lost weight[24]. Weight loss in severely obese individuals with impaired glucose tolerance reduces the progression to non-insulin-dependent diabetes 30-fold compared with non-dieted controls[25]. By contrast, in the Nurses' Health Study weight gain in excess of 10 kg during 16 years of follow-up was associated with a significant increase in mortality[26].

The evidence of increasing obesity with increasing risk of coronary heart disease in women provides further support for weight control programmes, especially in a group of women at increased risk of vascular disease from diabetes. Data from the Nurses' Health Study on 115 000 women followed for 16 years showed the lowest mortality was among women with a body mass index between 19 and 26.9 kg/m^2; when the body mass index exceeded 29 kg/m^2 death from coronary artery disease increased three-fold[26].

All evidence supports a policy that obese women with previous gestational diabetes should receive advice on weight loss, and non-obese women on weight maintenance. Emphasis should be made that this is to delay the progression of diabetes as well as to reduce the risk of heart disease.

Diet

Epidemiological studies in various populations have shown that high dietary intakes of saturated fats combined with low intakes of dietary fibre are associated with an increased incidence of diabetes[27]. The prevalence of non-insulin-dependent diabetes is highest in countries with a high fat intake and lower in those with a high carbohydrate intake[27]. Diets that have $>40\%$ of their total calories from fat are associated with decreased insulin sensitivity and an increased prevalence of non-insulin-dependent diabetes and other cardiovascular risk factors including hypertension, dyslipidaemia and obesity[28,29]. The protection offered by low-fat/high complex carbohydrate diets is likely to result from increased insulin sensitivity.

A diet needs to be considered in both quantitative and qualitative terms. The total energy content is important when advising about weight control and weight loss. Advocating healthy eating to all women with gestational diabetes should become a logical extension of the dietary advice they receive at the time of pregnancy.

Physical Activity

Short-term and long-term physical activity has a beneficial effect on insulin sensitivity, insulin secretion and carbohydrate metabolism in non-diabetic subjects[30]. Acute physical activity promotes glucose uptake into muscle.

Regular exercise increases the glucose transport response to insulin, thus increasing insulin sensitivity and reducing insulin response to oral glucose. Clamp studies have shown that insulin-stimulated glucose disposal increases approximately 30% with exercise in both diabetic and non-diabetic subjects[31].

Regular physical activity helps to prevent increasing adiposity with increasing age and reduces an individual's risk of developing non-insulin-dependent diabetes. The beneficial metabolic effects of exercise last as long as regular physical activity is maintained. Epidemiological studies have shown a lower prevalence amongst individuals with higher physical activity, an effect that is independent of weight and age[32-34]. Physical training programmes have been shown in prospective studies to reduce the prevalence of both impaired glucose tolerance and non-insulin-dependent diabetes[35,36]. A prospective study on 80 000 non-diabetic, middle-aged American women studied over eight years showed that regular exercise reduced the risk of developing non-insulin-dependent diabetes by a third, even in the presence of a positive family history[35]. Similar benefits from exercise were observed in a prospective study of 6000 male alumni students[36]. Both studies showed the greatest protection of exercise on maintaining glucose tolerance was conferred on those at greatest risk, namely those with a family history of non-insulin-dependent diabetes or obesity. Cross-sectional studies in populations with impaired glucose tolerance have shown that habitual physical activity reduces postprandial hyperinsulinaemia, independent of obesity, fat distribution and age, indicating that exercise is metabolically beneficial to this high-risk group[37]. The difference in levels of physical activity in Asian women in the UK compared to Caucasian women is believed to contribute to their earlier onset of non-insulin-dependent diabetes. Of the newly diagnosed women in the UK Prospective Diabetes Study the Asian women, despite being younger and less obese, were significantly less active than the Caucasian women, only 18% of the Asian women being classified as physically active compared with 41% of the Caucasian women[38].

In addition to any benefits on carbohydrate metabolism, regular physical exercise increases cardiovascular fitness and reduces cardiovascular risk factors, including lipid profiles, blood pressure and abdominal fat distribution[39]. Ongoing physical activity helps weight control, which can seldom be achieved without physical exercise. Physical activity is associated with increased longevity in men, even in the presence of obesity[40].

There is enough circumstantial evidence to recommend that all women with a history of gestational diabetes be encouraged to participate in regular exercise. The recommendation of the British Heart Foundation to reduce cardiovascular disease by exercising for 20 min or more three times a week, carried out at 50–60% of an individual's maximum aerobic capacity, is realistic and should be strongly encouraged[41]. For most women over the age of 45 years this level of exertion can be achieved by brisk walking.

ATTENTION TO CARDIOVASCULAR RISK FACTORS

Coronary heart disease is the commonest cause of death in women with diabetes[42]. Analysis of the Framingham data showed that women with diabetes had a three- to seven-fold higher risk of cardiovascular disease than non-diabetic women, compared with the two- to four-fold increased risk seen in diabetic men[42]. Impaired glucose tolerance itself is an important risk factor for cardiovascular disease[43]. Over the last 20 years in England and Wales there has been a fall in the death rate from coronary heart disease in women, which has been significantly greater in non-diabetic than diabetic women[44].

Health education for previous gestational diabetic women should focus not only on those modifiable risk factors pertaining to non-insulin-dependent diabetes but also those for heart disease, which include hypercholesterolaemia, hypertension and smoking.

Hypercholesterolaemia

Total cholesterol is an important established risk factor for coronary artery disease; in diabetic individuals for any level of cholesterol coronary heart mortality is increased four to five times that for non-diabetic subjects[45]. The benefits, however, of lowering cholesterol levels in women have been less studied than for men, in whom primary and secondary management of hypercholesteraemia has been shown to reduce coronary mortality[46,47]. Although none of the present trials have had adequate power definitively to show that lowering cholesterol levels in healthy women reduces the risk of coronary heart disease, observational data suggest that lowering the low-density lipoprotein cholesterol and raising high-density lipoprotein cholesterol should have similar benefit in women as in men[48]. It therefore seems prudent to encourage low-cholesterol diets in all women with previous gestational diabetes and to treat those with documented hypercholesterolaemia with appropriate drug therapy.

Hypertension

Hypertension is a common finding at the time of presentation of non-insulin-dependent diabetes, 54% of all newly diagnosed women being hypertensive on entry into the UK Prospective Diabetic Study[14]. The increased prevalence of hypertension in subjects with both non-insulin-dependent diabetes and impaired glucose tolerance is independent of age, weight and use of antihypertensive medication. Systolic hypertension increases with age and is a risk factor for the development of atherosclerotic vascular disease[49,50]. The frequency with which hypertension coexists with other cardiac risk factors in subjects with non-insulin-dependent diabetes has suggested to some investigators that a unifying metabolic aetiology exists to explain these associations[51].

Prospective studies on subjects with non-insulin-dependent diabetes demonstrate an increased risk of macrovascular disease in the presence of hypertension[52]. Hypertension also hastens the progression of diabetic microvascular disease. Systolic blood pressure correlates with the rate of decline in renal function in these subjects[53].

In the non-diabetic population the treatment of hypertension reduces mortality from stroke and to a lesser extent from coronary heart disease[54]. The degree to which treatment of hypertension in the non-insulin-dependent subject protects against premature coronary artery mortality is unknown[55]. Hypertension alongside other cardiovascular risk factors frequently precedes the diagnosis of non-insulin-dependent diabetes, and if the benefits of hypertensive treatment in these patients are to be realized, early diagnosis and treatment of hypertension will be required in the prediabetic stages[56]. This being so, women with previous gestational diabetes should have regular checks on their blood pressure and treatment commenced according to national guidelines.

Smoking

Smoking remains the leading preventable cause of death. Smoking greatly increases the risk of cardiovascular disease, and this is specially so in diabetic subjects[57]. In the last 15 years there has been an increase in the number of women who smoke. Of 1752 Caucasian women with newly diagnosed diabetes entering the UK Prospective Diabetes Study 29% were current smokers and a further 27% ex-smokers[38]. Women who smoke as little as four cigarettes a day have more than twice the risk of coronary artery disease[58]. The influence of cigarettes on the risk of myocardial infarction is greatest in young middle-aged adults. Women with previous gestational diabetes should be strongly encouraged not to smoke. The benefits of stopping smoking should also be stressed, as the risk of coronary heart disease in women falls to that of the background population within three to five years after cessation of smoking[59].

Hormone Replacement Therapy

Coronary artery disease in women increases after the menopause[60]. Hormonal replacement therapy in the form of unopposed oestrogen halves cardiovascular morbidity and mortality in the first 10 post-menopausal years[61]. The mechanisms by which oestrogen bestows cardiovascular protection are not fully understood, although a beneficial effect on lipid profiles, including a fall in low-density lipoproteins and rise in high-density lipoproteins, is believed to play a part[62]. Another beneficial effect on lipoprotein metabolism from oestrogen is thought to result from their antioxidant properties, inhibiting the formation of the more atherogenic moieties of the low-density lipoprotein[63]. Oestrogen usage has also been reported to reduce other metabolic cardiovascular risk factors, including platelet adhesiveness[64], fibrinolysis[65] and the activity of angiotensin converting enzyme[66]. The extent to which these favourable metabolic changes are negated by the addition of cyclical progesterone is an area of continuing research. Results from a three-year placebo-controlled randomized trial which compared the metabolic effects of unopposed oestrogen with those of oestrogen/progesterone showed both formulations to have similar beneficial effects on lipid profiles and fibrinogen activity without adversely affecting blood pressure or insulin concentrations[65]. However, this study did show that oestrogen usage alone was associated with higher high-density lipoproteins, and since this trial was not designed to look at cardiovascular endpoints it still has to be shown that these combined hormonal preparations provide a similar degree of cardiovascular protection. In addition, as there is a large variation in metabolic effects with the different progestational agents, it is likely that some combinations of oestrogen and progesterone are more cardioprotective than others.

The use of hormone replacement therapy for prophylaxis against heart disease and osteoporosis will remain a controversial subject. Publication of randomized trials with the power to examine both the long-term benefits and drawbacks are required. Oestrogen usage either alone or combined with progesterone significantly increases the risk of breast cancer by approximately 40% in women over 55 years who are currently taking, or who have taken, these hormone preparations for a period of five years or more[67]. This increased risk of breast cancer, which increases with increasing age, needs to be balanced against the cardioprotective effect of hormone replacement therapy. Even if these benefits are shown to outweigh the risk of breast cancer the use of post-menopausal hormone replacement therapy will remain an emotive subject for many women, as the fear of breast carcinoma is often greater than that of premature cardiovascular disease. Those women likely to benefit most from the cardioprotective effects of hormone replacement therapy are those at greatest risk for coronary artery disease. While hormone replacement therapy should be made readily available to women with previous gestational diabetes the final decision for its use must be taken on an individual basis, taking account of the woman's own wishes and fears.

THE POTENTIAL FOR THERAPEUTIC INTERVENTION

Three controlled published studies—two from the UK and the third from Sweden—using oral hypoglycaemic agents have looked at the rate of deterioration from impaired glucose tolerance to non-insulin-dependent diabetes. Neither of the two UK studies—the Bedford study[68] which used the sulphonylurea tolbutamide, or the Whitehall study[69] which used the biguanide pheformin—showed any benefit. In a 10-year study from

Molmöhus, Sweden[70], again no significant reduction in progression was seen with tolbutamide compared with placebo; however, estimates of compliance showed that less than half of those assigned to active treatment (23/49) actually continued to take tolbutamide over the 10-year period, and of the 23 subjects who did comply none actually developed non-insulin-dependent diabetes, compared with 15% in the placebo and diet-treated group. The benefit of these oral agents in delaying the progression of impaired glucose tolerance to non-insulin-dependent diabetes has therefore not been demonstrated.

The recent advent of the thiazolidinediones, a class of compounds that increase insulin sensitivity, provides the potential for a pharmacological approach to the primary prevention of non-insulin-dependent diabetes[71]. A recent study has shown that troglitazone, an oral thiazolidinedione, taken over a 3-month period improved glucose tolerance in 18 obese subjects with and without impaired glucose tolerance. In addition to increasing insulin sensitivity, systolic and diastolic blood pressure was also improved. This class of pharmacological agent that improves insulin insensitivity may prove beneficial not only for delaying the onset of non-insulin-dependent diabetes but also improving other metabolic components of cardiovascular risk.

EDUCATION AND EMPOWERMENT

Education support has become an integral part of diabetic care, with the realization that patient compliance with diet and lifestyle advice is only achieved with understanding of why it is important. Education must at all times be both comprehensible to the patient and culturally relevant. The success of education and patient compliance during the management of diabetic pregnancies is seen in women across all educational ranges. The high level of educational support provided by the diabetic-obstetric team to achieve this degree of compliance usually stops abruptly with delivery. Education on the likelihood of future diabetes and how this risk can be minimized should be part of the antenatal education these women receive.

While it is likely that weight control and physical exercise may prolong the period of normal glucose tolerance following a gestational diabetic pregnancy, the development of impaired glucose tolerance and later non-insulin-dependent diabetes is to be expected. Evidence suggests that this progression in previous gestational diabetic women occurs over a shorter period of time than in the background population[11]. All women with gestational diabetes should be made aware of the early symptoms of diabetes. Public awareness of the symptoms of diabetes is poor, and even in the presence of symptoms the diagnosis of non-insulin-dependent diabetes is often delayed by 10 years[72,73]; this delay is greater in ethnic minority groups, especially when literacy and language difficulties are present. It is this long period of undiagnosed and untreated diabetes that explains the high prevalence of micro- and macrovascular complications present at diagnosis, with 20% of newly diagnosed non-insulin-dependent diabetic patients having retinopathy and 18% electrocardiograph changes[74]. Early diagnosis of diabetes in women with previous gestational diabetes is essential if diabetic complications are to be reduced. These women should be encouraged to report symptoms of hyperglycaemia to their family physician, and to have their blood glucose checked on a regular basis.

FOLLOW-UP OF PREVIOUS GESTATIONAL DIABETIC WOMEN

Although most antenatal clinics organize a postpartum glucose tolerance test within the first three months of delivery, this is frequently poorly attended. In cases where no postpartum test has been undertaken the family physician should be informed, and encouraged to obtain a fasting or timed postprandial blood glucose to exclude diabetes. The handover of the medical responsibility for the long-term follow-up of gestational diabetic women is not usually well communicated to the family physician. Clear guidelines for postpartum screening of these women need to be drawn up by all obstetric clinics, defining who should be responsible and the recommended frequency for testing; all women should be informed of these follow-up arrangements. Guidelines for screening will need to reflect the population of women they serve, and in ethnic groups with high background prevalence rates of non-insulin-dependent diabetes an annual blood glucose test would be required for early diagnosis and treatment. In ethnic groups with low background prevalence rates and where other risk factors for an early onset of non-insulin-dependent diabetes are not present, a blood glucose test every two years may suffice, provided opportunistic testing is done in between if symptoms are present.

While we await the definitive studies to show whether non-insulin-dependent diabetes can be prevented or delayed through a combination of lifestyle behavioural modifications and possible pharmaceutical interventions, we should acknowledge that women with previous gestational diabetes are at heightened risk for both diabetes and cardiovascular disease and offer them the best advice available on today's studies. This includes the benefits of a low-fat diet, avoidance of obesity and the merits of regular exercise, in addition to general advice on cardiovascular protection with respect to smoking, blood pressure control and management of hypercholesterolaemia. This advice is similar to that we would give to a healthy middle-aged man, but the potential benefits are greater.

REFERENCES

1 King H, Rewers M. Global estimates for prevalence of diabetes mellitus and impaired glucose tolerance in adults. *Diabetes Care* 1993; **16**: 157–77.
2 Laing W, Williams R. *Diabetes: A Model for Health Care Management.* Office of Health Economics, London, 1989.
3 Eastman RC, Silverman R, Harris M *et al.* Lessening the burden of diabetes. *Diabetes Care* 1993; **16**: 1095–102.
4 Eriksson KF, Lindgarde F. Prevention of type 2 (non-insulin-dependent) diabetes mellitus by diet and physical exercise: the 6-year Malmo feasibility study. *Diabetologia* 1991; **34**: 891—8.
5 The Acropolis Affirmation. *IDF Bull* 1995; **40**(2): 44.
6 WHO Study Group. *Prevention of Diabetes Mellitus.* World Health Organization, Geneva, 1994.
7 Rose G. *The Strategy of Preventative Medicine.* Oxford University Press, Oxford, 1992.
8 Herman WH, Smith PJ, Thompson TJ *et al.* A new and simple questionnaire to identify people at increased risk for undiagnosed diabetes. *Diabetes Care* 1995; **18**: 382–7.
9 WHO Ad Hoc Diabetic Reporting Group. Diabetes and impaired glucose tolerance in women aged between 20 and 39 years. *World Health Stats Q* 1992; **45**: 321–7.
10 Motala AA, Omar MAK, Gouws E. High risk of progression to NIDDM in South-African Indians with impaired glucose tolerance. *Diabetes* 1993; **42**: 556–63.
11 Kjos SL, Peters RK, Xiang A *et al.* Predicting future diabetes in Latino women with gestational diabetes. *Diabetes* 1995; **44**: 586–91.
12 Henry OA, Beischer NA, Sheedy MT, Walstab JE. Gestational diabetes and follow-up among immigrant Vietnam-born women. *Aust NZ J Obstet Gynaecol* 1993; **33**: 109–14.
13 O'Sullivan JB. Body weight and subsequent diabetes mellitus. *JAMA* 1982; **248**: 949–52.
14 UK Prospective Diabetes Study VI. Complications in newly diagnosed type 2 diabetic patients and their association with different clinical and biochemical risk factors. *Diabetes Res* 1990; **13**: 1–11.
15 Colditz GA, Willett WC, Stampfer MJ. Weight as a risk for the clinical diabetes in women. *Am J Epidemiol* 1990; **132**: 501–13.
16 Buchanan TA, Metzger BE, Freinkel N, Bergman RN. Insulin sensitivity and b-cell responsiveness to glucose during late pregnancy in lean and moderately obese women with normal glucose tolerance or mild gestational diabetes. *Am J Obstet Gynecol* 1990; **162**: 1008–114.
17 Dornhorst A, Bailey PC, Anyaoku V *et al.* Abnormalities of glucose tolerance following gestational diabetes. *Q J Med* 1990; **284**: 1219–28.
18 Ryan EA, Imes S, Liu D *et al.* Defects in insulin secretion and action in women with a history of gestational diabetes. *Diabetes* 1995; **44**: 506–12.
19 Metzger BE, Cho NH, Roston SM, Radvany R. Prepregnancy weight and antepartum insulin secretion predict glucose tolerance five years after gestational diabetes mellitus. *Diabetes Care* 1993; **16**: 1598–605.
20 Casimirri F, Pasquali R, Cesari MP *et al.* Interrelationships between body weight, body fat distribution and insulin in obese women before and after hypocaloric feeding and weight loss. *Ann Nutr Metab* 1989; **33**: 79–87.
21 Dowse GK, Zimmet PZ, Gareeboo H *et al.* Abdominal obesity and physical activity as a risk factors for NIDDM and impaired glucose tolerance in Indian, Creole and Chinese Mauritians. *Diabetes Care* 1991; **14**: 271–82.
22 Lundgren H, Bengtsson C, Blohme G *et al.* Adiposity and adipose tissue distribution in relation to the incidence of diabetes in women: results from a prospective population study in Gothenburg, Sweden. *Int J Obstet* 1989; **13**: 413–23.
23 Goldstein DJ. Beneficial health effects of modest weight loss. *Int J Obesity* 1992; **16**: 397–415.
24 Chaturvedi N, Fuller JH. Mortality risk by body weight and weight change in people with NIDDM. The WHO Multinational Study of Vascular Disease in Diabetes. *Diabetes Care* 1995; **18**; 766–74.
25 Long SD, O'Brien K, MacDonald KG *et al.* Weight loss in severely obese subjects prevents

the progression of impaired glucose tolerance to type II diabetes: a longitudinal interventional study. *Diabetes Care* 1994; **17**: 372–5.

26 Manson JE, Willett WC, Stamfer MJ *et al*. Body weight and mortality among women. *N Engl J Med* 1995; **333**:677–85.

27 Zimmet P. Challenges in diabetes epidemiology: from West to the rest. *Diabetes Care* 1992; **15**: 232–52.

28 Marshall JA, Hamman RF, Baxter J. High-fat, low carbohydrate diet and the etiology of non-insulin-dependent diabetes: the San Louis Valley Diabetes Study. *Am J Epidemiol* 1991; **134**: 590–603.

29 O'Dea K. Westernisation, insulin resistance and diabetes in Australian Aborigines. *Med J Aust* 1991; **155**: 258–64.

30 Bjorntorp P, Fahlen M, Grimby G *et al*. Carbohydrate and lipid metabolism in middle-aged physically well-trained men: the effect of physical training on insulin production in obesity. *Metabolism* 1970; **19**: 631–8.

31 Sato Y, Iguchi A, Sakamoto N. Biochemical determination of training effects using insulin clamp technique. *Horm Metab Res* 1984; **16**: 483–6.

32 Taylor R, Ram P, Zimmet P *et al*. Physical activity and prevalence of diabetes in Melanesian and Indian men in Fiji. *Ann Nutr Metab* 1984; **27**: 578–82.

33 King H, Zimmet P, Raper LR, Balkau B. Risk factors for diabetes mellitus in three Pacific populations. *Am J Epidemiol* 1984; **119**: 396–409.

34 Taylor RJ, Bennett PH, LeGonidec G *et al*. The prevalence of diabetes mellitus in a traditional-living Polynesian population: the Wallis Island survey. *Diabetes Care* 1983; **6**: 334–40.

35 Manson JE, Rimm EB, Stampfer MJ *et al*. Physical activity and incidence of NIDDM women. *Lancet* 1991; **338**: 774–8.

36 Helmrich SP, Ragland DR, Leung RW, Paffenbarger RSJ. Physical activity and reduced occurrence of non-insulin-dependent diabetes mellitus. *N Engl J Med* 1991; **325**: 147–52.

37 Regensteiner JG, Shetterly SM, Mayer EJ *et al*. Relationship between habitual physical activity and insulin area among individuals with impaired glucose tolerance. *Diabetes Care* 1995; **18**: 490–7.

38 UK Prospective Diabetes Study Group. UK Prospective Diabetes Study XII: differences between Asian, Afro-Caribbean and White Caucasian type 2 diabetic patients at diagnosis of diabetes. *Diabetic Med* 1994; **11**: 670–7.

39 Zimmet P. The relationship of physical activity and cardiovascular risk factors in Mauritians. *Am J Epidemiol* 1991; **134**: 862–75.

40 Blair SN, Kohl HW III, Barlow CE *et al*. Changes in physical fitness and all-cause mortality: a prospective study on healthy and unhealthy men. *JAMA* 1995; **273**: 1093–8.

41 Hardman A. *Exercise and the Heart*. Report of a British Heart Foundation Working Group, British Heart Foundation, London, 1992.

42 Kannel WB, McGee DL. Diabetes and cardiovascular risk factors: the Framingham Study. *Circulation* 1979; **59**: 8–13.

43 Fontbonne A, Eschwege E, Cambien F *et al*. Hypertriglyceridemia as a risk factor of coronary heart disease mortality in subjects with impaired glucose tolerance and diabetes. *Diabetologia* 1989; **32**: 300–14.

44 Stephenson J, Swerdlow AJ, Devis T, Fuller JH. Recent trends in diabetic mortality in England and Wales. *Diabetic Med* 1992; **9**:417–21.

45 Fisher BM, Frier BM. Evidence for a specific heart disease of diabetes in humans. *Diabetic Med* 1990; **7**: 478–89.

46 Shepherd J, Cobbe SM, Ford I *et al*. Prevention of coronary heart disease with pravastatin in men with hypercholesterolemia. *N Engl J Med* 1995; **332**: 1301–7.

47 Scandinavian Simvastatin Survival Study Group. Randomised trial of cholesterol lowing in 4444 patients with coronary heart disease: the Scandinavian Simvastatin Survival Study. *Lancet* 1994; **344**: 1383–9.

48 Rich-Edwards JW, Manson JE, Hennekens CH, Burning JE. The primary prevention of coronary heart disease in women. *N Engl J Med* 1995; **332**: 1758–65.

49 Janka HU, Warram JH, Rand LI *et al*. Risk factors for the progression of background retinopathy in long standing IDDM. *Diabetes* 1989; **38**: 460–4.

50 Jarrett JR. Risk factors of macrovascular disease in diabetes mellitus. *Horm Metab Res* 1985; **15** (Suppl.): 1–3.

51 DeFronzo RA, Ferrannini E. Insulin resistance: a multifaceted syndrome responsible for NIDDM, obesity, hypertension, dyslipidemia and atherosclerotic cardiovascular disease. *Diabetes Care* 1991; **14**: 173–94.

52 Fuller JH, Haed J. WHO Study Group: Blood pressure, proteinuria and their relationship with circulatory mortality: the WHO multinational study of vascular disease in diabetics. *Diabete Metab* 1989; **15**: 273–7.

53 Nielsen S, Schmitz A, Rehling M, Mogensen CE. Systolic blood pressure relates to the rate of decline of glomerular filtration rate in type II diabetes. *Diabetes Care* 1993; **16**: 1427–32.

54 MacMahon S, Peto R, Culter J et al. Blood pressure, stroke, and coronary heart disease. Part I. Prolonged differences in blood pressure: prospective observational studies corrected for the regression dilution bias. *Lancet* 1990; **335**: 764–74.

55 Fuller J, Stevens L. Epidemiology of hypertension in diabetic patients and implications for treatment. *Diabetes Care* 1991; Suppl. **4**: 8–12.

56 Haffner SM, Stern MP, Hazuda HP et al. Cardiovascular risk factors in confirmed prediabetic individuals: does the clock for coronary heart disease start ticking before the onset of clinical diabetes? *JAMA* 1990; **263**: 2893–8.

57 Mulhauser I. Smoking and diabetes. *Diabetic Med* 1990; **7**: 10–15.

58 Willett WC, Green A, Stampfer MJ et al. Relative and absolute excess risks of coronary heart disease among women who smoke cigarettes. *N Engl J Med* 1987; **317**: 1303–9.

59 Rosenberg L, Palmer JR, Shapiro S. Decline in the risk of myocardial infarction among women who stop smoking. *N Engl J Med* 1990; **322**: 213–17.

60 Learner DJ, Kannel WB. Patterns of coronary heart disease morbidity and mortality in the sexes: a 26-year follow-up of the Framingham population. *Am Heart J* 1986; **111**: 383–90.

61 Grady D, Rubin SM, Petitt DB et al. Hormone therapy to prevent disease and prolong life in postmenopausal women. *Ann Intern Med* 1992; **117**: 1016–137.

62 Sacks FM, Walsh BW. The effects of reproductive hormones on serum lipoproteins: unresolved issues in biology and clinical practice. *Ann NY Acad Sci* 1990; **592**: 272–85.

63 Keaney JFJ, Shwaery GT, Xu A et al. 17 β-estradiol preserves endothelial vasodilator function and limits low-density lipoprotein oxidation in hypercholesterolemic swine. *Circulation* 1994; **18**: 1680–7.

64 Bar J, Tepper R, Fuchs J et al. The effects of estrogen replacement on platelet aggregation and adenosine triphosphate release in postmenopausal women. *Obstet Gynecol* 1993; **81**: 261–4.

65 Writing Group for the PEPI Trial. Effects of estrogen/progestin regimens on heart disease risk factors in postmenopausal women: the Postmenopausal Estrogen/Progestin Intervention (PEPI) Trial. *JAMA* 1995; **273**: 199–208.

66 Proudler AJ, Ahmed AIH, Crook D et al. Hormone replacement therapy and serum angiotensin-converting enzyme activity in post menopausal women. *Lancet* 1995; **346**: 89–90.

67 Colditz GA, Hankinson SE, Hunter DJ et al. The use of estrogens and progestins and the risk of breast cancer in postmenopausal women. *N Engl J Med* 1995; **332**: 1589–93.

68 Keen H, Jarrett RJ, McCartney P. The 10 year follow-up of the Bedford survey (1962–1972). *Diabetologia* 1982; **22**: 73–8.

69 Jarrett RJ, Keen H, Fuller JH, McCartney M. Worsening to diabetes in men with impaired glucose tolerance ('borderline diabetes'). *Diabetologia* 1979; **16**: 25–30.

70 Sartor G, Scherstén B, Carlström S et al. Ten-year follow-up of subjects with impaired glucose tolerance: prevention of diabetes by tolbutamide and diet regulation. *Diabetes* 1980; **29**: 41–4.

71 Nolan JJ, Ludvik B, Beerdsen P et al. Improvement in glucose tolerance and insulin resistance in obese subjects treated with troglitazone. *N Engl J Med* 1994; **331**: 1183–93.

72 Jackson DMA, Wills R, Davies J et al. Public awareness of the symptoms of diabetes mellitus. *Diabetic Med* 1991; **8**: 971–2.

73 Singh B, Jackson DMA, Wills R et al. Delayed diagnosis in non-insulin-dependent diabetes. *Diabetic Med* 1992; **304**: 1154–5.

74 United Kingdom Prospective Diabetes Study Group. UK Prospective Diabetes Study (UKDPS) V111. Study design, progress and performance. *Diabetologia* 1991; **34**: 877–90.

22

Diabetes in Subsequent Generations

DAVID J. PETTITT

National Institute of Diabetes and Digestive and Kidney Disease,
Phoenix, Arizona, USA

Diabetes begets diabetes. Numerous studies have reported higher rates of diabetes in the offspring of men and women who have diabetes than in the offspring of those who do not[1-8]. This is not surprising given that most of the major types of diabetes have a genetic basis, and genetic susceptibility may be a major reason for the familial occurrence of insulin-dependent diabetes mellitus[9,10], maturity onset diabetes of the young[11,12] and syndromes associated with mitochondrial DNA[13]. However, there are environmental influences as well and the legacy of the diabetic intrauterine environment cannot be ignored[14]. One of the major teratogenic effects of the diabetic intrauterine environment, observed in experimental animals as well as in human populations, is on the development of adipocytes and pancreatic beta cells[15]. The resulting effects on glucose metabolism may lead to the development of non-insulin-dependent diabetes. There are, of course, interactions between the intrauterine environment and genetics such that the effect of the former may be most apparent in populations with a high prevalence of diabetes because the offspring are more likely to be genetically susceptible.

GESTATIONAL AND NON-INSULIN-DEPENDENT DIABETES

Gestational diabetes and non-insulin-dependent diabetes mellitus have many characteristics in common and, in the absence of a pre-pregnancy glucose tolerance test, non-insulin-dependent diabetes is diagnosed as gestational diabetes. Therefore, these two types of diabetes will be considered together.

Diabetes and Pregnancy: An International Approach to Diagnosis and Management.
Edited by A. Dornhorst and D. R. Hadden.
© 1996 John Wiley & Sons Ltd.

Several populations have very high rates of non-insulin-dependent diabetes with onset before or during the childbearing years, so women in these populations will often have diabetes diagnosed before or during pregnancy. The Pima Indians of Arizona have the world's highest rate of non-insulin-dependent diabetes, which often develops at young ages. For the past 30 years, they have had oral glucose tolerance tests during pregnancy as well as on a routine basis approximately every two years, regardless of health[16,17]. Extensive data on diabetes are available for offspring of women who had diabetes during pregnancy as well as of those who remained normal or developed diabetes only after the pregnancy. Figure 22.1 shows the prevalence of diabetes by age group in offspring through 29 years of age in three categories of Pima Indians: (1) offspring of non-diabetic women, who have not developed diabetes during follow-up; (2) offspring of prediabetic women, who had normal glucose tolerance at the time of the pregnancy but who subsequently developed non-insulin-dependent diabetes; and (3) offspring of diabetic women, who had diabetes at the time of the pregnancy[18].

The strong effect of age as well as the differential effect of genes and environment can be seen. There was little diabetes before age 15 years, but when it was present it was found almost exclusively among the offspring of

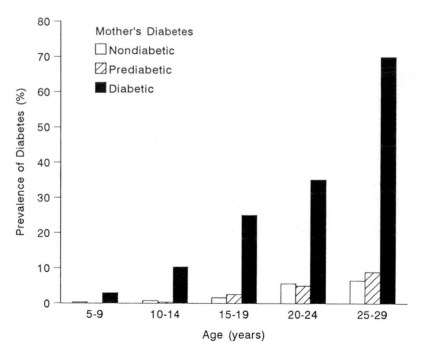

Figure 22.1. Prevalence of diabetes according to the mother's diabetes during and following pregnancy in 5–29-year-old Pima Indians (see text for description of groups, updated from Pettitt *et al.*[18])

diabetic women. In every age group, there was much more diabetes in the offspring of diabetic women than of non-diabetic or pre-diabetic women, and the rates in the offspring of the latter two groups were similar. These data indicate that the genetic predisposition, a factor for offspring of both diabetic and prediabetic women, is a much less important determinant of non-insulin-dependent diabetes in this population than is the intrauterine environment. This finding is reinforced by the much smaller effect of paternal than of maternal diabetes on the prevalence of diabetes in the offspring[18]. The small difference in diabetes prevalence between offspring of non-diabetic and prediabetic women is due, in large part, to the genetic differences these subjects inherited from their mothers, while the large difference in prevalence between the offspring of prediabetic and diabetic mothers is the lasting effect of the teratogenic diabetic intrauterine environment superimposed on the genetic predisposition.

The higher rate of diabetes may be mediated partially by the earlier development of obesity in the offspring of diabetic women, but this does not account for the magnitude of the difference seen[19]. Figure 22.2 shows the prevalence of severe obesity ($\geqslant 140\%$ relative weight for height) in the same three categories of offspring described above. Offspring of diabetic

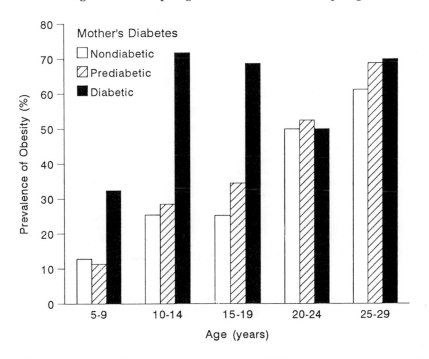

Figure 22.2. Prevalence of severe obesity (weight $\geqslant 140\%$ of age–sex–height specific standard) according to the mother's diabetes during and following pregnancy in 5–29-year-old Pima Indians (see text for description of groups, updated from Pettitt *et al.*[20])

women were much more obese before age 20 years[20], but thereafter there
was little difference[17]. In Pima Indians, obesity develops at a high rate in
early childhood and the diabetic intrauterine environment is an important
determinant of obesity during the first two decades of life. At older ages,
however, obesity is very prevalent regardless of maternal diabetes and an
additional effect of the intrauterine environment is no longer apparent.
Despite a similar prevalence of obesity after age 20 years, there was a big
difference in diabetes prevalence (Figure 22.1). On average, by 20 years of
age, the obese offspring of diabetic women will have been obese for a
longer period of time than the obese offspring of non-diabetic and

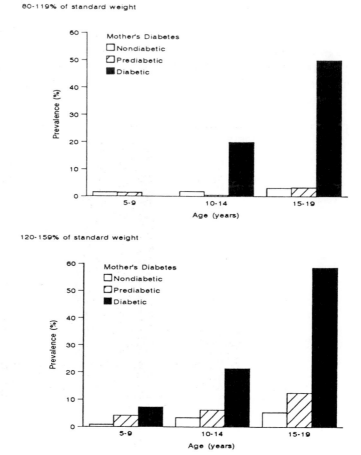

Figure 22.3. Prevalence of abnormal glucose tolerance (2 h glucose $\geqslant 7.8 \, \text{mmol/l}$)
according to the mother's diabetes during and following pregnancy in non-obese (top)
and obese (bottom) 5–19-year-old Pima Indians (see text for description of groups[19])

prediabetic women, and longer obesity duration is an important risk factor for non-insulin-dependent diabetes[21].

Figure 22.3 shows the prevalence of abnormal glucose tolerance (2 h glucose concentration ⩾7.8 mmol/l) according to maternal diabetes in non-obese (80–119% of standard weight for height) and obese (129–159% of standard weight) offspring aged 5–19 years. Even the non-obese offspring of diabetic women (top panel) have much higher rates of abnormal glucose tolerance[19] than the offspring of non-diabetic or prediabetic women. Among offspring of diabetic women, obesity (lower panel) adds little additional risk for non-insulin-dependent diabetes although it does add risk for the offspring of non-diabetic and prediabetic women.

Among populations in which non-insulin-dependent diabetes develops only rarely at young ages, possibly because of a lower genetic susceptibility, young offspring of women with diabetes during pregnancy are unlikely to develop non-insulin-dependent diabetes as defined by World Health Organization criteria[22]. However, these children are not immune to the effects of the intrauterine environment. Figure 22.4 shows the prevalence of impaired glucose tolerance in offspring of diabetic

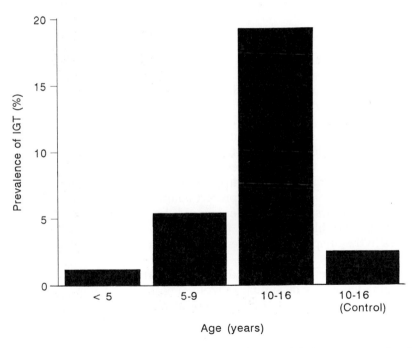

Figure 22.4. Prevalence of impaired glucose tolerance (IGT) by age in a racially mixed group of children of diabetic mothers followed from birth and in 10–16-year-old controls. Reproduced with permission from Silverman *et al.*[23]

women from a racially mixed population who were followed to adolescence[23]. The mothers were a mix of women with diabetes onset either before or during the pregnancy. Almost 20% of the offspring of diabetic women had impaired glucose tolerance by age 10–16 years—eight times the rate in 10–16-year-old children whose mothers did not have diabetes during pregnancy. As these children are otherwise apparently healthy, it is unlikely that they would undergo glucose tolerance tests in the course of routine health care. Even a fasting glucose drawn as part of a routine screening battery will miss the diagnosis of impaired glucose tolerance. Therefore, outside of the research setting, most abnormal glucose tolerance in adolescents and young adults will remain unidentified in most populations. Since impaired glucose tolerance is a strong risk factor for the development of non-insulin-dependent diabetes[17,24–27], routine glucose tolerance testing of the offspring of women who had gestational or pregestational diabetes might be warranted, even in the absence of other risk factors for non-insulin-dependent diabetes. Glucose tolerance tests would clearly be warranted if treatment of those with impaired glucose tolerance was shown to prevent the development of non-insulin-dependent diabetes. Studies are currently being planned to determine the effectiveness of diabetes prevention in persons with impaired glucose tolerance[28].

INSULIN-DEPENDENT DIABETES

The intrauterine effect of diabetes in the offspring of women with insulin-dependent diabetes mellitus is not as clear cut as for the offspring of women with non-insulin-dependent diabetes and it is not clear how much of the observed transmission is genetic and how much is due to the environment. Higher rates of insulin-dependent diabetes in the offspring of fathers than of mothers with insulin-dependent diabetes further complicates the situation[6]. This finding has several possible explanations: the transmission could be genetic with a differential susceptibility depending on which parent supplies the diabetes genes; the diabetic intrauterine environment could protect against insulin-dependent diabetes in susceptible offspring; or there could be selective perinatal loss of offspring susceptible to diabetes. Nevertheless, studies generally find more diabetes in the offspring of women with insulin-dependent diabetes than of those without[1–5].

The metabolic effects of the diabetic intrauterine environment on the developing fetus may be similar in women with insulin-dependent diabetes and in those with non-insulin-dependent diabetes. If so, some children whose mothers have insulin-dependent diabetes during pregnancy will, because it is so common, also inherit a susceptibility to non-insulin-dependent diabetes from either the mother or the father. Thus, even if much of the transmission of insulin-dependent diabetes is genetic, some of the offspring of the women with insulin-dependent diabetes will be susceptible to the metabolic disturbances found in the offspring of women with non-insulin-dependent diabetes because, in addition to having a mother with insulin-dependent diabetes, they will have inherited the susceptibility to obesity or non-insulin-dependent diabetes or both.

RARE TYPES OF DIABETES

Diabetes of any etiology that can affect fertile women can complicate pregnancy and, if diagnosed during gestation, may be diagnosed as gestational diabetes. More than a cursory mention of uncommon types of diabetes which may occur during pregnancy is beyond the scope of this chapter but there is currently much interest in maturity onset diabetes of the young[11,12] and maternally transmitted diabetes associated with certain types of mitochondrial DNA[13]. Although there is limited experience with pregnancy complicating either of these types of diabetes, which account for only a small fraction of all cases of diabetes, there is no reason to believe that the fetus of an affected woman will be any more or less susceptible to the teratogenic effects. Thus, special attention should also be paid to the pregnant woman with a family history of one of the rare types of diabetes, and if diabetes is identified during pregnancy the potential risk for the offspring should be recognized.

OTHER RISK FACTORS

Other risk factors for diabetes may predispose offspring to diabetes even in the absence of diabetes in pregnancy, or they may work in concert with the diabetic pregnancy to increase rates of diabetes in the offspring. Offspring of diabetic women tend to be macrosomic at birth and are at increased risk of subsequent obesity and diabetes, but even the normal birth weight offspring of diabetic women are at high risk of subsequent obesity[29]. High birth weight may be an associated risk factor caused by the same factors predisposing the child to obesity and diabetes in later life. Low birth weight is also a risk factor for diabetes in adulthood. This may be due to nutritional deprivation leading to impaired development of the fetal pancreas[30] or to the selective survival of low birth weight infants that are genetically susceptible to developing diabetes[31]. Among Pima adults, the risk of diabetes is just as high in those who had a very high birth weight as in those who had a low birth weight—a finding accounted for by maternal diabetes in pregnancy. Breastfeeding is also associated with less non-insulin-dependent diabetes[32] possibly because breastfed babies are less likely to be overfed and to become obese. Fetal and infant overnutrition predispose to obesity[33], which is a strong risk factor for diabetes[34], and any factors that can be controlled or prevented by lifestyle or environmental changes that will prevent obesity may subsequently prevent diabetes.

ANIMAL STUDIES

Animal studies are covered in previous chapters and are mentioned here only because they can help demonstrate the lasting effects of the diabetic intrauterine environment in the absence of genetically inherited diabetes. The developing fetal pups of genetically non-diabetic rats that are made hyperglycemic during pregnancy, either by pancreatic destruction with streptozotocin[35] or by glucose infusion[36], suffer problems typical of the diabetic pregnancy. As adults, the second generation rats have abnormal glucose tolerance tests[35,36]. In addition, the females have gestational diabetes so the third generation is affected as well[35]. Since these strains of animals are not genetically predisposed to diabetes and the experimental animals are raised under the same conditions as those not exposed to hyperglycemia *in utero*, the differences observed in the offspring can be attributed directly to the abnormal intrauterine environment.

THE VICIOUS CYCLE

The diabetic pregnancy can be thought of as a vicious cycle (Figure 22.5)[17,37]. As described in previous chapters, the woman with diabetes, whether pre-gestational or gestational, has a high-risk pregnancy with potential complications for herself and her developing fetus. The infant of a diabetic

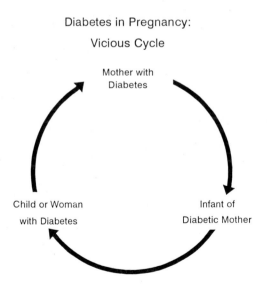

Figure 22.5. Diagram depicting the vicious cycle of diabetes in pregnancy. (Reproduced with permission from Knowler *et al.*[17])

woman is subject to complications during birth and in the newborn period. It has been recognized for decades that the problems for the woman with gestational diabetes do not end at delivery and that she is at high risk of developing diabetes in future years. It has become increasingly clear that the problems for the offspring are not over at birth either. The offspring are at a high risk of becoming obese during childhood and of developing non-insulin-dependent diabetes during adolescence or early adulthood. Hence, the young woman whose mother had diabetes during pregnancy is at risk of perpetuating the cycle by developing diabetes before or during her childbearing years. It remains to be seen if a degree of normalization of glucose metabolism can be achieved that will eliminate this risk, thus providing a lifelong benefit for the developing fetus and for future generations.

REFERENCES

1 White P. Childhood diabetes: its course, and influence on the second and third generation. *Diabetes* 1960; **9**: 345–55.
2 Simpson NE. Diabetes in the families of diabetics. *Can Med Assoc J* 1968; **98**: 427–32.
3 Yssing M. Long-term prognosis of children born to mothers diabetic when pregnant. In: Camerini-Davalos RA, Cole HS (eds), *Early Diabetes in Early Life*. Academic Press, New York, 1975; 575–86.
4 Bibergeil H, Godel E, Amendt P: Diabetes and pregnancy: early and late prognosis of children of diabetic mothers. In: Camerini- Davalos RA, Cole HS (eds), *Early Diabetes in Early Life*. Academic Press, New York, 1975; 427–34.
5 Köbberling J, Brüggeboes B. Prevalence of diabetes among children of insulin-dependent diabetic mothers. *Diabetologia* 1980; **18**: 459–62.
6 Warram JH, Krolewski AS, Gottlieb MS, Kahn CR. Differences in risk of insulin-dependent diabetes in offspring of diabetic mothers and diabetic fathers. *N Engl J Med* 1984; **311**: 149–52.
7 Dahlquist G, Blom L, Holmgren G et al. The epidemiology of diabetes in Swedish children 0–14 years: a six-year prospective study. *Diabetologia* 1985; **28**: 802–8.
8 Pettitt DJ, Aleck KA, Baird HR et al. Congenital susceptibility to NIDDM: role of intrauterine environment. *Diabetes* 1988; **33**: 835–51.
9 Rotter JI. The modes of inheritance of insulin-dependent diabetes mellitus. *Am J Hum Genet* 1981; **33**: 835–51.
10 Thompson G, Robinson WP, Kuhner MK et al. Genetic heterogeneity, modes of inheritance, and risk estimates for a joint study of caucasians with insulin-dependent diabetes mellitus. *Am J Hum Genet* 1988; **43**: 799–816.
11 Bell GI, Xiang K-S, Newman MV et al. The gene for non-insulin-dependent diabetes mellitus (maturity-onset diabetes of the young subtype) is linked to DNA polymorphism on human chromosome 20q. *Proc Natl Acad Sci USA* 1991; **88**: 1484–8.
12 Bowden DW, Gravius TC, Akots G, Fajans SS. Identification of genetic markers flanking the locus for maturity-onset diabetes of the young on human chromosome 20. *Diabetes* 1992; **41**: 88–92.
13 Ballinger SW, Shoffner JM, Hedaya EV et al. Maternally transmitted diabetes and deafness associated with a 10.4 kb mitochondrial DNA deletion. *Nature Genet* 1992; **1**: 11–15.
14 Pettitt DJ, Bennett PH. Long-term outcome of infants of diabetic mothers. In: Reece EA, Coustan D (eds), *Diabetes Mellitus in Pregnancy: Principles and Practice*, 2nd edn. 1995: Churchill Livingstone, New York, 379–88.
15 Freinkel N. Banting Lecture 1980: of pregnancy and Progeny. *Diabetes* 1980; **29**: 1023–35.
16 Bennett PH, Burch TA, Miller M. Diabetes mellitus in American (Pima) Indians. *Lancet* 1971; **ii**: 125–8.

17 Knowler WC, Pettitt DJ, Saad MF, Bennett PH. Diabetes mellitus in the Pima Indians: incidence, risk factors and pathogenesis. *Diabetes Metab Rev* 1990; **6**: 1–27.

18 Pettitt DJ, Aleck KA, Baird HR *et al*. Congenital susceptibility to NIDDM: role of intrauterine environment. *Diabetes* 1988; **37**: 622–8.

19 Pettitt DJ, Bennett PH, Everhart J et al. High plasma glucose concentrations in normal weight offspring of diabetic women. *Diabetes Res Clin Prac* 1985; Suppl. 1: S445 (Abstract).

20 Pettitt DJ, Baird HR, Aleck KA *et al*. Excessive obesity in offspring of Pima Indian women with diabetes during pregnancy. *N Engl J Med* 1983; **308**: 242–5.

21 Everhart JE, Pettitt DJ, Bennett PH, Knowler WC. Duration of obesity increases the incidence of NIDDM. *Diabetes* 1992; **41**: 235–40.

22 WHO Study Group. Prevention of Diabetes Mellitus. *World Health Organization Technical Report Series 844*, Geneva, 1994.

23 Silverman BL, Metzger BE, Cho NH, Loeb CA. Impaired glucose tolerance in adolescent offspring of diabetic mothers. *Diabetes Care* 1995; **18**: 611–17.

24 Lillioja S, Mott DM, Howard BV *et al*. Impaired glucose tolerance as a disorder of insulin action: longitudinal and cross-sectional studies in Pima Indians. *N Engl J Med* 1988; **318**: 1217–25.

25 Saad MF, Knowler WC, Pettitt DJ *et al*. The natural history of impaired glucose tolerance in the Pima Indians. *N Engl J Med* 1988; **319**: 1500–6.

26 Stern MP, Morales PA, Monterrosa A *et al*. Predicting diabetes: moving beyond impaired glucose tolerance. *Diabetes* 1993; **42**: 706–14.

27 Knowler WC, Narayan KMV, Hanson RL *et al*. Preventing non-insulin-dependent diabetes. *Diabetes* 1995; **44**: 483–8.

28 Diabetes Dispatch. Grants awarded for NIDDM prevention trial. *Diabetes Forecast* 1995; **48**: 60.

29 Pettitt DJ, Knowler WC, Bennett PH *et al*. Obesity in offspring of diabetic Pima Indian women despite normal birthweight. *Diabetes Care* 1987; **10**: 76–80.

30 Hales CN, Barker DJP. Type 2 (non-insulin-dependent) diabetes mellitus: the thrifty phenotype hypothesis. *Diabetologia* 1992; **35**: 595–601.

31 McCance DR, Pettitt DJ, Hanson RL *et al*. Birth weight and non-insulin-dependent diabetes: thrifty genotype, thrifty phenotype, or surviving small baby genotype? *Br Med J* 1994; **308**: 942–5.

32 Pettitt DJ, de Courten MP, Nelson RG *et al*. Lower prevalence of NIDDM in breast fed Pima Indians (Abstract). Diabetes 1994; 44 (Suppl. 1): 6A.

33 Brook CGD. Evidence for a sensitive period in adipose-cell replication in man. *Lancet* 1972; **ii**: 624–7.

34 Knowler WC, Pettitt DJ, Savage PJ, Bennett PH. Diabetes incidence in Pima Indians: contributions of obesity and parental diabetes. *Am J Epidemiol* 1981; **113**: 144–56.

35 Aerts L, Holemans K, Van Assche FA. Maternal diabetes during pregnancy: consequences for the offspring. *Diabetes/Metab Rev* 1990; **6**: 147–67.

36 Bihoreau MT, Ktorza A, Kinebanyan MF, Picon L. Impaired glucose homeostasis in adult rats from hyperglycemic mothers. *Diabetes* 1986; **35**: 979–84.

37 Pettitt DJ, Knowler WC. Diabetes and obesity in the Pima Indians: a cross-generational vicious cycle. *J Obes Weight Regul* 1988; **7**: 61–75.

23

Birth Weight and Adult Disease

JANIS BAIRD and DAVID I.W. PHILLIPS

MRC Environmental Epidemiology Unit, Southampton General Hospital,
Southampton, UK

Non-insulin-dependent diabetes is an important health problem accounting for an estimated 5% of the UK National Health Service annual expenditure. It is still poorly understood. While obesity and an inactive lifestyle are associated with a greater risk of acquiring it, these factors do not explain why some people but not others develop the disease. As non-insulin-dependent diabetes clusters in families, and its concordance in monozygotic twins is higher than in dizygotic twins, current opinion holds that the susceptibility to the disorder has a genetic basis. Recent studies, however, have now shown that impaired growth *in utero* leads to an increased risk of developing non-insulin-dependent diabetes and its precursor, impaired glucose tolerance, in adult life. These studies have led to a new hypothesis on the origin of non-insulin-dependent diabetes: that poor nutrition in fetal and infant life is detrimental to the development and function of the beta cells of the islets of Langerhans, and that altered development of tissues leads to insulin resistance. This chapter reviews the evidence for an association between the intrauterine environment, non-insulin-dependent diabetes and impaired glucose tolerance, and the potential mechanisms underlying this association.

EVIDENCE LINKING INTRAUTERINE ENVIRONMENT AND ADULT DISEASE

Early clues to the possible importance of early life in determining adult disease came from geographical studies. These studies were undertaken in an attempt to gain a better understanding of the aetiology of coronary heart

Diabetes and Pregnancy: An International Approach to Diagnosis and Management.
Edited by A. Dornhorst and D. R. Hadden.
© 1996 John Wiley & Sons Ltd.

disease, the epidemiology of which is poorly explained by known risk factors such as cigarette smoking, obesity and raised cholesterol levels. Coronary heart disease is a disease of affluence, with increasing rates of the disease being associated with increasing prosperity, and yet, paradoxically, its incidence is highest in poorer areas of the UK. Geographical studies revealed that mortality from coronary heart disease between 1968 and 1978 was highest in areas that had high infant mortality in 1921–5[1]. One possible explanation for this is that events in early life determine an individual's risk of developing heart disease. More detailed analysis revealed that neonatal mortality (deaths in the first month of life) seemed to have a stronger association with coronary heart disease mortality than did post-neonatal mortality (deaths from one month to one year of age), suggesting that factors associated with prenatal life played a greater part in determining the later risk of coronary heart disease[2]. This is also supported by migrant studies which have revealed that place of birth is strongly predictive of risk of dying from coronary heart disease regardless of place of death.

STUDIES IN ADULTS

The geographical clues to the link between the prenatal environment and adult disease led to a systematic search of archives and hospital record departments for birth records of subjects in middle and old age. A series of longitudinal studies were then undertaken in which birth measurements, used as a measure of fetal growth, were related to adult cardiovascular disease. In view of the association of cardiovascular disease with non-insulin-dependent diabetes, impaired glucose tolerance and insulin resistance, evaluation of glucose tolerance was an integral part of these studies.

The first set of records to be identified was in Hertfordshire. From 1911 onwards every baby born in the county was weighed at birth. They were then visited periodically throughout the first year of life and were weighed again at one year of age. The health visitor records used during this period have survived and have been used to trace men and women born 60 years ago.

The first group to be studied in Hertfordshire were 468 men aged 59 to 70 years who were born and were still living in east Hertfordshire[3]. Of the 408 men who had full glucose tolerance tests, complete blood measurements on all samples were obtained from 370. The percentage of men with impaired glucose tolerance (plasma glucose 7.8–11.0 mmol/1 at 2 h), or non-insulin-dependent diabetes ($\geq$11.1 mmol/1 at 2 h) fell progressively with increasing birth weight and increasing weight at one year of age. Table 23.1 shows that the relative risk of impaired glucose tolerance or non-insulin-dependent diabetes was six times higher in those who weighed $\leq$5.5 lb (2.5 kg) at birth than in those who weighed >9.5 lb (4.3 kg). Similar trends were seen for weight at one year. The prevalence of these disorders in men with birth

Table 23.1. Percentage of men aged 64 years with impaired glucose tolerance (2 h glucose 7.8–11.0 mmol/l) or diabetes, (2 h glucose ≥ 11.1 mmol/l) according to birth weight[3]

Birth weight (lb)[a]	Number of men	Percentage of men with 2 h glucose (mmol/l) of:			Odds ratio adjusted for body mass index (95% confidence interval)	
		7.8–11.0	≥11.1	≥7.8		
≤5.5	20	30	10	40	6.6	(1.5–28)
5.6–6.5	47	21	13	34	4.8	(1.3–17)
6.6–7.5	104	25	6	31	4.6	(1.4–16)
7.6–8.5	117	15	7	22	2.6	(0.8–8.9)
8.6–9.5	54	4	9	13	1.4	(0.3–5.6)
>9.5	28	14	0	14	1.0	–
All	370	18	7	25	*p* value for trend <0.001	

[a] 1 lb = 454 g.

weights of ≤2.5 kg was 40% compared to 14% in those in the highest birth weight group (>4.3 kg). The associations between weight at birth and at one year and glucose tolerance 60 years later were independent of the subjects' current body mass index, and were seen in each social class. When the subjects were divided according to weight at one year of age and current body mass index, 2 h plasma glucose was found to be highest in those who had the lowest weight at one year but the highest current body mass index. Conversely, the lowest 2 h plasma glucose was observed in those subjects with the highest weight at one year and lowest current body mass index. These findings suggest that fetal and infant growth protect against the effect of higher body mass in adult life, while lower body mass protects against the deleterious effects of reduced early growth.

A recent comparable study on east Hertfordshire women aged 60–71 years confirmed the association between impaired glucose tolerance and birth weight although the findings differed in some respects from those in the Hertfordshire men[4]. As in men plasma glucose and insulin concentrations decreased between women of lowest and highest birth weights. Strongest trends were seen, however, with fasting values rather than 2 h levels. It is unclear why these differences were observed although, since the picture observed in women is more likely to be seen in the presence of insulin resistance, one possible explanation is that low birth weight is more strongly associated with insulin resistance in women than in men.

The findings in Hertfordshire were substantiated by studies in other populations. In Preston, Lancashire, 140 men and 126 women aged between 46 and 54 years were studied[5]. This study was important because information relating to gestational age and more detailed anthropometric measurements at birth were available. Length, head circumference and placental weight had been recorded as well as birth weight. The prevalence of impaired glucose tolerance and non-insulin-dependent diabetes fell from 27% in those who weighed ≤2.5 kg at birth, to 6% in those of ≥3.41 kg. This trend was statistically significant and, as in Hertfordshire, remained so after allowing for current body mass index. Two-hour plasma glucose and insulin concentrations decreased with increasing birth weight ($p=0.004$ and $p=0.001$ respectively). In addition, low ponderal index at birth (weight/length³) and a high head circumference-to-length ratio were independently associated with raised 2 h plasma glucose and insulin concentrations, and individuals with impaired tolerance and non-insulin-dependent diabetes had a high ratio of placental weight to birth weight. This study confirmed the findings of the Hertfordshire study and demonstrated that the association between fetal growth and impaired glucose tolerance existed in both men and women. More importantly, by revealing that the association was independent of gestational age, the Preston study confirmed that it was mature growth-retarded infants rather than premature infants in whom the birth weight/glucose tolerance association was seen. A new observation was the association of particular patterns of fetal growth, thinness and shortness at birth, with increased risk of impaired glucose tolerance in adult life revealing that it was not merely retarded growth but disproportionate growth that was associated with increased risk of diabetes.

Robinson *et al.* studied a sample of men aged between 18 and 25 years in Southampton in order to investigate whether the relationship between fetal growth and impaired glucose tolerance could be observed at a younger age[6]. This would add further weight to the hypothesis that glucose tolerance is, in part, determined prenatally. Forty men with a mean age of 21 years who were born in Southampton General Hospital underwent an abbreviated 30 min glucose tolerance test. An association between 30 min plasma glucose levels and birth weight was observed. A 1 kg increase in birth weight corresponded to a 1.5 mmol decrease in 30 min plasma glucose (95% confidence intervals 0.4–2.6, $p = 0.01$). This trend was independent of gestational age. The confidence intervals indicate that this association may have arisen by chance, the small sample size giving inadequate statistical power. Nevertheless this study suggests that an association may exist at an early age and further work is needed in this age group to substantiate these findings.

McKeigue *et al.* confirmed the association observed in Preston between thinness at birth and impaired glucose tolerance in adult life[7]. They studied a cohort of men born between 1920 and 1924 in Uppsala, Sweden, who were still resident there in 1970. Glucose tolerance results were available in 1000 men in 1970 and 1065 men in 1980–4. The authors found an inverse relationship between birth weight and prevalence of non-insulin-dependent diabetes at 60 years (relative risk 1.4 for each standard deviation decrease at birth weight, $p=0.02$). There was a stronger inverse relationship between the ponderal index (kg/m³) at 60 years and the 60 min insulin level (relative risk 1.9 for one standard deviation decrease in ponderal index, $p<0.001$).

NON-EUROPEAN STUDIES

Other researchers have substantiated the association between birth weight and impaired glucose tolerance in non-European populations. Valdez *et al.* studied a large sample (*n* = 541) of young adults in San Antonio, Texas, in an attempt to generalize the findings from the UK studies to a new population[8]. The subjects were non-Hispanic Caucasians and Mexican Americans, the latter group having a high prevalence of non-insulin-dependent diabetes. Table 23.2 summarizes the results of glucose tolerance testing. The 2 h insulin and glucose values in different birth weight groups are shown. Birth weight was significantly inversely associated with fasting plasma insulin concentrations. Findings in relation to 2 h insulin showed a similar linear trend although they did not achieve statistical significance. These associations were independent of potential confounding factors such as social class and current body mass index. The findings of this study add weight to the evidence from the UK studies and are of particular note because the group studied were young adults amongst whom chronic diseases are still relatively infrequent.

Table 23.2. Age-adjusted mean values of selected variables by ethnicity and tertile of birth weight in men and women[8]

| | Tertile of birth weight for: | | | | | | | |
| | Mexican Americans | | | | Non-Hispanic whites | | | |
	1	2	3	*p* value	1	2	3	*p* value
Women								
n	78	74	76		20	22	20	
Birth weight (kg)	2.68	3.26	3.77		2.74	3.39	3.86	
2 h insulin (pmol/l)	478.4	407.3	372.2	0.184	273.4	350.1	228.7	0.245
2 h glucose (mmol/l)	5.74	5.62	5.52	0.696	5.37	5.09	5.19	0.839
Men								
n	61	62	62		22	22	22	
Birth weight (kg)	2.88	3.40	3.90		2.96	3.50	3.94	
2 h insulin (pmol/l)	330.2	300.04	255.9	0.505	207.9	196.9	184.1	0.944
2 h glucose (mmol/l)	5.06	5.16	5.08	0.920	4.86	5.19	4.78	0.562

McCance *et al.* looked for the association between impaired fetal growth and non-insulin-dependent diabetes in 1179 Pima Indians who were participating in an established cohort study[9]. Pima Indians have the highest reported prevalence (20–30%) of this form of diabetes which often begins at a relatively early age. Glucose tolerance was evaluated when participants in the cohort study were aged 20–39 years. The significance of differences in prevalence of diabetes and abnormal glucose tolerance at different birth weights was examined. A 'U'-shaped relationship between birth weight and glucose tolerance was found. Table 23.3 shows the prevalences of diabetes and impaired glucose tolerance according to age group and category of birth weight and it is clear that high prevalence of impaired glucose tolerance and non-insulin-dependent diabetes was associated with both the lowest and highest birth weights. Age-adjusted prevalence of diabetes at birth weights under 2.5 kg was 30%, while at birth weights of 3.5–4.49 kg it dropped to 17%, increasing to 32% at birth weights ≥ 4.5 kg. The group with the highest age-adjusted prevalence overall were those with lowest birth weight but highest current body mass index. The association between birth weights ≥ 4.5 kg and a raised prevalence of diabetes was not surprising in that previous work by Pettitt *et al.* had shown that maternal diabetes in pregnancy, which is known to be associated with macrosomia, can lead to increased prevalence of diabetes in successive generations[10]. By excluding the subjects whose mothers may have had gestational diabetes from the analysis the authors were able to demonstrate a significant reduction in the prevalence of diabetes in the high birth weight group. This study confirmed the findings of previous studies that low birth weight is associated with increased prevalence of non-insulin-dependent diabetes in adult life and that high body mass index further increases that risk. The observation of a U-shaped relationship had not been noted in the UK studies, probably because gestational diabetes is less prevalent, and the survival of infants of diabetic pregnancy born more than 60 years ago is likely to have been poor.

Table 23.3. Prevalences of diabetes and abnormal glucose tolerance according to age group and category of birth weight in 1179 Pima Indians at last biennial examination[9]

Age group (years)	Number (%) within birth weight groups (kg)			
	<2.50	2.50–3.49	3.50–4.49	≥4.50
Plasma glucose concentration at 2 h ≥ 11.1 mmol/l				
20–24	3/25 (12.0)	18/272 (6.6)	10/173 (5.8)	3/12 (25.0)
25–29	3/10 (30.0)	27/162 (16.7)	20/129 (15.5)	3/11 (27.3)
30–34	3/6 (50.0)	35/145 (24.1)	26/95 (27.4)	3/7 (42.9)
35–39	3/5 (60.0)	32/82 (39.0)	20/43 (46.5)	1/2 (50.0)
Total	12/46 (26.1)	112/661 (16.9)	76/440 (17.3)	10/32 (31.3)
Plasma glucose concentrations at 2 h ≥ 7.8 mmol/l				
20–24	7/25 (28.5)	45/272 (16.5)	24/173 (13.9)	5/12 (41.7)
25–29	3/10 (30.0)	56/162 (34.6)	34/129 (26.4)	3/11 (27.3)
30–34	5/6 (83.3)	58/145 (40.0)	46/95 (48.4)	3/7 (42.9)
35–39	4/5 (80.0)	46/82 (56.1)	29/43 (67.4)	1/2 (50.0)
Total	19/46 (41.3)	205/661 (31.0)	133/440 (30.2)	12/32 (37.5)

STUDIES IN CHILDREN

An early criticism of the work in adults was that the observed association may be due to unknown confounding factors occurring at some point during childhood or adult life. This led to studies of glucose tolerance in children.

Few studies in children had been performed due to the difficulties associated with investigating this age group. The results of two studies performed recently have, however, strengthened the evidence for a link between growth *in utero* and impaired glucose tolerance. Law *et al.* studied 250 seven-year-old children in Salisbury, Wiltshire[11]. Of the 250 subjects, 215 underwent an abbreviated 30 min oral glucose tolerance test. Children with low ponderal index (kg/m^3) at birth had higher plasma glucose concentrations at 30 min. The associations observed were independent of duration of gestation, gender, social class or current weight. For every unit fall in ponderal index 30 min plasma glucose concentrations rose by 0.07 mmol/1 (95% confidence intervals 0.00–0.14, $p = 0.04$). When children were divided into groups according to the distribution of ponderal index at birth, those in the lowest quarter (23 kg/m^3 or less) had a mean 30 min plasma glucose of 8.49 mmol/1 compared to a mean of 7.97 mmol/1 for those in the highest quarter (>27.5 kg/m^3). Although this study was not based on a full 2 h glucose tolerance test, it is the rapid (within 30 min) response of insulin to an oral glucose load that is crucial in determining glucose tolerance[11] and the findings of this study in a group of seven-year-old children therefore add support for the hypothesis that the pathogenesis of non-insulin-dependent diabetes is initiated in fetal life.

Yajnik *et al.* studied a younger age group in India[12]. They looked at the relationship between birth weight and glucose tolerance in children with a mean age of four years. Two groups were studied: 201 children who had been normal singelton births and 178 children who had been admitted to a special care unit as babies and whose birth weight had been less than 2.0 kg. No relation was found between fasting and 120 min glucose and birth weight in either group. An inverse relationship was observed, however, between birth weight and 30 min plasma glucose and insulin levels. In the normal birth group mean 30 min glucose and insulin concentrations were 8.1 mmol/1 and 321 pmol/1 in children whose birth weight was 2.4 kg or less compared with 7.5 mmol/1 and 289 pmol/1 in those who weighed more than 3 kg ($p = 0.01$ and 0.04 respectively). These findings were independent of their current size. Among the group who were of lower birth weight and had been looked after in the special care unit those with lowest birth weight also had higher plasma insulin concentrations at 30 min but there were no trends for plasma glucose. It was not possible to look at the association of glucose tolerance with ponderal index since length at birth was not measured routinely in these children.

These two studies performed in different populations of children suggest that the link between events *in utero* and non-insulin-dependent diabetes in adult life can be observed from an early age and that the associations between fetal growth and adult disease do not simply reflect the confounding influence of adverse environmental factors during childhood and adult life.

UNDERLYING MECHANISMS

PROGRAMMING

It is possible that the link between birth weight and diabetes can be explained by the effect of the environment *in utero* on the fetus. It is thought that the nutritional, hormonal and metabolic environment offered by the mother permanently affects the structure and function of the fetus, so programming it to develop diabetes in later life. The principle behind programming, as proposed by Lucas, is that a stimulus or insult at a critical period of development has lasting or lifelong significance[13].

Animal experiments offer numerous examples of programming. Young female rats injected with testosterone at a period shortly after birth developed normally until puberty but then failed to ovulate and exhibited abnormal sexual behaviour[14]. Similarly a critical period for development of sexual characteristics exists in humans where the secretion of testosterone by the fetal testis, at a critical period during gestation, leads to development of male internal genitalia.

Work on nutritional programming of carbohydrate metabolism has been carried out in both small animal models such as the rat and in larger models, namely the sheep and pig. Protein energy undernutrition of the pregnant ewe in mid to late gestation led to intrauterine growth retardation and reduced insulin secretion in response to glucose close to term[15]. Swenne *et al.* exposed young rats to a low-protein diet and found that this resulted in transient impaired glucose tolerance and persistent blunting of the insulin secretory response despite return to a normal diet later[16]. A later experiment by Dahri *et al.* showed that the offspring of rats fed on a low-protein diet during pregnancy showed reduction in pancreatic cell proliferation, reduction in islet size and vascularization and reduced pancreatic insulin content[17]. Eriksson and Swenne showed that the female rats fed with a low-protein diet developed subnormal insulin response and reduced beta-cell mass. These changes were maintained despite the resumption of normal diet and when these rats became pregnant their offspring were macrosomic with increased beta-cell mass and increased pancreatic insulin content[18]. Furthermore, Van Assche and Aerts were able to demonstrate that the effects of low-protein diet on female rats not only influenced carbohydrate metabolism in their offspring but also in future generations[19]. It has also been shown experimentally that pregnant sows, deprived of protein, give birth to viable but growth-retarded offspring[20]. In addition it has been demonstrated that piglets placed on a low-protein diet at weaning become glucose intolerant, and have abnormalities in pancreatic islet structures later in life[21].

INSULIN SECRETION AND INSULIN RESISTANCE

The mechanisms linking reduced fetal growth with diabetes in adult life are not fully understood. Insulin resistance is an early metabolic defect which predicts the disease but reduced beta-cell function is also characteristic of diabetes. If reduced fetal growth causes diabetes then associations between fetal growth and both insulin secretion and insulin resistance would be expected.

Insulin Secretion

There is evidence in humans linking malnutrition *in utero* or during early life with decreased insulin secretion: Van Assche and Aerts studied the fetal endocrine pancrease and showed that growth-retarded newborn infants had reduced numbers of beta cells and reduced insulin secretion[22]. Two studies of postnatally malnourished children have suggested that malnourishment leads to a permanent reduction of the insulin response to glucose[23,24]. As outlined above, these findings have been confirmed in animal experiments. Insulin secretion can be altered by subjecting either fetal or early postnatal animals to protein energy malnutrition or protein deficiency alone.

A recent study in Preston set out to confirm that insulin secretion was deficient in adults who had been growth retarded *in utero*[25]. Phillips *et al.* studied a subset of the original Preston cohort. Twenty-three subjects known to be glucose intolerant and 82 subjects with normal glucose tolerance were included in the study. Insulin secretion was measured following intravenous glucose tolerance testing. No relationship was found between insulin secretion and measurements of prenatal growth. These results argue against a major role for insulin secretion as a cause of impaired glucose tolerance in adults. They do not, however, exclude it. It is possible that the early growth/insulin secretion association could be obscured by the development of insulin resistance in the adult. This could be overcome by studies in younger subjects. In a recent study of 24 young men (mean age 26 years) in Southampton insulin secretion following an intravenous glucose tolerance test was measured[26]. Although insulin secretion was not found to relate to birth weight in this small sample, it was inversely related to the placental weight : birth weight ratio ($r = -0.48$, $p = 0.02$), which is known to be an indicator of poor fetal growth.

Insulin Resistance

While the evidence linking fetal growth with insulin secretion is contradictory, there is increasing evidence that reduced fetal growth leads to insulin resistance in adult life. Non-insulin-dependent diabetes and hypertension tend to occur in the same patients. People with both abnormalities often have abnormal serum lipids with raised triglyceride and low high-density lipoprotein concentrations. The combination of non-insulin-dependent diabetes, hypertension, raised serum triglyceride and reduced serum high density lipoprotein is known as syndrome X. Reaven has suggested that the primary defect in syndrome X is hyperinsulinaemia[27]. In the Hertfordshire study syndrome X (defined as a 2 h glucose of 7.7 mmol/l or more, a systolic blood pressure of 160 mmHg or more, or currently receiving antihypertensive treatment, and a serum triglyceride concentration equal to or above the median value of 1.4 mmol/l) was found to be more prevalent in those with birth weights of 5.5 lb (2.5 kg) or less[28]. The percentage of men with syndrome X, according to this definition, fell progressively from 30% in those who had birth weights of 5.5 lb (2.5 kg) or less to 6% in those who weighed 9.5 lb (4.3 kg) or more. A similar relationship was demonstrated in Preston and the finding has also been confirmed by Valdez *et al.* in a non-European population. These studies suggest a link between reduced fetal growth and insulin resistance. This led Phillips *et al.* to carry out a further study on a subset of the Preston cohort[29]. Twenty-two subjects known to be glucose intolerant and 81 subjects with normal glucose tolerance were included in the study. Insulin resistance was measured using a short insulin tolerance test where insulin is injected intravenously and the rate of detection of blood glucose is used as a measure of insulin resistance. Men and women who were thin at birth as indicated by a low ponderal index were more likely to be insulin resistant, as shown in Table 23.4. Men and women are subdivided according to ponderal index at birth and current body mass index. At each body mass, resistance was

Table 23.4. Mean insulin resistance (half-life of blood glucose in minutes) in men and women aged 50 years according to ponderal index at birth and adult body mass index[29]

Ponderal index (kg/m³)	Body mass index (kg/m²)				
	≤24.0	24.1–26.0	26.1–28.0	>28.0	All
≤20.6	17.9	18.0	23.1	30.7	20.6
	(8)	(8)	(4)	(6)	(26)
20.7–22.3	15.8	17.3	17.8	27.1	17.3
	(16)	(11)	(6)	(4)	(37)
22.4–25.0	14.4	20.7	21.0	20.4	17.9
	(8)	(4)	(3)	(8)	(23)
>25.0	14.1	16.1	17.8	18.5	16.6
	(4)	(4)	(3)	(6)	(17)
All	15.6	17.7	19.5	22.6	18.0
	(36)	(27)	(16)	(24)	(103)

Figures in parenthesis are number of people.

greatest in those with low ponderal index. Conversely, at each ponderal index, resistance was greater in those with high body mass, and the greatest mean resistance was therefore seen in those with low ponderal index at birth and high current body mass index. It would appear then that individuals who are thin at birth and obese as adults are the most resistant to insulin and therefore at greatest risk of developing diabetes.

THRIFTY PHENOTYPE HYPOTHESIS

The evidence for an association between fetal nutrition and carbohydrate metabolism in later life led Hales to propose the thrifty phenotype hypothesis: the undernourished fetus and infant are programmed to become nutritionally thrifty[30]. Their beta-cell complement is reduced and they develop insulin resistance. It is proposed that provided such an individual remains undernourished their carbohydrate metabolism is adequate. A sudden move to overnutrition, however, will result in diabetes because of deficiencies in beta-cell function and tissue sensitivity to insulin. This hypothesis, therefore, explains the links between obesity and the development of diabetes in predisposed individuals. It also sheds light on the epidemiology of non-insulin-dependent diabetes. Wide variations in prevalence are seen in different populations, with prevalence of 1–10% in European populations compared with prevalence as high as 20–30% in Pima Indians and Nauruan Islanders. Prior to the 1940s non-insulin-dependent diabetes was virtually unknown in these two groups. It is believed that a rapid transition from subsistence living to a more Westernized diet led to these trends.

CONCLUSIONS

There is now substantial evidence that poor fetal growth leads to a greater risk of impaired glucose tolerance and diabetes in adult life. The association between size at birth and glucose tolerance has been demonstrated in a number of populations. It has a strong and graded nature and is independent of social class and adult lifestyle factors. There is accumulating evidence from animal experiments that poor maternal nutrition may result in programming of metabolic pathways in the fetus which place it at higher risk of developing disease. Observations in humans suggest that the same occurs in the undernourished human fetus, resulting in a nutritionally thrifty individual who will develop diabetes if exposed to overnutrition in later life.

Further work is needed to characterize more precisely the aspects of the environment *in utero* that lead to programming of carbohydrate metabolism in the fetus. It is clear, however, that in the future strategies for the prevention of diabetes will need to focus on the health of mothers and babies as well as on adult lifestyle.

REFERENCES

1 Barker DJP, Osmond C. Infant mortality, childhood nutrition, and ischaemic heart disease in England and Wales. *Lancet* 1986 **i**: 1077–81.
2 Barker DJP, Osmond C, Law CM. The intrauterine and early postnatal origins of cardiovascular disease and chronic bronchitis. *J Epidemiol Community Health* 1989; **43**: 237–40.
3 Hales CN, Barker DJP, Clark PMS *et al*. Fetal and infant growth and impaired glucose tolerance at age 64. *Br Med J* 1991; **303**: 1019–22.
4 Fall CHD, Osmond C, Barker DJP *et al*. Fetal and infant growth and cardiovascular risk factors in women. *Br Med J* 1995; **310**: 428–31.
5 Phipps K, Barker DJP, Hales CN *et al*. Fetal growth and impaired glucose tolerance in men and women. *Diabetologia* 1993; **36**: 225–8.
6 Robinson SM, Walton RJ, Clark PMS *et al*. The relation of fetal growth to plasma glucose in young men. *Diabetologia* 1992; **35**: 444–6.
7 McKeigue PM, Leon DA, Berglund L *et al*. Relationship of birthweight and ponderal index to non-insulin dependent diabetes and insulin response to glucose challenge in men aged 50–60 years. *Diabetic Med* 1994; **11**: S17.
8 Valdez R, Athens MS, Thompson GH *et al*. Birthweight and adult health outcomes in a biethnic population in the USA. *Diabetologia* 1994; **37**: 624–31.
9 McCance DR, Pettitt DJ, Hanson RL *et al*. Birth weight and non-insulin dependent diabetes: thrifty genotype, thrifty phenotype, or surviving small baby genotype? *Br Med J* 1994; **308**: 942–5.
10 Pettitt DJ, Aleck KA, Baird HR *et al*. Congenital susceptibility to NIDDM: role of intrauterine environment. *Diabetes* 1988; **37**: 622–8.
11 Law CM, Gordon GS, Shiell AW *et al*. Thinness at birth and glucose tolerance in seven year old children. Unpublished, 1993.
12 Yajnik CS, Fall CHD, Vaidya U *et al*. Fetal growth and glucose and insulin metabolism in four-year-old Indian children. *Diabetic Med* 1995; **12**: 330–6.
13 Lucas A. Programming by early nutrition in man. In: Bock GR, Whelan J (eds), *The Childhood Environment and Adult Disease (CIBA Foundation Symposium 156)*. Wiley, Chichester, 1991; 38–55.
14 Barraclough CA. Production of anovulatory sterile rats by single injection of testosterone proprionate. *Endocrinology* 1961; **68**: 62–7.
15 Fowden A. Effects of arginine and glucose on the release of insulin in the sheep fetus. *J Endocrinol* 1980; **85**: 121–9.
16 Swenne I, Crace CJ, Milner RDG. Persistent impairment of insulin secretory response to glucose in adult rats after limited period of protein-calorie malnutrition early in life. *Diabetes* 1987; **36**: 454–8.
17 Dahri S, Snoeck A, Reusens-Billen B *et al*. Islet function in offspring of mothers on low-protein diet during gestation. *Diabetes* 1991; **40**: 115–20.
18 Eriksson UJ, Swenne I. Diabetes in pregnancy: fetal macrosomia, hyperinsulinism, and islet hyperplasia in the offspring of rats subjected to temporary protein-energy malnutrition early in life. *Pediatr Res* 1993; **34**: 791–5.
19 Van Assche FA, Aerts L. Long term effects of diabetes and pregnancy in the rat. *Diabetes* 1985; **34** (Suppl. 2): 116–18.
20 Pond WG, Maurer RR, Klindt J. Fetal organ response to maternal protein deprivation during pregnancy in swine. *J Nutr* 1991; **121**: 504–9.
21 Heard CRC. Effects of severe protein-calorie deficiency on the endocrine control of carbohydrate metabolism. *Diabetes* 1966; **15**: 78–89.
22 Van Assche FA, Aerts L. The fetal endocrine pancreas. *Contrib Gynaecol Obstet* 1979; **5**: 44–57.
23 James WPT, Coore HG. Persistent impairment of insulin secretion and glucose tolerance after malnutrition. *Am J Clin Nutr* 1970; **23**: 386–9.
24 Milner RDG. Metabolic and hormonal responses to glucose and glucagon in patients with infantile malnutrition. *Pediatr Res* 1971; **5**: 33–9.
25 Phillips DIW, Hirst S, Clark PMS *et al*. Fetal growth and insulin secretion in adult life.

Diabetologia 1994; **37**: 592–6.

26 Wills J, Watson JM, Hales CN, Phillips DIW. The relation of fetal growth to insulin secretion in young men. *Diabetic Med* 1996 (in press).

27 Reaven GM. Role of insulin resistance in human disease. *Diabetes* 1988; **37**: 1595–607.

28 Barker DJP, Hales CN, Fall CHD *et al.* Type 2 (non-insulin dependent) diabetes mellitus, hypertension and hyperlipidemia (syndrome X): relation to reduced fetal growth. *Diabetologia* 1993; **36**: 62–7.

29 Phillips DIW, Barker DJP, Hales CN *et al.* Thinness at birth and insulin resistance in adult life. *Diabetologia* 1994; **37**: 150–4.

30 Hales CN, Barker DJP. Type 2 (non-insulin dependent) diabetes mellitus: the thrifty phenotype hypothesis. *Diabetologia* 1992; **35**: 595–601.

24

The Perspective of a Mother with Diabetes

Name:	Hayley J. Blanchard		
Age:	25 years		
Past medical history:	Developed insulin-dependent diabetes at age eight years. No family history of diabetes		
Obstetric history:	First baby. No miscarriages		
Pre-pregnancy insulin dosage	am52 Insulatard pm44 Insulatard	Before breakfast Before lunch Before dinner	12 Actrapid 14 Actrapid 14 Actrapid
End of pregnancy dosage	am34 Protophane pm36 Protophane	Before breakfast Before lunch Before dinner	32 Actrapid 30 Actrapid 28 Actrapid
Post-pregnancy insulin dosage	am22 Protophane pm22 Protophane	Before breakfast Before lunch Before dinner	12 Actrapid 16 Actrapid 18 Actrapid

PREPARATIONS FOR PREGNANCY

When I was very young I seem to remember hearing it was very dangerous for diabetic women to have children—at the time this did not concern me. It was about 12–18 months pre-conception that I started to do my own research on diabetic pregnancy. I was pleased to discover that having diabetes during pregnancy should not make a pregnancy difficult or mean

Diabetes and Pregnancy: An International Approach to Diagnosis and Management.
Edited by A. Dornhorst and D. R. Hadden.
© 1996 John Wiley & Sons Ltd.

that I could not produce a normal, healthy baby. I found out that as long as I maintained good glucose control before conception and throughout the pregnancy any complications associated with diabetes could be avoided. I knew that my condition would be closely managed with the help of the obstetrician and diabetic physician. My personal aims were to achieve good glucose control and to give up my smoking habit of 20 cigarettes per day. One of the main apprehensions at the back of my mind was whether my child would be born with or go on to develop diabetes. I discussed this with my diabetic physician and was assured that this was unlikely especially as my diabetes was not hereditary. I was told that the chances of my child going on to develop diabetes were about the same as anyone else. My husband and I were reassured by this news and we felt confident about trying for a baby once I had my blood sugars well controlled and had managed to stop smoking.

I was meticulous about my pre-conception preparations and made sure that my diabetes was assessed in full beforehand. I was given the all clear. I managed to stop smoking three months before conception. It only took about four weeks to conceive and my husband and I were both delighted. My blood sugar control was A1 apart from one week of sky-high results that refused to drop even with extra insulin. This was due to an emotional upset, the sad loss of my grandmother. I was, however, reassured that such a short period of raised sugars would not cause any damage. I consulted my diabetic physician to tell him a home pregnancy testing kit had indicated I was pregnant and I had a hospital test to confirm the result. It too came back positive. At this stage I was keen to seek any advice regarding what I should be doing to ensure the first trimester's control was good. I was told to record my blood glucose results and that I would see the obstetrician in conjunction with my diabetic physician at 12 weeks.

FIRST TRIMESTER

During the first 12 weeks of pregnancy I found that I did not require any more insulin but I was prepared for the fact that later on the extra demands of pregnancy and the maternal production of hormones with anti-insulin effects may necessitate my dosage being increased considerably. During my pregnancy I felt highly motivated to achieve excellent control and to attend the antenatal clinics frequently. I knew the reality of poor glucose control for the baby and me. Luckily I escaped the added complication of regular morning sickness and was only sick once during the first trimester. I suffered from occasional episodes of nausea and headaches but these were short lived. The main problem I had was the extreme tiredness from lunchtime every day for the first three months. This did result in a change of my insulin therapy. I had always taken my evening insulin before I went to bed and as I was falling asleep at about 8.00 p.m. I was taking it at this time. I was therefore suffering from hypos at about 1.00 a.m. when the long- and short-acting insulins were working together. This was remedied by setting my alarm clock for 11.00 p.m. and giving my long-acting insulin at this time. I would eat my dinner at about 6.40 p.m. and be asleep by about 8.00 p.m. As you can imagine it was not long before I began to suffer from heartburn and Gaviscon came to my rescue.

From 12 weeks on I received regular fortnightly checks at the hospital where I was given advice on the management of my diabetes. At every visit there were always about five people in the consulting room and to begin with this was a bit daunting, but as the pregnancy progressed it was reassuring to have the whole team of experts there to advise where necessary. The target glucose levels I was given to achieve were <5.5 mmol/l before breakfast and <7.5 mmol/l after each meal.

SECOND TRIMESTER

As the weeks went by my insulin requirements increased in fits and bursts. I suspect that it was easier to achieve my target glucose results because I was using a Novopen and the flexibility of this insulin administration was a very important aspect in my diabetic care. I became obsessive about keeping my blood sugars low. The frequent hypos were a pain but I felt safer with the knowledge that this would not harm the baby. The main problem associated with my hypos was that I had no signals that one was on the way. My husband regularly had to remedy my hypos and make sense of my senseless talk. This was an extremely worrying time for him and it was the first occasion that he had seen me going hypoglycaemic so regularly and so frequently without signals. I became very reliant upon him at this time and his support was priceless. A useful aid at this time was recommended by the diabetic health visitor. This was Hypostop—a glucose gel that could be squeezed into the mouth, and this did the trick quickly if I was obliging. We had a supply of glucagon injections in case of emergencies but we did not need to use them. However, the knowledge that they were on hand was a reassurance to both of us. My non-diabetic mother-to-be friends were also experiencing periods where they needed to snack on sweet bars at sudden and regular intervals so I did not feel I was having too bad a time of it. The distressing aspect for me was that frequently I knew I was going hypo but I did not seem to be able to tell my hand to get my glucose tablets out of my desk or bag and yet I knew where they were.

Throughout the pregnancy I had regular scans to check on the baby's growth and the amount of amniotic fluid around the baby. At 32 weeks I had a scan to look at the development of the heart. This proved normal, much to our relief. I certainly felt very well looked after throughout the pregnancy and this was very important to us. I realized that I was fortunate to see the same people on every occasion and this was a clear advantage over non-diabetic mothers-to-be. I would stress that explanation of all additional scans to the mother-to-be is extremely important; not all mothers are brave enough to ask why these are necessary and if they are routine in diabetic care during pregnancy. There were never many people in the same situation as me in the waiting area so I did feel I missed out on the chit-chat aspect. Joining an antenatal class remedied this problem to some extent. It would have been useful to talk to someone with established diabetes who had been through the whole process to ask those questions you really did not want to waste your consultant/surgeon's time asking.

THIRD TRIMESTER

A scan showed that the baby weighed approximately 6 lb at 30 weeks and repeat scans were then carried out every two weeks to check on the growth rate. These showed that the baby was gaining about half a pound a week. I was deeply upset at this news and although I knew I had maintained the very best control I could I felt it had not been good enough and that I had failed in some way. At this stage the medical team were extremely supportive and for this I was very grateful. The rate of growth did slow down slightly at the very end but it was agreed that a caesarean section with epidural anaesthetic would be advisable. The baby weighed approximately 8½ lb at my last scan taken at 36 weeks. As an established diabetic I knew I was prone to a number of disorders while pregnant, owing to fluctuations in blood sugar levels. I did suffer from mild pre-eclamptic toxaemia from 36 weeks onwards and this was monitored closely at a day unit, but luckily I escaped any other complications. At this point my husband and I agreed that the doctors/surgeons were the experts and we would do what they suggested for the safe delivery of the baby and for my health too.

At 37 weeks a date was set for the 3rd August 1994 for the caesarean. This was two weeks early. In a way it was nice to see a light at the end of the tunnel. By this stage I had put on nearly three stones in weight and getting around was becoming increasingly difficult—the weather was also extremely hot and I felt very uncomfortable. I felt hypo a lot of the time and kept eating to prevent this occurring. During the last week I seemed to be able to eat something sweet and still have a very low glucose result afterwards. I found it very hard to achieve stable glucose control towards the end of the pregnancy. It was a frightening time as my hypo signs were reduced and this meant I had to rely on family and friends. In turn I felt rather vulnerable and a burden as well. The baby was pressing on a nerve and causing me intermittent loss of feeling on my left hip/thigh region and I could not move any distance without pain. This restriction was an additional annoyance as I am fiercely independent. However, at this stage I knew I had to relent and accept help to ensure that if a hypo happened no harm would come to the baby and me.

THE BIRTH

I went into hospital the night before to ensure all necessary preparations were performed. I was first on the list for the following morning. The midwives and doctors were all very friendly and keen to see if there was anything I wanted to know. However, it's very hard to know what to ask when you don't know where to start. Therefore I didn't really ask anything and instead stayed awake all night in anticipation of what was going to happen. I think an informative discussion where the patient is given an outline of what happens rather than being asked what they want to know before the Caesarean would be helpful.

The following morning the doctor came bright and early to put my lines in for the glucose and insulin pumps that were to be my control for the next stage. I was slightly worried about the pump control. However, on this occasion the control was good as the staff were not rigid about the doses written in the notes and the flexibility they displayed avoided an unnecessary hypo. My husband was with me from about 6.30 a.m. and he looked just as exhausted and excited as I felt. My operation was delayed because there were several emergencies to be carried out. Eventually it was my turn to go up to the delivery suite and my husband was taken away to put on his surgical gown. We were introduced one by one to the whole team and they were all fantastic. We entered the theatre to be delighted by a background of classical music—a pleasant distraction for myself. My husband was keen to make sure I was comfortable and the combination of this with the humour of the theatre staff was of paramount importance. I had an additional drip inserted for the epidural and was all set within about 20 min, legs and abdomen numb and green screen in place. I had my blood pressure automatically checked at regular intervals. My husband found the operation and work of the theatre staff fascinating but I was happy to stay behind the green screen.

Jamie was born at 10.08 a.m. Everyone laughed and said he looked just like me. He screamed and I cried. His Apgar score at birth was 9/10 and at 5 min was 9/10 as well. He weighed 9 lb 4 oz. Jamie was put to the breast as soon as I was out of theatre and topped up with some formula milk. He stayed with me until about 2.30 the following morning when his blood sugar suddenly dropped quite low after having remained stable for about 16 h, and he did not seem to have the energy to drink the milk. He was then taken to special care where he was monitored closely for the rest of the day and returned to me the day after. This unavoidable early separation was a particularly emotional time for me, especially as I did not anticipate it would happen. His blood sugar did go back to normal fairly quickly and this was a relief. The stay in special care did not really help me to establish breastfeeding. At the time the most important thing was to keep Jamie's blood sugar levels stable. It was not really fair to expect him to exert any more energy than was necessary to get the required! I did, however, attempt to establish the breast at every feed but it was only when he left special care that my attempts began to pay off, thanks to the help of the midwives.

I remained in hospital for five days and needless to say was pleased to go home to a more comfortable and relaxed atmosphere. With the help of my midwife I was able to become comfortable with my breastfeeding technique and establish some sort of routine. My caesarean scar healed well and the stitch was removed by the midwife at home on the sixth day.

My insulin requirements dropped to a similar amount to that pre pregnancy the day after the birth. It took about three days before my glucose results stabilized. I only needed to adjust the evening Protophane dosage due to night feeding and subsequent night eating. Apart from that adjustment I have not really needed to change my insulin dramatically apart from an extra six units of Actrapid per day.

Six months on I have managed to lose all the weight I gained during pregnancy—now I need to lose that stone I gained pre pregnancy when I gave up smoking! Incidentally I have not recommenced smoking, so it should be easier to achieve any pre-pregnancy aims next time round and to start the pregnancy at a weight that will allow for a substantial increase!

On reflection I would say that any diabetic pregnancy can be a successful one so long as it is entered into closely with the health care team, be it at the hospital or general practice. The pregnancy certainly does require extra care to achieve the necessary balances but I think the motivation of the mother-to-be is quite strong, and this helps. The diabetic mother also requires a network of support from family, friends and colleagues, especially when those hypo signs say goodbye! However, I am sure family support is not always possible, due to social circumstances, and therefore it is even more important for the diabetic health care team to be aware of these needs. It is important for all health care workers involved to be aware that diabetic mothers have worries specific to diabetes on top of the routine ones that all pregnant women have and that these may not always be obvious. It is very important for the diabetic mother to be aware of the fact that the baby may require monitoring in a special care unit after birth and to be prepared for this outcome. Where possible a separation of this kind should be avoided, with the ultimate aim to keep mother and baby together. I hope to avoid some of the problems I experienced in this pregnancy in the next one but even if I can't I feel they were a small price to pay compared to such a wonderful reward at the end. Jamie is doing well now and his development is in no way different from that of any other child his age (Figure 24.1).

I need to say a big thank you to the obstetric physician, the obstetrician and their respective teams at Queen Charlotte's Hospital, London, who were extremely supportive throughout my pregnancy and afterwards.

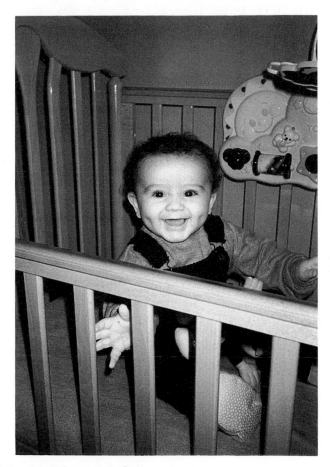

Figure 24.1. Jamie aged nine months

Epilogue: The Way Forward

Diabetes and Pregnancy: An International Approach to Diagnosis and Management by Dr Anne Dornhorst and Professor David Hadden highlights both the clinical aspects of diabetes and pregnancy, and the scientific approach which has to guide the proper management of this biological challenge. The international team of authors, experts in their own domains, has endeavoured with success to foster the interdisciplinary attitude needed to provide proper health care to mother and neonate. It has achieved more by highlighting the need for creating awareness and education at all levels. This is germane to developed countries, but even more so to less privileged countries and societies where conditions remain life threatening for the unborn and the offspring in early childhood.

A special feature warrants further consideration and action. World Health Organization experts have raised major issues when they indicated that young females of childbearing potential in less privileged countries have a greater prevalence of impaired glucose tolerance than males. Why should young females be more affected than males, and would their own metabolic framework during pregnancy affect the developing fetal endocrine pancreas, with consequences such as diabetes later in their progeny? In view of the epidemiology of diabetes throughout the world and especially in developing countries, the maternal transmission of diabetes has to be eagerly scrutinised. Clinical observations and investigational data which demonstrate the possible vertical transmission of non-insulin-dependent diabetes from the mother to her progeny in relation to her high blood sugar during pregnancy have been discussed in this book. Further action has to be called for to implement proper preventive interventions during pregnancy which may hinder this diabetes epidemic.

Another issue relates to the fetal and infant origin of chronic degenerative diseases later in life, which have become a main concern of public health. There is a further need to specify that as well as high maternal blood sugar, the impact of the mother's health and poor nutrition on fetal organ development will have consequences later. Not only large for dates infants born to mothers with disturbed carbohydrate metabolism but small for dates infants of mothers with or without diabetes have a greater likelihood to become diabetic themselves, and to develop cardiovascular diseases later.

Future progress in developmental biology should unravel the mechanisms involved in the early genesis of diabetes and cardiovascular diseases and provide further substantiation of the clinical epidemiological data. Securing the appropriate quantity and quality of food, including specific proteins or amino acids to young females of childbearing potential and to pregnant mothers, should offer better health for the unborn child.

This textbook is an inspiration for the clinician, the epidemiologist and the investigator in developmental biology, and hopefully through its implementation will lead to a new and assured prevention of chronic degenerative diseases.

Professor Joseph J. Hoet

Université Catholique de Louvain, Faculté des Sciences, et Organization Mondiale de la Sante, Centre Collaborateur pour le Développement de la Biologie du Pancreas endocrine, Place Croix du Sud, 5 B-1348 Louvain-la-Neuve, Belgium.

Index

Index compiled by Geoffrey C. Jones